The Cerebral Cortex in Neurodegenerative and Neuropsychiatric Disorders

The Cerebral Cortex in Neurodegenerative and Neuropsychiatric Disorders

Experimental Approaches to Clinical Issues

Edited by

David F. Cechetto
Nina Weishaupt
University of Western Ontario,
London, ON, Canada

AMSTERDAM • BOSTON • HEIDELBERG • LONDON
NEW YORK • OXFORD • PARIS • SAN DIEGO
SAN FRANCISCO • SINGAPORE • SYDNEY • TOKYO

Academic Press is an imprint of Elsevier

Academic Press is an imprint of Elsevier
125 London Wall, London EC2Y 5AS, United Kingdom
525 B Street, Suite 1800, San Diego, CA 92101-4495, United States
50 Hampshire Street, 5th Floor, Cambridge, MA 02139, United States
The Boulevard, Langford Lane, Kidlington, Oxford OX5 1GB, United Kingdom

Notices
Knowledge and best practice in this field are constantly changing. As new research and experience
broaden our understanding, changes in research methods, professional practices, or medical treatment
may become necessary.

Practitioners and researchers may always rely on their own experience and knowledge in
evaluating and using any information, methods, compounds, or experiments described herein.
In using such information or methods they should be mindful of their own safety and the safety
of others, including parties for whom they have a professional responsibility.

To the fullest extent of the law, neither the Publisher nor the authors, contributors, or editors,
assume any liability for any injury and/or damage to persons or property as a matter of products
liability, negligence or otherwise, or from any use or operation of any methods, products,
instructions, or ideas contained in the material herein.

Library of Congress Cataloging-in-Publication Data
A catalog record for this book is available from the Library of Congress

British Library Cataloguing-in-Publication Data
A catalogue record for this book is available from the British Library

ISBN: 978-0-12-801942-9

For information on all Academic Press publications
visit our website at https://www.elsevier.com

Working together
to grow libraries in
developing countries

www.elsevier.com • www.bookaid.org

Publisher: Mara Conner
Acquisition Editor: Natalie Farra
Editorial Project Manager: Kathy Padilla
Production Project Manager: Karen East and Kirsty Halterman
Designer: Matthew Limbert

Typeset by TNQ Books and Journals

Contents

Part I
Introductory Chapters

1. Anatomy of the Cerebral Cortex
K.S. Rockland

2. Cortical Plasticity in Response to Injury and Disease
N. Weishaupt

Part II
The Cerebral Cortex in Neurodegenerative Disorders

4. **Alzheimer's Disease**
    J.H.K. Tam and S.H. Pasternak

10. Cortical Involvement in Multiple Sclerosis
P. Bannerman

Part III
The Cerebral Cortex in Neuropsychiatric Disorders

11. Prefrontal Cortical Abnormalities in Cognitive Deficits of Schizophrenia
N. Rajakumar

12. Role of the Prefrontal Cortex in Addictive Disorders
J. Renard, L. Rosen, W.J. Rushlow and S.R. Laviolette

List of Contributors

A.E. Arrant University of Alabama at Birmingham, Birmingham, AL, United States

P. Bannerman Shriners Hospital for Children, Sacramento, CA, United States

R. Bartha University of Western Ontario, London, ON, Canada

D.F. Cechetto University of Western Ontario, London, ON, Canada

R.L.M. Faull University of Auckland, Auckland, New Zealand

M. Jog University of Western Ontario, London, ON, Canada

E.H. Kim University of Auckland, Auckland, New Zealand

S.R. Laviolette University of Western Ontario, London, ON, Canada

T.-Y. Lee University of Western Ontario, London, ON, Canada; St. Joseph's Health Centre, London, ON, Canada

N. Mehrabi University of Auckland, Auckland, New Zealand

A.J. Moszczynski Western University, London, ON, Canada

D.G. Munoz University of Toronto, Toronto, ON, Canada

S.H. Pasternak Western University, London, ON, Canada

N. Rajakumar University of Western Ontario, London, ON, Canada

J. Renard University of Western Ontario, London, ON, Canada

E.D. Roberson University of Alabama at Birmingham, Birmingham, AL, United States

K.S. Rockland Boston University School of Medicine, Boston, MA, United States

L. Rosen University of Western Ontario, London, ON, Canada

W.J. Rushlow University of Western Ontario, London, ON, Canada

M.J. Strong Western University, London, ON, Canada

J.H.K. Tam Western University, London, ON, Canada

L.J. Tippett University of Auckland, Auckland, New Zealand

H.J. Waldvogel University of Auckland, Auckland, New Zealand

N. Weishaupt University of Western Ontario, London, ON, Canada

Foreword

Knowledge accrues in pieces, but it is understood in patterns. As subspecialties grow, so do the gaps between them. The greatest gap of all occurs between experimental research and clinical application, within and among fields. This book goes a long way in bridging these gaps. It begins with an introductory chapter on the cerebral cortex, stressing the similarities and differences among species, particularly between humans and rodents, the favorite experimental species. Next comes a chapter on cortical plasticity and response to injury, setting out the dynamics of injury and repair that underpin most brain conditions. The chapter on imaging outlines how it is increasingly possible to study pathological and repair mechanisms in vivo both in humans and in animals. This is followed by a section on seven common neurodegenerative disorders, ending with a section on neuropsychiatric disorders, the other set of manifestations of a disordered brain.

A remarkable feature of this book lies in the joint coauthorship of basic scientists and clinicians accustomed to working with each other. This provides a coherent and unique understanding of how integrated, experimental, and clinical work can move forward together.

This volume should have a broad appeal to clinicians trying to understand experimental methodologies, techniques, and approaches; to basic scientists in seeing the clinical relevance of their work; and to all those interested in the brain who want to know how a myriad of little pieces coalesce to make up increasingly understandable patterns.

Vladimir Hachinski, CM MD DSc FRCPC FRSC
Dr Hon causa (X4)
Distinguished University Professor
University of Western Ontario
London, Ontario, Canada

Introduction

The cerebral cortex has approximately 10 billion neurons that provide an inordinate amount of high-level processing. It is the neurons in the cerebral cortex in humans that is responsible for the cognitive processing or the conscious mind. The final site of termination for sensory signals is the cerebral cortex, leading to an awareness of the external and internal milieu. Complex processing using several different cortical networks leads to the generation of simple movements or even very complex executive functions, such as decision making and setting goals.

The cerebral cortex plays an important part in some of the most prevalent neurological diseases and neuropsychiatric disorders in our society. For some conditions, involvement of the cerebral cortex has only recently been emerging. Experimental research into the role of the cortex in disease has contributed greatly to our current knowledge, and further advances are needed. This book focuses on how preclinical investigations are addressing the clinical issues surrounding the involvement of the cerebral cortex in selected conditions of the nervous system. Each chapter has been written by an expert in his/her field in an effort to provide a comprehensive review of the clinical manifestations of cortical involvement, and a resource on leading animal models and experimental techniques currently available to tackle cortical issues in disease. Thus this book provides a link between cortical clinical problems and investigational approaches that we hope will help foster future research with high translational value.

Textbook resources on the cerebral cortex are abundant. The intent of this volume is to contribute cutting-edge insights into how the cerebral cortex functions in disease states, and how it is affected by individual neurological and neuropsychiatric disorders. What makes this book unique is the link it provides between clinical issues and preclinical research related to the cerebral cortex. The focus on animal models and experimental techniques is aimed at providing a practical resource on modeling clinical issues to be useful for researchers from students to principal investigators. A resource of this kind, covering major neurological and neuropsychiatric diseases and the role of the cerebral cortex, has not been previously available.

In this book, we have provided three general topics of particular importance to understanding and undertaking experimental investigations of diseases of the cerebral cortex. The remaining chapters are devoted to particular neurological or neuropsychiatric conditions and the role of the cerebral cortex. These chapters have some common themes related to pathology, as well as to the associated imaging technologies and the type of models used to investigate each condition.

The first chapter provides an excellent overview of the anatomy of the cerebral cortex. In particular, this chapter eloquently describes the similarities in the cerebral cortex between species, as well as the areas in which species have developed specialized components for specific behaviors. It is clear that there are many organizational similarities in the cerebral cortex of humans and animal models, even rodents. This chapter specifically states, "the primary cortical areas are recognizable across species, as are the basic cortical layers and cell types, and the main neurochemical transmitter and neuromodulatory systems." However, the description of the differences emphasizes one of the major limitations in using animal models to examine important neurological and neuropsychiatric conditions. Unlike many subcortical sites, in animal models there is some degree of diversion from the patterns and cytoarchitecture seen in the human that may complicate the interpretation of results.

Chapter 2 deals with one of the unique features of the cerebral cortex that has major implications for the cerebral cortex in response to disease. This chapter emphasizes the importance of plasticity in CNS injury and disease, particularly in the cerebral cortex, in spite of the inability of cortical neurons to undergo adult neurogenesis. Of particular importance for some neurodegenerative and neuropsychiatric diseases is the impact of experience in plasticity in the cerebral cortex, especially as it relates to sensory input, using key examples from visual and auditory deprivation. Thus experience may begin to restore the loss of function caused by altered connections or chemistry of the cerebral cortex. On the other hand, after brain trauma or cerebral infarcts caused by stroke, part of the brain recovery process for function may be relocated in adjacent cortical areas, compensating for the loss of tissue. There are several means by which innate cortical plasticity may be manipulated to play a therapeutic role in neurodegenerative and neuropsychiatric diseases, many of which are described in other chapters. Some of the possible means may include maximizing cognitive reserve and cognitive training, transcranial magnetic stimulation to induce plasticity, and use of growth factors such as insulinlike growth factor (IGF), ciliary neurotrophic factor (CNTF), glial cell–derived neurotrophic factor (GDNF), and brain-derived neurotrophic factor (BDNF) that are proving to be important in cortical plasticity.

As many of the chapters on specific cortical conditions indicate, neuroimaging experts continue to develop essential tools for early identification, experimental investigations, and assistance in therapeutic approaches. Chapter 3 does an excellent job of summarizing all of the recent imaging approaches available for neurodegenerative diseases and provides an excellent overview directly related to some of the discussion found in individual chapters on specific conditions of neurodegenerative diseases. The information provided listing the latest approaches, methods, and agents that are available for imaging the cerebral cortex can be very helpful to scientists intending to undertake new investigations. Furthermore, of particular interest is the discussion on the increased role that imaging is playing in the management of patients with neurodegenerative disease. For example, in Alzheimer disease (AD), neuroimaging can be used as a biomarker in the presymptomatic phase, to identify the etiology, establish pathophysiological changes, and predict progression.

This discussion on the role of imaging for cerebral cortex conditions is supported by many of the chapters on specific neurological and neuropsychiatric conditions affecting the cerebral cortex, indicating that imaging is becoming increasingly important. Many of these chapters indicate that new approaches are being used to monitor the progress of the disease or even may be critical biomarkers in early, treatable stages of cortical diseases.

For example, in Chapter 3 on brain imaging, the resting brain networks are described and it is stated that the default mode network (DMN) is the most relevant in AD because it is involved in episodic memory formation and attention. The DMN is composed of cortical regions such as the cingulate, precuneus, inferior parietal cortex, medial prefrontal cortices, and the hippocampus. Chapter 4 indicates how the DMN regions are involved in AD using the Pittsburgh-B (PiB) compound and positron emission tomography (PET) for imaging amyloid. PET has also been effective in neuropsychiatric conditions. Chapter 12 indicates that PET has demonstrated addiction-related effects in multiple cortical regions.

Functional magnetic resonance imaging (fMRI) is becoming particularly useful in several conditions because it is capable of demonstrating changes in the neural networks associated with cortical activity. Chapters 4 and 6 describe how fMRI is used to demonstrate a lower connectivity in the DMN in AD and frontotemporal dementia (FTD). Chapter 9 describes how a number of fMRI studies have been effective in showing that amyotrophic lateral sclerosis (ALS) produces changes in neural networks. In particular, this chapter describes how resting state fMRI has shown the impact of ALS on three different neural networks, including the salience network, the DMN, and the central executive network. Chapters 11 and 12 also indicate how the neural networks are affected in neuropsychiatric conditions using fMRI. Schizophrenic patients are unable to deactivate the DMN network during cognitive tasks, and regions such as the anterior cingulate cortex, orbitofrontal cortex, and dorsolateral prefrontal cortex have altered functional activity as a result of addiction.

In addition, Chapter 4 on AD suggests how fMRI techniques might be a very useful approach as an early biomarker of cortical changes. The role of fMRI as a biomarker is particularly emphasized in Chapter 6 on FTD, in which reduced connectivity of the DMN is seen 10–15 years before the neurological symptoms. This potential biomarker role is also described in Huntington disease, Chapter 8, in which impairments in the functional connections between the anterior cingulate and lateral prefrontal cortices are observed before the onset of symptoms. Furthermore, fMRI has demonstrated possible plasticity in Huntington disease because it has shown compensatory brain responses and reorganization of circuits.

In addition to imaging, there are some common themes that appear in the chapters on specific neurodegenerative and neuropsychiatric conditions. For example, several chapters refer to the role that tau and amyloid play in the pathology of the disease. The role of tau and amyloid is relatively well known in dementia, as described in Chapters 4, 5, and 6. For example, Chapter 4 describes how neurofibrillary tangles (NFTs) and insoluble aggregates of amyloid present different patterns of progression of AD pathology in the cerebral cortex, even though both of these were previously thought to be integral pathological components of the disease. Chapter 4 indicates that this discrepancy in disease progression may be resolved by an examination of the pattern of soluble oligomeric forms of amyloid. However, Chapter 9 has a very interesting discussion on the controversy surrounding alterations in tau metabolism in the frontotemporal dysfunction associated with ALS.

Another defining condition that appears to be important in many of the cerebral cortex disorders is neuroinflammation. This is emphasized in Chapters 4, 5, and 6 on AD, vascular dementia, and FTD. In Chapter 10 on multiple sclerosis (MS) the deleterious effects of inflammatory cytokines are described with effects that can include direct damage by the disruption of synaptic transmission leading to excitotoxicity and even demyelination or inhibition of remyelination. In Chapter 6 there is a discussion on antiinflammatory therapies for FTD. In Chapter 9 it is also indicated that immunoreactive glia are a significant feature of ALS. The discussion surrounding the role of neuroinflammation in multiple conditions suggests that the cerebral cortex may be particularly vulnerable to degeneration resulting from neuroinflammation. It also suggests that an antiinflammatory regimen developed for one condition may in fact be relevant for other degenerative conditions of the cerebral cortex. Of particular interest in this regard is the new methodologies provided by neuroimaging. As described in Chapter 3, it is now possible to use PET with benzodiazepine receptor ligands to visualize activated microglia in the cerebral cortex. This is permitting clinical investigations to be run in parallel with experimental studies to confirm some basic mechanisms related to neuroinflammatory changes in neurodegenerative diseases. Thus although the cerebral cortex is a very complex and differentiated structure anatomically and damage to specific cortical structures results in very different clinical expression of neurodegenerative disease, some common pathological mechanisms remain, including tau, amyloid, and neuroinflammation, that may be exploited for the purpose of understanding the diseases and designing therapeutic strategies.

Because of the large area of the cerebral cortex and the diverse regions all with different functions, it is difficult to create animal models that are based on making lesions, occluding blood vessels, stimulation of cortical sites, or other surgical techniques. As can be seen from multiple chapters, many experimental models for AD, FTD, ALS, and MS have focused on genetic changes associated with the condition. Often, because of the molecular heterogeneity of the cerebral cortex, transgenic or gene knockout models permit relatively specific molecular cortical disruptions that closely align with the neurodegenerative or neuropsychiatric condition. The exception to this approach, almost by definition, is that of the role of the prefrontal cortex in addictive disorders. In this case, as described in Chapter 12, animal models are based on the administration of drugs to induce animal concomitants of clinical addictive syndromes.

The last 2 chapters focus on conditions that can be considered neuropsychiatric. Chapter 12 on addiction examines in detail the role of the prefrontal cortex, similar to the focus of Chapter 11 on schizophrenia. Given that the overwhelming bulk of our understanding of how the prefrontal cortex controls reward and addiction-related behaviors comes from rodent-based basic neuroscience research approaches, a critical question concerns whether the rodent prefrontal cortex can actually serve as an effective analog for the complexity of the primate prefrontal cortex, an issue that was addressed to some extent in Chapter 1 in the examination of comparative cortical anatomy. It seems that both of these chapters indicate that current experimental models are very useful in our understanding of cortical mechanisms in neuropsychiatric conditions, as was also seen in the use of rodent models in neurodegenerative diseases.

Thus this volume provides the necessary information to understand the role of the cerebral cortex in a number of neurodegenerative and neuropsychiatric diseases, as well as a reference to important information on cortical anatomy, plasticity, and neuroimaging for context to these conditions. It is hoped that these chapters form the basis to assist those working in clinical settings, and early or advanced experimental investigators. In particular, the common themes, as well as the peculiar differences seen in the various diseases, suggest excellent opportunities for novel experimental and therapeutic approaches.

David F. Cechetto
Nina Weishaupt

Part I

Introductory Chapters

Chapter 1

Anatomy of the Cerebral Cortex

K.S. Rockland

Boston University School of Medicine, Boston, MA, United States

INTRODUCTION

The distinctive core features of neocortical anatomy were already recognized by the early architectonic investigators; namely, layers, verticality, and regional differences in cellular and myelin distribution, defined as *discrete areas.* In the 100 years or so since the first maps of the Vogts and Brodmann, cortical research has forged ahead, especially in terms of cell types, intraareal and interareal connectivity, and, most recently, gene expression. Needless to say, given the complexity of brain structure and function, the overall cortical organization is at best only partially understood, and almost every feature (layers, cell types, verticality or "columns," and areas) remains under active investigation and debate. As just one example, a popular proposal of cortical uniformity (Rockel, Hiorns, & Powell, 1980) has been replaced, after the introduction of different counting techniques, by new data more supportive of systematic, cross-cortex and cross-species variation (Charvet, Cahalane, & Finlay, 2015; DeFelipe, Alonso-Nanclares, & Arellano, 2002).

The present chapter, while keeping in mind the open questions on cortical anatomy, aims to provide general orientation and background. Given the prominence of animal models in experimental approaches to disease, special attention is given to differences between human and rodent cortical anatomy. Finer species specializations are not considered, although these are increasingly attracting attention (in rodents, eg, Beaudin, Singh, Agster, & Burwell, 2013; Krubitzer, Campi, & Cooke, 2011). Some of the obvious specializations are briefly discussed in this introductory section, followed by more extensive discussion of areas, layers, verticality, cell types, and connections. A substantial body of longer reviews and chapters is available for further detail (eg, Douglas, Markram, & Martin, 2004; Kirkcaldie, 2012; Zilles, 2004, Chapter 27; Zilles & Wree, 1995).

An obvious distinction of the cerebral cortex in humans is the expansion, considered as a hallmark of human evolution. The human cortex is thicker, has more cells than the smaller brains of rats and mice, and has more areas. It has

The Cerebral Cortex in Neurodegenerative and Neuropsychiatric Disorders.
http://dx.doi.org/10.1016/B978-0-12-801942-9.00001-X

more white matter, in contrast with rodents, where connections often travel through the deeper cortical layers and not through the relatively shallow white matter. The human brain is gyrencephalic (ie, highly folded), albeit not uniquely so, because this property is shared with other species such as cats, dogs, nonhuman primates, and the large-brained elephant and cetaceans.

Gyrencephaly, whether in human or other large brains, has important consequences for differential architectonics and connectivity (Mota & Herculano-Houzel, 2012; Sun & Hevner, 2014). The laminar thickness and spatial arrangement are altered at the gyral crown, sulcal walls, and sulcal depths. The sulcal depths are preferentially associated with the short-distance U-fiber connections. Several causal mechanisms have been proposed for cortical folding (Zilles, Palomero-Gallagher, & Amunts, 2013), including an important role for the proliferative cycle in early development. Current ideas raise the possibility that gyrencephaly should be accepted as the ancestral mammalian trait (Lewitus, Kelava, Kalinka, Tomancak, & Huttner, 2014).

Hemispheric laterality, both functional and anatomical, is a pronounced feature of the human neocortex, although laterality effects have been reported in other species; for example, in aquatic mammals, unihemispheric sleep and hemispheric independence of eye movements (Mortensen et al., 2014). Hippocampal asymmetry in a long-term memory task has been reported in mice (Shipton et al., 2014).

With few exceptions, the same neuron types are found in primates and rodents, although there are differences in degree of dendritic branching and density of dendritic spines (Ballesteros-Yanez, Benavides-Piccione, Elston, Yuste, & DeFelipe, 2006; Benavides-Piccione, Ballesteros-Yanez, DeFelipe, & Yuste, 2002; Elston, Benavides-Piccione, Elston, Manger, & DeFelipe, 2011). Area distribution is variable, especially of interneurons (DeFelipe, Gonzalez-Albo, Del Rio, & Elston, 1999, DeFelipe, Ballesteros-Yanez, Inda, & Munoz (2006); Roux & Buzsaki, 2015). Narrow spindle cells (ie, Von Economo cells) are not found in rodents but do occur in other species besides humans (Butti, Santos, Uppal, & Hof, 2013; Evrard, Forro, & Logothetis, 2012; Seeley et al., 2012). Similarly, giant cells in the motor or visual cortex do not occur in rodents but do occur in other species besides humans. Astrocytes are disproportionately larger in humans than in mice, and their processes are more complex (Oberheim, Wang, Goldman, & Nedergaard, 2006).

An important difference between primates and rodents relates to the thalamus and, by extension, to the organization of thalamocortical connections. With the exception of the visual thalamus, there are significantly fewer inhibitory neurons in the rodent thalamus (Jones, 2010), and the reticular nucleus of the thalamus, composed of inhibitory neurons, is enlarged. The extent and density of axons immunoreactive (denoted by the suffix-*ir*) for the dopamine transporter (DAT) is remarkably greater in the macaque dorsal thalamus (and, by extension, presumably in humans), with the mediodorsal association nucleus and the ventral motor nuclei having the densest immunolabeling (Fig. 1.1). Ultrastructural

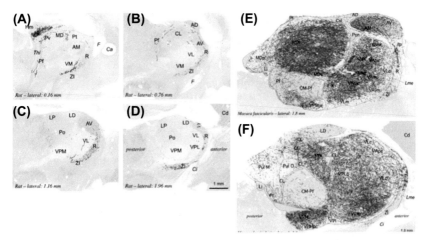

FIGURE 1.1 Distribution of dopamine transporter immunoreceptive (DAT-ir) axons *(red)* in parasagittal sections of the rat (A–D) and macaque monkey thalamus (E, F). Note differential distribution and greater density in the macaque thalamus. *Reproduced with permission from Oxford University Press, Garcia-Cabezas et al., (2009). Dopamine innervation in the thalamus: monkey vs rat.* Cerebral cortex 19 *(2), 424–434.*

analysis of the macaque mediodorsal nucleus reveals that thalamic interneurons (which are absent in the rodent) are a main postsynaptic target of DAT-ir axons (Garcia-Cabezas, Martinez-Sanchez, Sanchez-Gonzalez, Garzon, & Cavada, 2009).

Almost as notable as species differences are the many conserved features of cortical organization between primates and rodents. The primary cortical areas are recognizable across species, as are the basic cortical layers and cell types, and the main neurochemical transmitter and neuromodulatory systems. Despite the previously mentioned differences in thalamic organization, both primates and rodents have a conspicuous parallel system of driving corticothalamic projections from layer 5 and modulatory corticothalamic projections from layer 6 (Rouiller & Welker, 2000).

CORTICAL AREAS

In the general mammalian plan, the cerebral cortex is parcellated into discrete motor, primary sensory, and association areas (Zilles, 2004, Chapter 27). The number of cortical areas, exclusive of the primary sensory and motor areas, is species-dependent. Individual areas are specified by the interplay of intrinsic genetic mechanisms and extrinsic information conveyed by thalamocortical input (O'Leary, Chou, & Sahara, 2007). The primary areas are topographically organized (in terms of peripheral visual, auditory, and somatosensory fields) and are interconnected with primary thalamic nuclei. The degree of specialization of the primary areas is also species-dependent and correlated with dominant sensory modality and behaviors. In the highly visual primates, the primary visual cortex, although comparatively thin, has distinctive sublaminar structure as well as modular organization for ocular dominance and orientation selectivity. For rodents, the somatosensory barrel cortex is a highly specialized representation of the snout vibrissae.

Historically, areas were delineated on the basis of differences in cell and myelin density. More recently, gene expression profiles to some extent have confirmed area parcellations (Fig. 1.2), although only a very few area-specific genes have so far been reported (Bernard et al., 2012; Watakabe et al., 2007; Yamamori, 2011; Yamamori & Rockland, 2006). More common is the occurrence of gradient-wise gene expression across primary and association cortices. The distribution of various receptors ("receptor fingerprints") is another marker for area boundaries (Zilles, Palomero-Gallagher, & Schleicher, 2004). Some areas have "sharp" boundaries (especially specialized primary sensory and limbic areas), but the majority seem to have less sharp borders (Rosa & Tweedale, 2005).

How are areas organized as networks? A popular view has emphasized a hierarchical organization, where primary sensory areas are at the lowest level, with progressive serial projections emanating through the association areas (Graziano & Aflalo, 2007; Markov & Kennedy, 2013). There have, however, been extensive discussions about "reverse hierarchies," where connections proceed into the sensory areas (Hochstein & Ahissar, 2002); "alternative hierarchies" derived from properties such as reaction times (Petroni, Panzeri, Hilgetag, Kotter, & Young, 2001); and supraareal clusters based on functional imaging (Buckner & Yeo, 2014).

The great cortical sensory systems are largely, but not exclusively, modality specific. The primary sensory areas in rodents are mutually interconnected by a network of border-crossing, long-range connections (eg, Mongolian gerbil, Henschke, Noesselt, Scheich, & Budinger, 2014; rat, Stehberg, Dang, & Frostig, 2014). In rats, direct connections have been reported from the retrosplenial cortex, a higher order limbic association cortex, to the primary visual cortex (Vogt & Miller, 1983). Cross-sensory connections have been reported in primates (Borra & Rockland, 2011; Falchier, Clavagnier, Barone, & Kennedy, 2002; Rockland & Ojima, 2003), but appear to be sparser than in rodents. In monkeys, projections from parahippocampal areas to the primary visual cortex have been repeatedly verified (Doty, 1983; Kennedy & Bullier, 1985; Rockland & Van Hoesen, 1994).

The association areas receive converging cortical inputs from other association areas and sensory cortices, and from nonprimary thalamic nuclei, and are substantially expanded in human and nonhuman primate brains. Their organization is much less understood than is the case for primary and early association areas. Below is a walk-through of four classical cortical domains. This is very brief, and also noncomprehensive, leaving out the auditory cortex, insula, motor cortex, and other major areas. For the insula cortex, an important association area excluded because of space considerations, see Butti & Hof (2010)

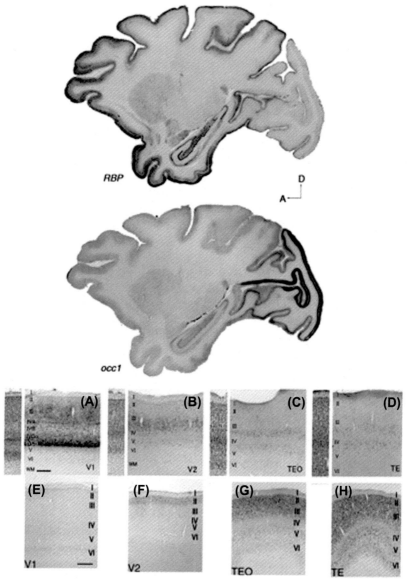

FIGURE 1.2   Expression of *occ1* (predominantly in area V1) and *RBP* (predominantly in association cortex) in the macaque neocortex, sagittal sections. *Bottom*: Higher magnification to show laminar distribution in selected areas. *Reproduced from Elsevier, Yamamori & Rockland, (2006). Neocortical areas, layers, connections, and gene expression.* Neuroscience Research 55, *11–27.*

and Craig (2010). Primary areas are less directly implicated in neurodegenerative and neuropsychiatric disorders and have accordingly not been included, as well as for the sake of conciseness (see General Reviews, such as Zilles, 2004, Chapter 27).

Frontal Cortex

In primates, three broad subdivisions of the frontal cortex are dorsolateral, medial, and orbital (Fig. 1.3). Each of these have further subdivisions, definable by cellular, myelin, or receptor architectonics and by differential connectivity with other cortical areas, mediodorsal and midline thalamic nuclei, striatum, amygdala, hypothalamus, and periaqueductal gray (Ongur & Price, 2000). In humans, monkeys, and, to some extent, rodents, separable networks have been associated with visceromotor or sensory functions (respectively, medial frontal or lateral orbital regions).

Several articles have discussed whether rodents have a frontal cortex (Krubitzer et al., 2011; Preuss, 1995; Uylings, Groenewegen, & Kolb, 2003). A main argument against, aside from the obviously smaller territory in rodents, has been that frontal areas in the rodent are agranular, without a layer 4. In favor has been the argument that in both primates and rodents, frontal areas have reciprocal connections with the mediodorsal thalamus. The general agreement seems to be that the granular, lateral prefrontal regions of primates are without homologues in the rodent, but that the medial and orbital regions can be viewed as approximately homologous. Specifically, the rodent infralimbic cortex has connections consistent with a role in the control of visceral/autonomic activity, as does the orbitomedial prefrontal cortex (PFC) of primates, and the rodent prelimbic cortex has connections consistent with a role in limbic–cognitive functions (Vertes, 2004). Worth noting in regard to cross-species homologies is that there are direct projections from hippocampal *cornu Ammonis* (CA) region 1 to both primate and rodent frontal areas, selectively targeting medial regions (Barbas & Blatt, 1995; Cavada, Company,

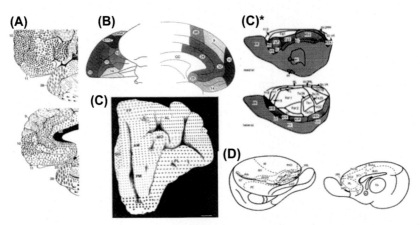

FIGURE 1.3   Architectonic maps of the prefrontal cortex, according to (A) the classical map of Brodmann in humans; (B) Petrides and Pandya (1994), in humans; (C) the orbital frontal map of Hof, Mufson, and Morrison (1995) in humans, (C*) medial *(top)* and lateral *(bottom)* surfaces in rat (Zilles & Wree, 1995), and (D) lateral *(left)* and medial *(right)* surfaces of the rat brain (Krettek & Price, 1977). *Reproduced with permission (from Figs. 1.1 and 1.3) from Oxford University Press, Ongur & Price, (2000). The organization of networks within the orbital and medial prefrontal cortex of rats, monkeys and humans. Cerebral Cortex 10(3), 206–219.*

Tejedor, Cruz-Rizzolo, & Reinoso-Suarez, 2000; Hoover & Vertes, 2007; Zhong, Yukie, & Rockland, 2006).

In rodents, motor areas are considered part of the frontal region, as is the *cingulate cortex* dorsomedially. The cingulate cortex [Brodmann areas (BAs) 24 and 32] is identifiable by gross location, overlying the anterior two-thirds of the corpus callosum and wrapping around this anteriorly (Fig. 1.4). In rodents, two subdivisions of BA32 and four subdivisions of BA24 are distinguished on the basis of gross location, cytoarchitecture, receptor binding patterns, and intracingulate connectivity (Vogt et al., 2013; Vogt & Paxinos, 2014). The posterior cingulate (BA23) in primates is lacking in rodents, where instead there is an expanded retrosplenial region (BA29). The anterior cingulate is associated with mood disorders, shows preferential loss of interneurons in variants of Huntington disease (see Chapter 8 and Kim et al., 2014), and has been reported to exhibit cytoarchitectural disorder in some cases of autism (Simms, Kemper, Timbie, Bauman, & Blatt, 2009).

Parietal Cortex

The parietal region in rodents is identifiable by gross location (posterior and lateral to the primary somatosensory cortex), by receptor binding (Caspers et al., 2013), and by patterns of thalamic and cortical connectivity (Kamishina et al., 2009; Wilber et al., 2015). In rats it has been subdivided into three (Zilles, 2004,

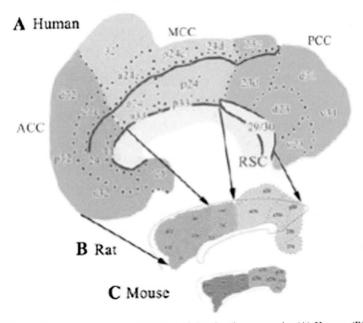

FIGURE 1.4 Summary maps of subdivisions of the cingulate cortex in: (A) Human, (B) Rat, and (C) Mouse. *ACC,* Anterior cingulate cortex; *MCC,* midcingulate cortex; *PCC,* posterior cingulate cortex; *RSC,* retrosplenial cortex. *Reproduced with permission from Springer, Vogt & Paxinos, (2014). Cytoarchitecture of mouse and rat cingulate cortex with human homologies.* Brain Structure & Function 219, *185–192.*

Chapter 27) or four regions (Wilber et al., 2015), in contrast with at least three large domains in the macaque (BAs 5, 7a, and 7b) and seven larger domains in the inferior parietal lobule of humans (Caspers et al., 2013). In both primates and rodents, there are dense parietofrontal connections (Graziano & Cooke, 2006). In general terms, the parietal cortex is associated with spatial awareness, orientation, and motor control (Reep & Corwin, 2009). In primates, some subdivisions contribute to corticospinal projections (Rozzi et al., 2006).

Temporal Cortex

The temporal lobe has undergone substantial expansion in humans, accompanied by ventral migration and reorganization of the hippocampus, and immediately adjoining subicular fields. The temporal pole is considered unique to human and non-human primates, and is closely involved in declarative memory (Insausti, 2013). In primates, the temporal lobe encompasses the inferotemporal visual association cortex, the primary and association auditory cortex, the parahippocampal region, the perirhinal cortex and, medial to the rhinal sulcus, the entorhinal cortex (EC).

The EC is reciprocally interconnected with the hippocampal formation and is of further interest because of its early pathology in Alzheimer's disease (AD) (see Chapter 4, and Braak & Braak, 1998; Braak, Rub, Schultz, & Del Trecici, 2006). In both human and nonhuman primates (Hevner & Wong-Riley, 1992), seven fields have been distinguished on the basis of differential cytoarchitectonics and (in monkeys) connectivity (Fig. 1.5). In rats and mice, two fields have been identified: the lateral EC and the medial EC (MEC). Grid cells, implicated in spatial navigation, are concentrated in the MEC (Moser et al., 2014; Witter, Canto, Couey, Koganezawa, & O'Reilly, 2013).

Laterally adjacent to the EC, the perirhinal region (BAs 35 and 36) has been subject to considerable debate as to whether it is best viewed as part of the medial temporal lobe memory system or as a perceptual region (De Curtis & Pare, 2004; Murray, Bussey, & Saksida, 2007; Suzuki & Naya, 2014). Anatomically, it is interconnected with the EC, but because it shares this property with other cortical regions, may not best be viewed in an exclusive "gatekeeper" role between the rest of neocortex and the EC.

CORTICAL LAYERS

By convention, the neocortex is described as having six layers. Allocortices (olfactory cortex and the hippocampus) are three-layered. Classically, the six neocortical layers were defined by differences in cell size and cell packing density (cytoarchitectonics). Myelin distribution, angioarchitectonics, and receptor-binding fingerprints also show layer-distinct patterns. The relative thickness of the individual layers varies by cortical area and by species. In rodents, the deeper, infragranular layers (below layer 4) are thicker, but in primates it is the supragranular layers (above layer 4) that are thicker (Fig. 1.6). This reflects differences in the proliferative cycles during development and is thought to have

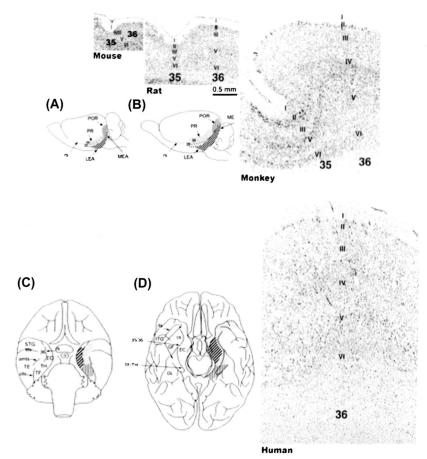

FIGURE 1.5 Schematic maps of the entorhinal and perirhinal areas in mouse (A), rat (B), monkey (C), and human (D). Top: Photomicrographs of Nissl-stained coronal sections through perirhinal cortex (areas 35 and 36) of the mouse, rat, macaque monkey, and human. The laminar pattern is indicated by Roman numerals. *Reproduced with permission from John Wiley and Sons, Burwell, (2000). The parahippocampal region: corticocortical connectivity.* Annals of the New York Academy of Sciences 1225, 47–58.

consequences for the proportion of cortical versus subcortical projections. Subcortical projections, in both rodents and primates, originate almost exclusively from the deeper cortical layers (see section: Layers and Outputs).

Layer 1 is cell-sparse, containing distal dendrites of many, but not all, underlying pyramidal cells, myelinated and unmyelinated fiber systems, and inhibitory interneurons and their associated microcircuitry (Jiang, Wang, Lee, Stornetta, & Zhu, 2013; Lee et al., 2014). Layers 2–6 all have a mix of excitatory pyramidal cells and inhibitory interneurons. Layer 2 is about the same thickness as layer 1 and in many areas can be distinguished as slightly more cell

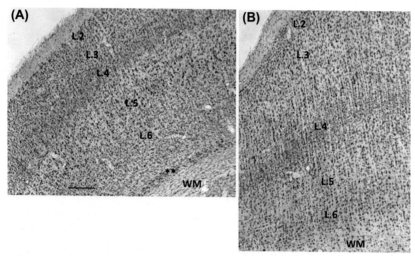

FIGURE 1.6   Nissl-stained sections of (A) rat somatosensory cortex, and (B) macaque monkey temporal cortex. The cortical thickness is greater in monkey, and layer 4 is more deeply situated. **, Layer seven, or residual subplate below layer 6; *L*, layer; *WM*, white matter (Scale bar = 200 μm).

dense than the underlying layer 3. Layer 4 (the granular layer) is a cell-dense band of small cells between layers 3 and 5. Layer 4 contains spiny stellate cells in the primary sensory areas, but small pyramids without extrinsic projections in other areas. Layers 5 and 6 lie between layer 4 and the white matter and, in many, but not all, areas are easily distinguishable. Layer 5 is typically less cell-dense and often has scattered large pyramidal cells. Below layer 6, there is a scattering of inhibitory and excitatory neurons (subgriseal, interstitial, or white matter neurons). In rodents, this population forms a thin sublayer. In humans, this layer is reported to be more neuron-dense in certain pathological conditions (Connor, Crawford, & Akbarian, 2011; Kanold & Luhmann, 2010; Yang, Fung, Rothwell, Tianmei, & Weickert, 2011). Some white matter neurons have corti-cothalamic projections (Giguere & Goldman-Rakic, 1988).

   The six-layer division, although useful as a standard reference and nomen-clature, has always been recognized as to some extent confusing. That is, layers have uneven borders, which are more scalloped than straightedge; incursion of neurons into immediately adjacent layers is common; and neurons with soma in one layer send their dendrites and local axons into overlying or underlying layers. An important further distinction is between granular and agranular areas, corresponding respectively to sensory and associational areas versus motor and limbic areas (Garcia-Cabezas & Barbas, 2014; Shipp, Adams, & Friston, 2013). Both cortical types occur in rodents and primates, but the agranular type is more abundant in rodents. In some species, such as dolphins and whales, the entire cortex is agranular, lacking in the small-celled layer 4 (Butti, Raghanti, Sherwood, & Hof, 2011).

The EC is distinguished by prominent cell islands in layer 2 (Fig. 1.5), a layer 4 that is cell-poor, and, especially in primates, a layer 6 characterized by a number of thin cellular lamellae ("onion skin"). Different subdivisions can be established on the basis of distinctness of the cell islands (Hevner & Wong-Riley, 1992).

A small number of genes are expressed in a layer-specific manner. These include *Cux2* (upper layers), *Rorbeta* (layer 4), *ERB81* (layer 5), and *Nurr1* (layer 6) (Arion, Unger, Lewis, & Mimics, 2007; Hevner, 2007; Molnar & Cheung, 2006; Watakabe et al., 2012). *Fez1* is specific for corticospinal neurons in layer 5. Patterns of gene expression vary across species (Fig. 1.7) and areas (Yamamori, 2011). There is a high degree of variability in gene expression profiles of individual neurons within a given layer, which is presumed to relate to a high diversity of neuronal subtypes, as yet poorly understood (Sorensen et al., 2015). Gene expression patterns are proving useful in assessing alterations in conditions such as human nodular heterotopia (Garbelli et al., 2009), epileptogenic focal cortical dysplasia (Hadjivassiliou et al., 2010; Rossini et al., 2011), and schizophrenia (Arion, Horvath, Lewis, & Mimics, 2010).

Layers and Outputs (Fig. 1.8)

Discussions of long-distance, extrinsic connections (ie, those beyond the home area of the projecting neuron) often summarize the supragranular layers as

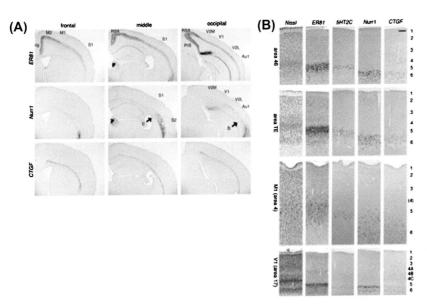

FIGURE 1.7   (A) In situ hybridization patterns of layer-specific genes in mouse cortex. (B) Layer-specific genes in four areas of macaque monkey cortex. *Reproduced with permission from Oxford University Press, Watakabe et al., (2007). Comparative analysis of layer-specific genes in mammalian neocortex. Cerebral Cortex 17(8), 1918–1933.*

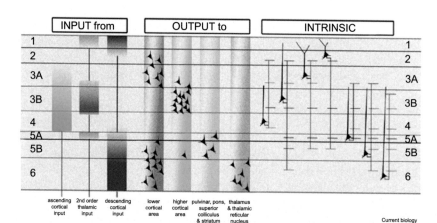

FIGURE 1.8 Summary schematic of inputs, outputs, and intrinsic excitatory connections of a generic, nonprimary area of primate cerebral cortex. *Reproduced with permission from Elsevier, Shipp, (2007). Structure and function of the cerebral cortex.* Current Biology 17, R443–R449.

projecting to various cortical targets, whereas the infragranular project subcortically. This is strictly correct for the upper layers, except for a small population of layer 3 neurons that project to the striatum in both primates and rodents. The deeper layers, however, in all areas and in both rodents and primates, contain projection neurons that target both cortical and subcortical structures. The proportion of neurons projecting to the various potential targets is area-dependent, and, although often overlooked, some pyramidal neurons have only local axonal collaterals without long-distance projections. This has been repeatedly reported for neurons in layer 6 (Thomson, 2010), but is likely to be true for those in other layers as well.

Neurons in layer 6 project to the thalamus (especially from layer 6B), to other cortical areas (from 6A), and to the claustrum (Thomson, 2010). Neurons projecting to these three different targets have distinguishable dendritic arbors, local axon collateralization (Katz, 1987), and differential gene expression profiles (Harris & Shepherd, 2015). Neurons in layer 5 have widespread connections, projecting subcortically to the thalamus, colliculi, pons, and striatum, and to other ipsilateral and contralateral cortical areas (Harris & Shepherd, 2015; Molnar & Cheung, 2006; Shipp, 2007).

An important point is that projections to a given target often originate from neurons in different layers. Corticothalamic projections originate from neurons in layers 5 and 6 in both primates and rodents; callosal and corticocortical projections originate from neurons in layers 3 and 5 in an area dependent manner; and feedback cortical projections originate from neurons in layers 2, upper 3, and 6. The reason for the bilaminar distribution is unclear, but may be related to a need for differential combinations of extrinsic and intrinsic circuitry and/or factors of temporal delays.

Layers and Inputs

Main inputs to cortical areas are from the thalamus (specific and/or associational), hypothalamus, amygdala, zona incerta (inhibitory to layer 1), other cortical areas, and serotonergic, dopaminergic, or noradrenergic neuromodulatory projections. Inputs from the thalamus (Jones, 2001) are mainly to layer 4 (core inputs from primary sensory and associational thalamic nuclei) or to layer 1 (matrix inputs from intralaminar and associational thalamic nuclei), from the hypothalamus to layer 6, and from the amygdala to layer 1 and other layers except layer 4. Cortical inputs are either to layer 4 and adjoining layers ("feedforward") or to layer 1 and other layers except layer 4 ("feedback") (Markov & Kennedy, 2013; Rockland, 1997, 2004; Shipp, 2007). Numerically, the main source of inputs to an individual pyramidal cell is intrinsic (ie, from neurons within the same area as the neuron of interest). In layer 3 of primates but not rodents, these form conspicuous patches over 2–3 mm from the parent soma (Boucsein, Nawrot, Schnepel, & Aertsen, 2011; Gilbert & Wiesel, 1983; Martin, Roth, & Rusch, 2014).

Extrinsic inputs commonly target one or more cortical layers; for example, thalamocortical terminations to the primary visual cortex in monkeys terminate densely in layer 4, but also in layers 6 and 1. This termination pattern is especially clear from visualization of geniculocortical terminations at single-axon resolution (Blasdel & Lund, 1983). Similarly, feedback cortical connections in the macaque terminate densely in layer 1, but also in layer 6. In rodents, these observe less of a laminar segregation, but consistently avoid layer 4.

Because dendrites usually extend through multiple layers, identifying the layer of termination for inputs is only a first step and not very informative unless there is also identification of the postsynaptic neurons. This identification has been difficult, and relatively few circuitry-level input maps are available for neocortex, unlike for the more simply stratified hippocampus (Megias, Emri, Freund, & Gulyas, 2001). Investigation of target localization and specificity is now rapidly advancing, especially in the mouse, where optogenetics and two-photon microscopy can be easily applied. So far, these studies are supportive of target specificity, even at the level of individual dendrites. Synaptic efficacy, however, depends not only on dendritic location, but rather on a combination of location, postsynaptic spine morphology, and channel and receptor distribution (eg, for layer 2 of mouse frontal cortex; Little & Carter, 2012). A reasonable conclusion, extrapolating from these results in rodents, is that pathology-related changes in spine density and/or morphology will have dramatic effects on specific individual inputs (see Chapter 2).

Interlaminar intrinsic circuitry is complex and likely to incorporate multiple potential routings. Circuitry will not necessarily be homogeneous within a single area; for example, the subdivisions of the somatosensory barrel cortex in the rodent (barrels or septa) have differential connectivity (Alloway, 2008; Lee, Alloway, & Kim, 2010).

CORTICAL VERTICALITY (COLUMNS)

The neocortex has a pronounced verticality that is obvious in cell stains, as noted by the early architectonic researchers. The vertical arrangements of cell bodies and, in particular, regional variability in the degree of verticality, were basic criteria in area identification (see Fig. 81 in Von Economo, 1927/2009). The cellular verticality is more pronounced in primates than in rodents, and is in part related to the radial glia scaffolding in early development and to the larger volume of neuropil-filled extracellular space in primates (Kirkcaldie, 2012; Spocter et al., 2012). Cellular columnarity implies a clear row of cell bodies from layers 2–6. In fact, however, this is rarely the case. More typically, cellular columns are only segments of about 400 µm in length (Fig. 1.9). Further, narrow columns in the upper layers can overlay wider cell aggregates in the immediately underlying deeper layers ("huddles"; Casanova, El-Baz, Vanbogaert, Narahari, & Trippe, 2009; Von Economo, 1927/2009). In nonprimate species, there is a dramatic range of patterns, including distinct cell aggregates or short columns in layer 5 of the bottlenose dolphin, but thin, pencil-like columns in layers 5 and 6 of the somatosensory cortex in the gray seal and manatee (Butti et al., 2011).

Several investigators have reported differences in size, shape, or cellular composition in cellular "minicolumns" (see Cell Types) in normal and autistic brains (eg, Casanova, El-Baz, Vanbogaert, Narahari, & Switala, 2010; review in Buxhoeveden, 2012). These investigators report average core width for normal brains as 11.5 µm in upper layers, 14.3 µm in layer 4, and 20.6 µm in deeper layers, but 8.7, 11.8, and 16.0 µm, respectively, for autistic brains (see, among others, Chance, Casanova, Switala, & Crow, 2008 on altered minicolumn spacing in auditory cortex of schizophrenic brains). These reports have been based on standard two-dimensional preparations, which often cut slantwise through the cortical thickness, with subsequent distortions to any apparent columnarity. As an assay and possible therapeutic target, changes in columnarity can be useful, but further investigation using global three-dimensional tissue specimens will be desirable.

Several other components besides cell bodies have a vertical organization. There are vertical fascicles of myelinated axons, from outgoing pyramidal cell axons and/or some incoming afferents (Peters & Sethares, 1996). Double-bouquet interneurons have narrow, vertically oriented axons (Yanez et al., 2005). Apical dendrites of some pyramidal cells cluster in small bundles. These, like the cellular columns, are often called minicolumns, and contrast with larger scale "macrocolumns" (respectively, ~50–80 and ~250 µm in diameter; Jones, 2000; Rockland & Ichinohe, 2004). Macrocolumns are associated with afferent input, as best established for thalamocortical input to the rodent somatosensory barrel cortex and ocular dominance columns in primates, but molecular factors may also have a significant role (Assali, Gaspar, & Rebsam, 2014; Crowley & Katz, 2002; Nakazawa, Koh, Kani, & Maeda, 1992).

To date, there has been only limited success toward any unified view of cortical columnar organization. In part, there is considerable regional variability,

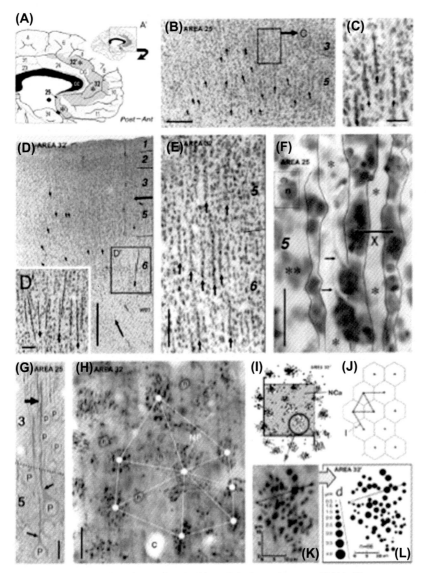

FIGURE 1.9 Cellular (B–F) and dendritic (G–L) minicolumns from area 32 (A) of human cortex. (H–K) are tangential sections to illustrate dendritic composition of the minicolumns. *Reproduced with permission from Gabbott, (2003). Radial organization of neurons and dendrites in human cortical areas 25, 32, and 32′.* Brain Research 992, *298–304.*

with only some areas (ie, temporal and extrastriate occipital in humans) having a conspicuous verticality. Further, as remarked, the candidate structures are neither identical in scale nor referenced to a common dimension; that is, basal dendrites of pyramidal cells, oblique dendrites, and apical dendritic tufts all extend beyond the dimension of a minicolumn and abundantly invade what would be adjacent columnar territories (Jones, 2000; Molnar, 2013; Rockland & Ichinohe, 2004). More particularly, there have been direct experimentally based challenges to the popular hypothesis of uniform cortical organization, based on comparative counts of narrow cellular columns (Rockel et al., 1980). At the macro scale, a study of rat barrel cortex found a 2.5-fold increase in the number of neurons per barrel, dorsal to ventral, and a concurrent increase in cortical thickness by 0.5 mm (Meyer et al., 2013).

For dendritic minicolumns, tangential sectioning has facilitated visualization and quantification (eg, Gabbott, 2003; Peters, Cifuentes, & Sethares, 1997); but because these are best demonstrated by immunohistochemistry for microtubule associated protein 2, a major problem is adequate quality of human postmortem tissue. The basic characterization, carried out in rodent sensory cortices, is that a core of apical dendrites of layer 5 pyramidal neurons is joined and encased by dendrites of layer 3 pyramids. In monkey visual cortex, the bundles were calculated as 23 μm across, and associated with 64 pyramidal neurons and 16 γ-aminobutyric acid (GABA) transmitting (GABAergic) neurons (Fig. 19 in Peters & Sethares, 1996). Some layer 5 neurons (solitons) do not join bundles. Dendrites of layer 4 and layer 6 neurons are also separate. In rat visual cortex and to some extent monkey cortical areas, layer 2 neurons join in pronounced dendritic bundles that interdigitate with apical dendrites from layer 5 (Ichinohe, Fujiyama, Kaneko, & Rockland, 2003; Ichinohe & Rockland, 2004).

Dendritic minicolumns vary across areas and species. In the retrosplenial cortex of rats, but not mice or primates, callosally projecting neurons in layer 2 form distinctive dendritic bundles (Wyss, Van Groen, & Sripanidkulchai, 1990). In macaque monkeys, the layer 5–based dendritic minicolumns that have been demonstrated in visual area (V) 1 are less prominent in area V2 and do not extend much above layer 4 (Peters et al., 1997).

One histological study in medial PFC (BAs 25, 32, and 32′) of humans has presented evidence for a radial organization of minicolumns (Gabbott, 2003). The author reports a range of 51 to 62 dendrites per cluster, dendritic diameters as 0.5–4.0 μm, and average intercluster center-to-center spacing of 55 μm. Short vertical stacks of 15–19 somata, reminiscent of cellular columns, were also reported (see Fig. 1.9).

Environmentally induced changes in dendritic minicolumns have been reported in rat visual cortex after visual deprivation (Gabbott & Stewart, 2012). Whereas the number of clusters remained constant, there was a significant reduction in the mean number of medium- and small-sized dendritic profiles. Other studies have investigated molecular influences in bundle formation. Reduced expression of *Satb2* in layer 2/3 neurons resulted in abnormal clumps of neuronal somata and dendritic fascicles in mouse visual cortex and, to a lesser extent, in somatosensory and motor areas (ie, in an anteroposterior gradient; Zhang et al., 2012). Dendritic bundles in the somatosensory cortex of $5-HT_{3A}$ receptor knockout mice are more dispersed compared with wildtype mice (Smit-Rigter, Wadman, & van Hooft, 2011). Overexpression of *NT3* in E18 rats resulted in abnormally distinct dendritic bundles in layer 2 of somatosensory cortex (Miyashita et al., 2010).

CELL TYPES

Pyramidal Neurons

Pyramidal neurons, the main cortical cell type, are excitatory glutamatergic neurons. In general, they have a pyramid-shaped soma and a pyramid-shaped dendritic tree. There is, however, considerable diversity on morphological grounds alone (DeFelipe & Farinas, 1992). The soma can be oval rather than pyramidal. One of the basal dendrites can be asymmetrically accentuated (compass cells of Von Economo) and almost as extensive as the main apical dendrite. The apical dendrite can be single or forked. For most pyramidal cells, the apical dendrite extends toward or into layer 1, but for a small number of pyramids (inverted), the apical dendrite extends toward or into the white matter. In primates, there are several populations of giant pyramidal neurons: Betz cells in motor cortex are a major source of corticospinal projections, and Meynert cells in the primary visual cortex project to the extrastriate middle temporal/V5 area and, often by collaterals, to the pulvinar and superior colliculus (Rockland, 2013).

In vitro studies and, to a lesser extent, intracellular filling in vivo of identified projection neurons, have provided a wealth of evidence for pyramidal subtypes as defined by correlated features such as firing properties, dendritic morphology, intrinsic interlaminar axonal collaterals, and extrinsic axon or extrinsic target structures (Fig. 1.10). One exhaustive study in rat PFC identified "more than 10" different pyramidal subtypes on the basis of dendritic morphology and firing properties (Van Aerde & Feldmeyer, 2014).

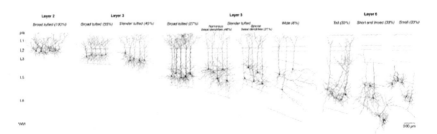

FIGURE 1.10 Overview of pyramidal subtypes in the rat medial prefrontal cortex (mPFC). Morphological reconstruction of soma and dendrites of five example cells for each morphological subtype. Cortical layers are indicated with *dashed lines. L,* Layer; *WM,* white matter. *Reproduced with permission from Oxford University Press, van Aerde & Feldmeyer, (2015). Morphological and physiological characterization of pyramidal neuron subtypes in rat medial prefrontal cortex.* Cerebral Cortex 25(3), 788–805.

Neurons in layer 6 (early born developmentally) show the greatest heterogeneity. A seminal early in vitro study in cat visual cortex (Katz, 1987) identified morphological criteria that distinguished three populations in layer 6: namely, corticoclaustral, corticothalamic, and intrinsic corticocortical. In areas except for primary sensory areas, corticocortical feedback neurons (Rockland, 1994) are located in layer 6. These four subtypes are likely to occur widely in other cortices.

In layer 5, two broad classes of projection neurons have been identified (Fig. 1.11) as intracephalic, having projections only to cortical and striatal targets (ie, within the telencephalon), and pyramidal tract, projecting to the brainstem but with collaterals to the thalamus, striatum, and several other regions (Harris & Shepherd, 2015; Molyneaux, Arlotta, Menezes, & Macklis, 2007; Reiner, Hart, Lei, & Deng, 2010).

Corticothalamic neurons (Rockland, 1996; Rouiller & Welker, 2000; Sherman & Guillery, 2002) are distinguished by home layer of the soma (layer 5 or 6), by dendritic morphology (respectively, tufted or slender), and by extrinsic axon features. Neurons in layer 5 have small terminal arbors with a small number of big synapses located proximally at the thalamic postsynaptic neuron. Neurons in layer 6 have spatially divergent arbors with a large number of small terminal specializations located distally on the thalamic postsynaptic neurons. Layer 6 corticothalamic neurons, but usually not those in layer 5, have collaterals to the reticular nucleus of the thalamus.

Neurochemical Features

A small number of glutamatergic pyramidal cells have a colocalized calcium-binding protein. A group of calretinin-positive (CR^+) pyramidal cells has been identified in layer 5A of the anterior cingulate cortex in humans and, to a lesser degree, the great apes (Hof, Nimchinsky, Perl, & Erwin, 2001). In humans and macaques, some large neurons in layer 5 are parvalbumin-positive (PV^+): namely, Betz cells in the motor cortex, Meynert cells in the visual cortex, and some large neurons in parietal areas (Constantinople, Disney, Maffie, Rudy, & Hawken, 2009; Ichinohe et al., 2004; Preuss & Kaas, 1996). Some of these are also positive for KV3.1b, a potassium channel more usually associated with rapid firing interneurons. In mice, PV^+ pyramidal cells have been reported in layer 5 of visual, motor, and, especially numerous, in somatosensory areas.

Calbindin-positive (CB^+) pyramidal neurons are common in the rodent cortex. In monkeys, there are several reports of CB^+ neurons, mainly in layer 3 of the PFC (Gabbott & Bacon, 1996) and in an increasing gradient from area V1 to temporal cortical regions (Kondo, Hashikawa, Tanaka, & Jones, 1994). This trend continues into hippocampal CA1, where a sizable subpopulation of neurons in the superficial sublayer is CB^+. These CA1 neurons are also positive for the synaptic zinc, an activity-related neuromodulator (Slomianka, Amrein, Knuesel, Sorensen, & Wolfer, 2011). Comparable data are not available for neocortical CB^+ pyramids.

(A) Commissural; callosal projection neurons

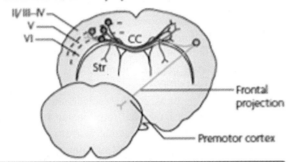

- Callosal neurons (layers II/III, V, VI)
- Callosal neurons with ipsilateral frontal projections (layer V)
- Callosal neurons with striatal projections (layer Va)

(B) Corticofugal; corticothalamic neurons

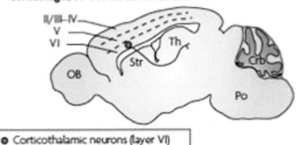

- Corticothalamic neurons (layer VI)

(C) Corticofugal; subcerebral projection neurons

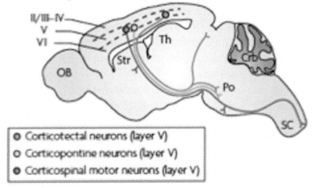

- Corticotectal neurons (layer V)
- Corticopontine neurons (layer V)
- Corticospinal motor neurons (layer V)

FIGURE 1.11 Subtypes of projection neurons within the neocortex, shown for rodent. *CC*, corpus callosum; *Po*, pons; *Sc*, superior colliculus; *Str*, striatum; *Th*, thalamus. *Reproduced with permission from Macmillan Publishers Ltd., Molyneaux et al., (2007). Neuronal subtype specification in the cerebral cortex.* Nature Reviews Neuroscience 8, 427–437.

The cytoskeletal marker SMI32 (antibody against nonphosphorylated neurofilaments) is selectively expressed in subpopulations of pyramidal neurons, in both primates and rodents. Finer correlation, however, with specific feedforward or feedback connections has not yielded a clear association (Hof et al., 1996). In temporal areas of patients with AD, loss of SMI32 expression is paralleled by an increase in neurofibrillary tangles and antibody AT8 reactivity (Thangavel, Sahu, Van Hoesen, & Zaheer, 2009).

A subset of pyramidal neurons in both rodents and primates uses synaptic zinc. These include some corticostriatal, corticoclaustral, and corticocortical neurons, but specifically not corticothalamic neurons. One study in monkeys found that feedback neurons in layer 6, but seemingly not those in layers 2 and 3, were more likely to use synaptic zinc than feedforward projecting neurons. This is consistent with dense labeling for zinc-positive terminations in parts of layers 1 and 6 (preferentially targeted by feedback projections) but not layer 4 (zone of thalamocortical and feedforward cortical terminations; Ichinohe, Matsushita, Ohta, & Rockland, 2010). Zinc dyshomeostasis has been associated with neuronal injury and death in major human neurological disorders such as stroke, epilepsy, and AD (Sensi et al., 2011).

Interneurons

Functionally significant interneuron diversity is firmly established (Fig. 1.12) based on morphological features such as dendritic morphology, neurochemistry, postsynaptic target domains, and, to some extent, firing properties (DeFelipe, 2002; Kepecs & Fishell, 2014; Kubota, 2014). Early work in the 1990s commonly subdivided GABAergic interneurons on the basis of colocalized neuropeptides or expression of the calcium-binding proteins, calbindin (CB), parvalbumin (PV), or calretinin (CR), as correlated with other features (Kawaguchi & Kubota, 1997). These three broad categories occur in both rodents and primates, but with significant quantitative differences between species and across areas (DeFelipe et al., 1999, 2002; Gabbott, Jays, & Bacon, 1997; Yanez et al., 2005). More recently, investigators working with mice have preferred a modified classification, according to expression of PV, somatostatin, or the ionotropic serotonin receptor, 5HT3a. This is in accord with embryological origins of these subpopulations and accounts for nearly 100% of the GABAergic neurons (Rudy, Fishell, Lee, & Hjerling-Leffler, 2011). The literature on interneuron types and circuitry is substantial and only a very few specific examples are covered here, as representative of the role of interneuron circuitry.

Parvalbumin-Positive Interneurons

PV^+ interneurons are the most abundant category and are further subdivided into two large subtypes. Basket cells preferentially target cell bodies and proximal dendrites of pyramidal and nonpyramidal neurons, and chandelier cells (axoaxonic

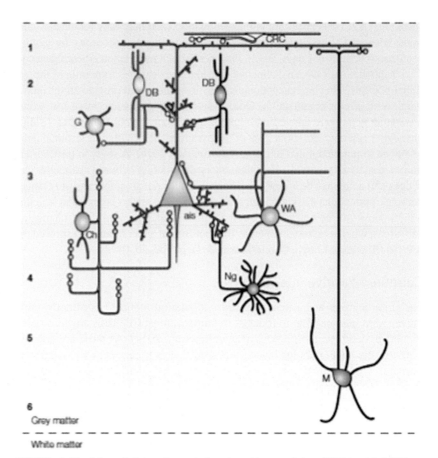

FIGURE 1.12 Subpopulations of γ-aminobutyric acid transmitting (GABAergic) inhibitory interneurons and the location of their synaptic inputs to a generic postsynaptic pyramidal cell *(green)*. *ais*, axon initial segment; *CB/red*, calbindin; *Ch*, chandelier; *CR/yellow*, calretinin; *CRC*, Cajal-Retzius cell; *DB*, double bouquet cell; *M*, Martinotti cell; *Ng*, neurogliaform; *PV/ blue*, parvalbumin; *WA*, wide-arbor basket cell. *Reproduced with permission from Macmillan Publishers Ltd., Lewis et al., (2005). Cortical inhibitory neurons and schizophrenia.* Nature Reviews Neuroscience 6, *312–324.*

cells) have terminations directed to the pyramidal cell axon initial segment (DeFelipe, 1997). Basket cells are either large, with an extensive horizontal axon, or small and with a more localized axon territory (Kisvarday, 1992). Some basket cells express cholecystokinin (CCK) instead of PV. This distinction is important because postmortem studies have established multiple molecular alterations in the two neurochemical subtypes that are associated with schizophrenia (see Chapter 11, and Curley & Lewis, 2012; Lewis, Hashimoto, & Volk, 2005): namely, lower expression of glutamic acid decarboxylase (GAD) by CCK basket cells, and lower $GABA_A$ receptor α_1 subunit in pyramidal cells postsynaptic to PV basket cells. Generally speaking, CCK basket cells are implicated in mood and necessary for theta oscillations, whereas PV basket cells are implicated in timing and necessary for gamma oscillations (Curley & Lewis, 2012). Thus pericellular innervation is heterogeneous.

Chandelier cells have a distinctive cartridgelike "candle" formation of the terminal boutons. They are exceptionally easy to identify and provide an intriguing window to circuit organization. One study using a transgenic mouse in which chandelier cells were labeled with green fluorescent protein found that a single chandelier cell contacts about 20% of the pyramidal cells within its terminal field, and does so nonrandomly (Blazquez-Llorca et al., 2014). A study in postmortem human tissue has reported a complementary distribution between chandelier cartridges and what may be a subtype of basket cell termination, forming very dense, complex pericellular basket endings. Sensory-motor areas (except area V1) had a high density of complex basket cell formations and low density of chandelier cartridges, whereas association areas (but not frontal areas 13 and 47) showed the reverse (Blazquez-Llorca, Garcia-Marin, & DeFelipe, 2010).

Calretinin-Positive Interneurons

CR$^+$ interneurons are a heterogeneous population, which is distinctly more prevalent in humans than in rodents. In humans, most CR$^+$ cells are considered bipolar in dendritic morphology (Radonjic et al., 2014). As these are concentrated in the supragranular layers, the zone that is preferentially expanded in primates, CR$^+$ interneurons have been discussed as specifically associated with primate-specific corticocortical processing.

Layer 1 Interneurons

Layer 1 harbors a heterogeneous mix of GABAergic neurons, including CR$^+$ Cajal-Retzius cells in development. An excellent example of circuit complexity is a study of slices of rat sensorimotor cortex, which identified and minutely reported the elements of two interneuronal circuits and how these impact on firing properties of layer-5 pyramidal cells (Jiang et al., 2013). Single bouquet cells appeared designed for disinhibition. These formed unidirectional inhibitory connections on seven discernible subtypes of interneurons in layers 2 and 3, which themselves inhibited the entire dendritic–somatic–axonal axis of a small number of layer 5 pyramids. Elongated neurogliaform neurons, in contrast, mediated pyramidal cell inhibition by having mutual inhibitory and electrical interneuronal connections. These results were interpreted in the context of possible attentional tasks, in part because of the mix of extrinsic cholinergic and feedback inputs to layer 1 (Larkum, 2013), and also have implications for the overall excitatory–inhibitory balance.

Nitric Oxide Producing γ-Aminobutyric Acid Transmitting Interneurons

These neurons comprise a small, heterogeneous subtype that colocalizes neuropeptide Y or somatostatin, and occurs mainly in layers 1, 2, and 6 and white matter in rodents and primates. Nitric oxide (NO) neurons have pleiotropic actions, among which is an important role in activity-related cycles of vasodilation and vasoconstriction (Barbaresi, Fabri, & Mensa, 2014; Tricoire, Kubota, & Cauli, 2013). Given the diffusion properties of NO, these neurons are estimated to have a sphere of influence extending over a radius of 100 μm.

CONNECTIONS

Cortical areas participate in a dense network of intrinsic and extrinsic connections (Harris & Shepherd, 2015; Markov & Kennedy, 2013; Rockland, 1997; Shipp, 2007). Intrinsic connections (ie, local connections, within the same area as the parent neuron) consist of a variety of intralaminar, interlaminar, and very local inhibitory and excitatory connections. Intralaminar (horizontal) connections can be extensive, extending over a radius of 2.0–3.0 mm from the parent soma. These consist of collaterals of extrinsically projecting pyramidal neurons, and in primates, but not rodents, form patchy aggregates of terminations. The few studies that have quantified the number of collaterals per neuron suggest that these vary up to about nine (Gilbert & Wiesel, 1983; Martin et al., 2014; Yabuta & Callaway, 1998).

Extrinsic connections originate mainly from pyramidal cells, although a very small number of GABAergic cells have extrinsic cortical projections in both primates and rodents (Tomioka & Rockland, 2007). As summarized, pyramidal neurons in the infragranular layers project to multiple subcortical structures (colliculi, pons, periaqueductal gray) and thereby participate in multisynaptic loops, which eventually return to the cortex. There are only few data on the relative number of intrinsic and extrinsic synapses for any pyramidal neuron, but there is some evidence that for corticocortical and perhaps corticothalamic projecting neurons, the number of intrinsic synapses is greater.

Extrinsic cortical connections can be subdivided as feedforward (originating mainly from layer 3 or layers 3 and 5) and feedback (originating mainly from layers 2, 3A, and 6). This implies a more or less serial progression of connections from the primary sensory and early association areas, to association areas in the frontal, parietal, and temporal lobes, but, although a convenient distinction, it is important not to overemphasize the duality (Rockland, 1997, 2004). For one thing, there is strong evidence for iterative, nonserial interareal interactions. Simultaneous recordings from area V1 and extrastriate area V4 in awake monkeys show that visual information about global contours in a cluttered background emerges initially in V4, approximately 40 ms sooner than in V1, and continues to develop in parallel in both areas (Chen et al., 2014). Moreover, there are clearly further subtypes based on differences in axon caliber (Anderson & Martin, 2002; Innocenti, Vercelli, & Caminiti, 2014), density of terminal specializations (Anderson & Martin, 2009), and whether or not the neurons use synaptic zinc (Ichinohe et al., 2010). A study in auditory cortex describes both feedforward and feedback projections as including multiple strands that target neurons in different layers (Hackett et al., 2014).

The primate cortical visual system has been depicted as sequential processing "streams" proceeding through extrastriate areas from the primary area. These were originally conceived as dual dorsal and ventral steams (respectively associated with motion-processing and object recognition). More recently, the idea of two streams in primates has been revisited as having a more complex organization, constrained by at least six distinct cortical and subcortical systems (Kravitz, Saleem, Baker, Ungerleider, & Mishkin, 2013). In the mouse, recent studies have identified at least five extrastriate areas associated with primary visual cortex, with some indication of functionally specialized streams (Glickfeld, Reid, & Andemann, 2014; Marshel, Garrett, Nauhaus, & Callaway, 2011; Wang, Sporns, & Burkhalter, 2012).

Connections are inherently complex, by definition linking multiple structures that operate through flexible roles and flexible routes in different behaviors. Ongoing discussions stress task-modulated response and a "picture of functional neuronal networks in which local circuits dealing with different valences interact to transfer information across different brain areas" (Luthi & Luscher, 2014). The terminology and representations fall far short of conveying the actual complexity. The arrows commonly used in summary diagrams or the tabular connectivity matrices tend to imply a point-to-point organization. In reality, connections are divergent (one neuron projecting to hundreds or thousands of others), convergent (one neuron receiving thousands of synapses from hundreds of other neurons), and often branched (Rockland, 2004, 2013).

Arrows or double-headed arrows are a convenient representation of reciprocal connectivity, but this is almost always an idealization. At the cell-to-cell level, there are no data about direct reciprocity; and a reasonable assumption would be that any direct cell-to-cell reciprocating connections would be only a small subset of a neuron's synaptic inputs. At the structure-to-structure level, corticothalamic, corticoamygdala, and most corticocortical connections are reciprocal; corticostriatal, corticocollicular, and other corticosubcortical connections are not.

The strength or efficacy of projections (connectional "weights") depends not only on the number of synapses but also on factors such as the strength of individual synapses, in relation to number of presynaptic vesicles and the assortment of activated postsynaptic receptors, as well as the location of the synapse in relation to the postsynaptic target and neighboring synapses (Glickfeld et al., 2014). A case in point is the thalamocortical projection to primary sensory areas. Multiple studies report that these comprise only a small proportion of the synaptic input to layer 4 neurons, but nevertheless strongly excite the postsynaptic targets (da Costa & Martin, 2011; Latawiec, Martin, & Meskenaite, 2000; Peters & Payne, 1993). One aspect of this seeming discrepancy, as demonstrated in rat somatosensory cortex, is that thalamocortical and corticocortical synapses are both weak, but thalamic synapses are sufficiently convergent and coincidentally active to exert an outsized influence (Schoonover et al., 2014).

CONCLUDING REMARKS

The cerebral cortex has been under investigation with increasingly powerful techniques for over a century. As put forth in this chapter, there is general agreement as to the basic anatomical features, but at the same time, it is widely acknowledged that key organizational components remain to be discovered (Bargmann & Marder, 2013). This is not a negative, but more a call for a new surge in research endeavors, as is in fact happening. The present excitement in the field, backed with significantly improved technical developments, is a promising scenario for important new insights and therapeutic strategies.

REFERENCES

Alloway, K. D. (2008). Information processing streams in rodent barrel cortex: the differential functions of barrel and septal circuits. *Cerebral Cortex, 18*, 979–989.

Anderson, J., & Martin, K. A. C. (2002). Connection from cortical area V2 to MT in macaque monkey. *Journal of Comparative Neurology, 495*, 709–721.

Anderson, J., & Martin, K. A. C. (2009). The synaptic connections between cortical areas V1 and V2 in macaque monkey. *The Journal of Neuroscience: The Official Journal of the Society for Neuroscience, 29*, 11283–11293.

Arion, D., Horvath, S., Lewis, D. A., & Mimics, K. (2010). Infragranular gene expression disturbances in the prefrontal cortex in schizophrenia: signature of altered neural development? *Neurobiology of Disease, 37*, 738–746.

Arion, D., Unger, T., Lewis, D. A., & Mimics, K. (2007). Molecular markers distinguishing supragranular and infragranular layers in the human prefrontal cortex. *The European Journal of Neuroscience, 25*, 1843–1854.

Assali, A., Gaspar, P., & Rebsam, A. (2014). Activity dependent mechanisms of visual map formation: from retinal waves to molecular regulators. *Seminars in Cell and Developmental Biology, 35*, 136–146.

Ballesteros-Yanez, I., Benavides-Piccione, R., Elston, G. N., Yuste, R., & DeFelipe, J. (2006). Density and morphology of dendritic spines in mouse neocortex. *Neuroscience, 138*, 403–409.

Barbaresi, P., Fabri, M., & Mensa, E. (2014). Characterization of NO-producing neurons in the rat corpus callosum. *Brain and Behavior, 4*, 317–336.

Barbas, H., & Blatt, G. J. (1995). Topographically specific hippocampal projections target functionally distinct prefrontal areas in the rhesus monkey. *Hippocampus, 5*, 511–533.

Bargmann, C. L., & Marder, E. (2013). From the connectome to brain function. *Nature Methods, 10*, 483–490.

Beaudin, S. A., Singh, T., Agster, K. L., & Burwell, R. D. (2013). Borders and comparative cytoarchitecture of the perirhinal and postrhinal cortices in an F1 hybrid mouse. *Cerebral Cortex, 23*, 460–476.

Benavides-Piccione, R., Ballesteros-Yanez, I., DeFelipe, J., & Yuste, R. (2002). Cortical area and species differences in dendritic spine morphology. *Journal of Neurocytology, 31*, 337–346.

Bernard, A., Tanis, K. Q., Luo, R., Podtelezhnikov, A. A., Finney, E. M., McWhorter, M. M. E., et al. (2012). Transcriptional architecture of the primate neocortex. *Neuron, 73*, 1083–1099.

Blasdel, G. G., & Lund, J. S. (1983). Termination of afferent axons in macaque striate cortex. *The Journal of Neuroscience: The Official Journal of the Society for Neuroscience, 3*, 1389–1413.

Blazquez-Llorca, L., Garcia-Marin, V., & DeFelipe, J. (2010). GABAergic complex basket formations in the human neocortex. *Journal of Comparative Neurology, 518,* 4917–4937.

Blazquez-Llorca, L., Woodruff, A., Inan, M., Anderson, S. A., Yuste, R., DeFelipe, J., et al. (2014). Spatial distribution of neurons innervated by chandelier cells. *Brain Structure and Function* (Epub ahead of print).

Borra, E., & Rockland, K. S. (2011). Projections to early visual areas V1 and V2 in the calcarine fissure from parietal association areas in the macaque. *Frontiers in Neuroanatomy, 5* (article 35).

Boucsein, C., Nawrot, M. P., Schnepel, P., & Aertsen, A. (2011). Beyond the cortical column: abundance and physiology of horizontal connections imply a strong role for inputs from the surround. *Frontiers in Neuroscience, 5* (article 32).

Braak, H., & Braak, E. (1998). Evolution of neuronal changes in the course of Alzheimer's disease. *Journal of Neural Transmission. Supplement, 53,* 127–140.

Braak, H., Rub, U., Schultz, C., & Del Trecici, K. (2006). Vulnerability of cortical neurons to Alzheimer's and Parkinson's diseases. *Journal of Alzheimer's Disease, 9,* 35–44.

Buckner, R. L., & Yeo, B. T. T. (2014). Borders, map clusters, and supra-areal organization in visual cortex. *Neuroimage, 93,* 290–297.

Burwell, R. D. (2000). The parahippocampal region: corticocortical connectivity. *Annals of the New York Academy of Sciences, 911,* 25–42.

Butti, C., & Hof, P. R. (2010). The insular cortex: a comparative perspective. *Brain Structure and Function, 214,* 477–493.

Butti, C., Raghanti, M. A., Shrwood, C. C., & Hof, P. R. (2011). The neocortex of cetaceans: cytoarchitecture and comparison with other aquatic and terrestrial species. *Annals of the New York Academy of Sciences, 1225,* 47–58.

Butti, C., Santos, M., Uppal, N., & Hof, P. R. (2013). Von Economo neurons: clinical and evolutionary perspectives. *Cortex: A Journal Devoted to the Study of the Nervous System and Behavior, 49,* 312–326.

Buxhoeveden, D. P. (2012). Minicolumn size and human cortex. *Progress in Brain Research, 195,* 219–235.

Casanova, M. F., El-Baz, A., Vanbogaert, E., Narahari, P., & Switala, A. (2010). A topographic study of minicolumnar core width by lamina comparison between autistic subjects and controls: possible minicolumnar disruption due to an anatomical element in-common to multiple laminae. *Brain Pathology, 20,* 451–458.

Casanova, M. F., El-Baz, A., Vanbogaert, E., Narahari, P., & Trippe, J. (2009). Minicolumnar width: comparison between supragranular and infragranular layers. *Journal of Neuroscience Methods, 184,* 19–24.

Caspers, S., Schleicher, A., Bacha-Trams, M., Palomero-Gallagher, N., Amunts, K., & Zilles, K. (2013). Organization of the human inferior parietal lobule based on receptor architectonics. *Cerebral Cortex, 23,* 615–628.

Cavada, C., Company, T., Tejedor, J., Cruz-Rizzolo, R. J., & Reinoso-Suarez, F. (2000). The anatomical connections of the macaque monkey orbitofrontal cortex: a review. *Cerebral Cortex, 10,* 220–242.

Chance, S. A., Casanova, M. F., Switala, A. E., & Crow, T. J. (2008). Auditory cortex asymmetry, altered minicolumn spacing and absence of ageing effects in schizophrenia. *Brain: A Journal of Neurology, 131,* 3178–3192.

Charvet, C. J., Cahalane, D. J., & Finlay, B. L. (2015). Systematic, cross-cortex variation in neuron numbers in rodents and primates. *Cerebral Cortex, 25,* 147–160.

Chen, M., Yan, Y., Gong, X., Gilbert, C. D., Liang, H., & Li, W. (2014). Incremental integration of global contours through interplay between visual cortical areas. *Neuron, 82,* 682–694.

Connor, C. M., Crawford, B. C., & Akbarian, S. (2011). White matter neuron alterations in schizophrenia and related disorders. *International Journal of Developmental Neuroscience, 29*, 325–334.

Constantinople, C. M., Disney, A. A., Maffie, J., Rudy, B., & Hawken, M. J. (2009). Quantitative analysis of neurons with Kv3 potassium channel subunits, Kv3.1b and Kv3.2, in macaque primary visual cortex. *Journal of Comparative Neurology, 516*, 291–311.

da Costa, N. M., & Martin, K. A. (2011). How thalamus connects to spiny stellate cells in the cat's visual cortex. *The Journal of Neuroscience: The Official Journal of the Society for Neuroscience, 31*, 2925–2937.

Craig, A. D. (2010). The sentient self. *Brain Structure & Function, 214*, 563–577.

Crowley, J. C., & Katz, L. C. (2002). Ocular dominance development revisited. *Current Opinion in Neurobiology, 12*, 104–109.

Curley, A. A., & Lewis, D. A. (2012). Cortical basket cell dysfunction in schizophrenia. *Journal of Physiology, 590*, 715–724.

De Curtis, M., & Pare, D. (2004). The rhinal cortices: a wall of inhibition between the neocortex and the hippocampus. *Progress in Neurobiology, 74*, 101–110.

DeFelipe, J. (1997). Types of neurons, synaptic connections and chemical characteristics of cells immunoreactive for calbindin-D28K, parvalbumin and calretinin in the neocortex. *Journal of Chemical Neuroanatomy, 14*, 1–19.

DeFelipe, J. (2002). Cortical interneurons: from Cajal to 2001. *Progress in Brain Research, 136*, 215–238.

DeFelipe, J., Alonso-Nanclares, L., & Arellano, J. I. (2002). Microstructure of the neocortex: comparative aspects. *Journal of Neurocytology, 31*, 299–316.

DeFelipe, J., Ballesteros-Yanez, I., Inda, M. C., & Munoz, A. (2006). Double-bouquet cells in the monkey and human cerebral cortex with special reference to areas 17 and 18. *Progress in Brain Research, 154*, 15–32.

DeFelipe, J., & Farinas, I. (1992). The pyramidal neuron of the cerebral cortex: morphological and chemical characteristics of the synaptic inputs. *Progress in Neurobiology, 39*, 563–607.

DeFelipe, J., Gonzalez-Albo, M. C., Del Rio, M. R., & Elston, G. N. (1999). Distribution and patterns of connectivity of interneurons containing calbindin, calretinin, and parvalbumin in visual areas of the occipital and temporal lobes of the macaque monkey. *Journal of Comparative Neurology, 412*, 515–526.

Doty, R. W. (1983). Non geniculate afferents to striate cortex in macaques. *Journal of Comparative Neurology, 218*, 159–173.

Douglas, R., Markram, H., & Martin, K. (2004). Neocortex. In G. M. Shepherd (Ed.), *The synaptic organization of the brain* (5th ed.) (pp. 499–558). New York: Oxford University Press.

Elston, G. N., Benavides-Piccione, R., Elston, A., Manger, P. R., & DeFelipe, J. (2011). Pyramidal cells in the prefrontal cortex of primates: marked differences in neuronal structure among species. *Frontiers in Neuroanatomy, 5*, 764 (article 2).

Evrard, H., Forro, T., & Logothetis, N. (2012). Von Economo neurons in the anterior insula of the macaque monkey. *Neuron, 74*, 482–489.

Falchier, A., Clavagnier, S., Barone, P., & Kennedy, H. (2002). Anatomical evidence of multimodal integration in primate striate cortex. *The Journal of Neuroscience: The Official Journal of the Society for Neuroscience, 22*, 5749–5759.

Gabbott, P. L. A. (2003). Radial organization of neurons and dendrites in human cortical areas 25, 32, and 32′. *Brain Research, 992*, 298–304.

Gabbott, P. L. A., & Bacon, S. J. (1996). Local circuit neurons in the medial prefrontal cortex (areas 24a,b,c, 25 and 32) in the monkey. II. Quantitative areal and laminar distributions. *Journal of Comparative Neurology, 364*, 609–636.

Gabbott, P. L. A., Jays, P. R. L., & Bacon, S. J. (1997). Calretinin neurons in human medial pre-frontal cortex (Areas 24a, b, c, 32', and 25). *Journal of Comparative Neurology, 381,* 389–410.

Gabbott, P. L., & Stewart, M. G. (2012). Visual deprivation alters dendritic bundle architecture in layer 4 of rat visual cortex. *Neuroscience, 207,* 65–77.

Garbelli, R., Rossini, L., Moroni, R. F., Watakabe, A., Yamamori, T., Tassi, L., et al. (2009). Layer-specific genes reveal a rudimentary laminar pattern in human nodular heterotopia. *Neurology, 73,* 746–753.

Garcia-Cabezas, M. A., & Barbas, H. (2014). Area 4 has layer IV in adult primates. *The European Journal of Neuroscience, 39,* 1824–1834.

Garcia-Cabezas, M., Martinez-Sanchez, P., Sanchez-Gonzalez, M. A., Garzon, M., & Cavada, C. (2009). Dopamine innervation in the thalamus: monkey versus rat. *Cerebral Cortex, 19,* 424–434.

Giguere, M., & Goldman-Rakic, P. S. (1988). Mediodorsal nucleus: areal, laminar, and tangential distribution of afferents and efferents in the frontal lobe of rhesus monkeys. *Journal of Comparative Neurology, 277,* 195–213.

Gilbert, C. D., & Wiesel, T. N. (1983). Clustered intrinsic connections in cat visual cortex. *The Journal of Neuroscience: The Official Journal of the Society for Neuroscience, 3,* 1116–1133.

Glickfeld, L. L., Reid, R. C., & Andermann, M. L. (2014). A mouse model of higher visual cortical function. *Current Opinion in Neurobiology, 24,* 28–33.

Graziano, M. S. A., & Aflalo, T. N. (2007). Rethinking cortical organization: moving away from discrete areas arranged in hierarchies. *The Neuroscientist: A Review Journal Bringing Neurobiology, Neurology and Psychiatry, 13,* 138–147.

Graziano, M. S. A., & Cooke, D. F. (2006). Parieto-frontal interactions, personal space, and defensive behavior. *Neuropsychologia, 44,* 845–859.

Hackett, T. A., de la Mothe, L. A., Camalier, C. R., Falchier, A., Lakatos, P., Kajikawa, Y., et al. (2014). Feedforward and feedback projections of caudal belt and parabelt areas of auditory cortex: refining the hierarchical model. *Frontiers in Neuroscience, 8* (article 72).

Hadjivassiliou, G., Martinian, L., Squier, W., Blumcke, I., Aronica, E., Sisodiya, S. M., et al. (2010). The application of cortical layer markers in the evaluation of cortical dysplasias in epilepsy. *Acta Neuropathologica, 120,* 517–528.

Harris, K. D., & Shepherd, G. M. G. (2015). The neocortical circuit: themes and variations. *Nature Neuroscience, 18,* 170–181.

Henschke, J. U., Noesselt, T., Scheich, H., & Budinger, E. (2014). Possible anatomical pathways for short-latency multisensory integration processes in primary sensory cortices. *Brain Structure and Function* (Epub ahead of print).

Hevner, R. F. (2007). Layer-specific markers as probes for neuron type identity in human neocortex and malformations of cortical development. *Journal of Neuropathology & Experimental Neurology, 66,* 101–109.

Hevner, R. F., & Wong-Riley, M. T. (1992). Entorhinal cortex of the human, monkey, and rat: metabolic map as revealed by cytochrome oxidase. *Journal of Comparative Neurology, 326,* 451–469.

Hochstein, S., & Ahissar, M. (2002). View from the top: hierarchies and reverse hierarchies in the visual system. *Neuron, 36,* 791–804.

Hof, P. R., Mufson, E. J., & Morrison, J. H. (1995). Human orbitofrontal cortex: cytoarchitecture and quantitative immunohistochemical parcellation. *Journal of Comparative Neurology, 359,* 48–68.

Hof, P. R., Nimchinsky, E. A., Perl, D. P., & Erwin, J. M. (2001). An unusual population of pyramidal neurons in the anterior cingulate cortex of hominids contains the calcium-binding protein calretinin. *Neuroscience Letters, 307,* 139–142.

Hof, P. R., Ungerleider, L. G., Webster, M. J., Gattass, R., Adams, M. M., Saailstad, C. A., et al. (1996). Neurofilament protein is differentially distributed in subpopulations of corticocortical projection neurons in the macaque monkey visual pathways. *Journal of Comparative Neurology*, *376*, 112–127.

Hoover, W. B., & Vertes, R. P. (2007). Anatomical analysis of afferent projections to the medial prefrontal cortex in the rat. *Brain Structure and Function*, *212*, 149–179.

Ichinohe, N., Fujiyama, F., Kaneko, T., & Rockland, K. S. (2003). Honeycomb-like mosaic at the border of layers 1 and 2 in the cerebral cortex. *The Journal of Neuroscience: The Official Journal of the Society for Neuroscience*, *23*, 1372–1382.

Ichinohe, N., Matsushita, A., Ohta, K., & Rockland, K. S. (2010). Pathway-specific utilization of synaptic zinc in the macaque ventral visual cortical areas. *Cerebral Cortex*, *20*, 2818–2831.

Ichinohe, N., & Rockland, K. S. (2004). Region specific micromodularity in the uppermost layers in primate cerebral cortex. *Cerebral Cortex*, *14*, 1173–1184.

Ichinohe, N., Watakabe, A., Miyashita, T., Yamamori, T., Hashikawa, T., & Rockland, K. S. (2004). A voltage-gated potassium channel, Kv3.1b, is expressed by a subpopulation of large pyramidal neurons in layer 5 of the macaque monkey cortex. *Neuroscience*, *129*, 179–185.

Innocenti, G. M., Vercelli, A., & Caminiti, R. (2014). The diameter of cortical axons depends both on the area of origin and target. *Cerebral Cortex*, *24*, 2178–2188.

Insausti, R. (2013). Comparative neuroanatomical parcellation of the human and nonhuman primate temporal pole. *Journal of Comparative Neurology*, *521*, 4163–4176.

Jiang, X., Wang, G., Lee, A. J., Stornetta, R. L., & Zhu, J. (2013). The organization of two new cortical interneuronal circuits. *Nature Neuroscience*, *16*, 210–219.

Jones, E. G. (2000). Microcolumns in the cerebral cortex. *Proceedings of the National Academy of Sciences USA*, *97*, 5019–5021.

Jones, E. G. (2001). The thalamic matrix and thalamocortical synchrony. *Trends in Neurosciences*, *24*, 595–601.

Jones, E. G. (2010). The thalamus. In G. M. Shepherd, & S. Grillner (Eds.), *Handbook of brain microcircuits* (pp. 59–74). Oxford Univ. Press.

Kamishina, H., Conte, W. L., Patel, S. S., Tai, R. J., Corwin, J. V., & Reep, R. L. (2009). Cortical connections of the rat lateral posterior thalamic nucleus. *Brain Research*, *1264*, 36–56.

Kanold, P. O., & Luhmann, H. J. (2010). The subplate and early cortical circuits. *Annual Review of Neuroscience*, *33*, 23–48.

Katz, L. C. (1987). Local circuitry of identified projection neurons in cat visual cortex brain slices. *The Journal of Neuroscience: The Official Journal of the Society for Neuroscience*, *7*, 1223–1249.

Kawaguchi, Y., & Kubota, Y. (1997). GABAergic cell subtypes and their synaptic connections in rat frontal cortex. *Cerebral Cortex*, *7*, 476–486.

Kennedy, H., & Bullier, J. (1985). A double-labeling investigation of the afferent connectivity to cortical areas V1 and V2 of the macaque monkey. *The Journal of Neuroscience: The Official Journal of the Society for Neuroscience*, *5*, 2815–2830.

Kepecs, A., & Fishell, G. (2014). Interneuron cell types are fit to function. *Nature*, *505*, 318–326.

Kim, E. H., Thu, D. C., Tippett, L. J., Oorschot, D. E., Hogg, V. M., Roxburgh, R., et al. (2014). Cortical interneuron loss and symptom heterogeneity in Huntington disease. *Annals of Neurology*, *75*, 717–727.

Kirkcaldie, M. T. K. (2012). Neocortex. In C. Watson, G. Paxinos, & L. Puelles (Eds.), *The mouse nervous system* (pp. 52–111). Elsevier, Academic Press.

Kisvarday, Z. F. (1992). GABAergic networks of basket cells in the visual cortex. *Progress in Brain Research*, *90*, 385–405.

Kondo, H., Hashikawa, T., Tanaka, K., & Jones, E. G. (1994). Neurochemical gradient along the monkey occipito-temporal cortical pathway. *Neuroreport, 5*, 613–616.

Kravitz, D. J., Saleem, K. S., Baker, C. I., Ungerleider, L. G., & Mishkin, M. (2013). The ventral visual pathway: an expanded neural framework for the processing of object quality. *Trends in Cognitive Sciences, 17*, 26–49.

Krettek, J. E., & Price, J. L. (1977). Projections from the amygdala complex to the cerebral cortex and thalamus in the rat and cat. *Journal of Comparative Neurology, 172*, 687–722.

Krubitzer, L., Campi, K. L., & Cooke, D. F. (2011). All rodents are not the same: a modern synthesis of cortical organization. *Brain, Behavior and Evolution, 78*, 51–93.

Kubota, Y. (2014). Untangling GABAergic wiring in the cortical microcircuit. *Current Opinion in Neurobiology, 26*, 7–14.

Larkum, M. (2013). A cellular mechanism for cortical associations: an organizing principle for the cerebral cortex. *Trends in Neurosciences, 36*, 141–151.

Latawiec, D., Martin, K. A., & Meskenaite, V. (2000). Terminations of the geniculocortical projection in the striate cortex of macaque monkey: a quantitative immunoelectron microscopic study. *Journal of Comparative Neurology, 419*, 306–319.

Lee, T., Alloway, K. D., & Kim, U. (2010). Interconnected cortical networks between primary somatosensory cortex septal columns and posterior parietal cortex in rat. *Journal of Comparative Neurology, 519*, 405–419.

Lee, A. J., Wang, G., Jiang, X., Johnson, S. M., Hoang, E. T., Lante, F., et al. (2014). Canonical organization of layer 1 neuron-led cortical inhibitory and disinhibitory interneuronal circuits. *Cerebral Cortex* Feb 18. (Epub ahead of print).

Lewis, D. A., Hashimoto, T., & Volk, D. W. (2005). Cortical inhibitory neurons and schizophrenia. *Nature Reviews Neuroscience, 6*, 312–324.

Lewitus, E., Kelava, I., Kalinka, A. T., Tomancak, P., & Huttner, W. B. (2014). An adaptive threshold in mammalian neocortex evolution. *PLoS Biology, 12*, e1002000.

Little, J. P., & Carter, A. G. (2012). Subcellular synaptic connectivity of layer 2 pyramidal neurons in the medial prefrontal cortex. *The Journal of Neuroscience: The Official Journal of the Society for Neuroscience, 32*, 12808–12819.

Luthi, A., & Luscher, C. (2014). Pathological circuit function underlying addiction and anxiety disorders. *Nature Neuroscience, 17*, 1635–1643.

Markov, N. T., & Kennedy, H. (2013). The importance of being hierarchical. *Current Opinion in Neurobiology, 23*, 187–194.

Marshel, J. H., Garrett, M. E., Nauhaus, I., & Callaway, E. M. (2011). Functional specialization of seven mouse visual areas. *Neuron, 72*, 1040–1054.

Martin, K. A., Roth, S., & Rusch, E. S. (2014). Superficial layer pyramidal cells communicate heterogeneously between multiple functional domains of cat primary visual cortex. *Nature Communications, 5*, 5252.

Megias, M., Emri, Z. S., Freund, T. F., & Gulyas, A. I. (2001). Total number and distribution of inhibitory and excitatory synapses on hippocampal CA1 pyramidal cells. *Neuroscience, 102*, 527–540.

Meyer, H. S., Egger, R., Guest, J. M., Foerster, R., Reissl, S., & Oberlaender, M. (2013). Cellular organization of cortical barrel columns is whisker-specific. *Proceedings of the National Academy of Sciences of the USA, 110*, 19113–19118.

Miyashita, T., Wintzer, M., Kurotani, T., Konishi, T., Ichinohe, N., & Rockland, K. S. (2010). Neurotrophin-3 is involved in the formation of apical dendritic bundles in cortical layer 2 of the rat. *Cerebral Cortex, 20*, 229–240.

Molnar, Z. (2013). Cortical columns. In J. L. R. Rubenstein, & P. Rakic (Eds.), *Neural circuit development and function in the healthy and diseased brain* (Vol. 3) (pp. 109–129). Amsterdam: Elsevier.

Molnar, Z., & Cheung, A. F. P. (2006). Towards the classification of subpopulations of layer V pyramidal projection neurons. *Neuroscience Research, 55*, 105–115.

Molyneaux, B. J., Arlotta, P., Menezes, J. R. L., & Macklis, J. D. (2007). Neuronal subtype specification in the cerebral cortex. *Nature Reviews Neuroscience, 8*, 427–437.

Mortensen, H. S., Pakkenberg, B., Dam, M., Dietz, R., Sonne, C., Mikkelsen, B., et al. (2014). Quantitative relationships in delphinid neocortex. *Frontiers in Neuroanatomy, 8*, 132.

Moser, E. I., Roudi, Y., Witter, M. P., Kentros, C., Bonhoeffer, T., & Moser, M. B. (2014). Grid cells and cortical representation. *Nature Reviews Neuroscience, 15*, 466–481.

Mota, B., & Herculano-Houzel, S. (2012). How the cortex gets its folds: an inside-out, connectivity-driven model for the scaling of mammalian cortical folding. *Frontiers in Neuroanatomy, 6* (article 3).

Murray, E. A., Bussey, T. J., & Saksida, L. M. (2007). Visual perception and memory: a new view of medial temporal lobe function in primates and rodents. *Annual Review of Neuroscience, 30*, 99–122.

Nakazawa, M., Koh, T., Kani, K., & Maeda, T. (1992). Transient patterns of serotonergic innervation in the rat visual cortex: normal development and effects of neonatal enucleation. *Brain Research. Developmental Brain Research, 66*, 77–90.

Oberheim, N. A., Wang, X., Goldman, S., & Nedergaard, M. (2006). Astrocytic complexity distinguishes the human brain. *Trends in Neurosciences, 29*, 547–553.

O'Leary, D. D. M., Chou, S.-J., & Sahara, S. (2007). Area patterning of the mammalian cortex. *Neuron, 56*, 252–269.

Ongur, D., & Price, J. L. (2000). The organization of networks within the orbital and medial prefrontal cortex of rats, monkeys, and humans. *Cerebral Cortex, 10*, 206–219.

Peters, A., Cifuentes, J. M., & Sethares, C. (1997). The organization of pyramidal cells in area 18 of the rhesus monkey. *Cerebral Cortex, 7*, 405–421.

Peters, A., & Payne, B. R. (1993). Numerical relationships between geniculocortical afferents and pyramidal cell modules in cat primary visual cortex. *Cerebral Cortex, 3*, 69–78.

Peters, A., & Sethares, C. (1996). Myelinated axons and the pyramidal cell modules in monkey primary visual cortex. *Journal of Comparative Neurology, 365*, 232–255.

Petrides, M., & Pandya, D. N. (1994). Comparative architectonic analysis of the human and the macaque frontal cortex. In F. Boller, & J. Grafman (Eds.), *Handbook of neuropsychology* (p. 17e58). Amsterdam: Elsevier.

Petroni, F., Panzeri, S., Hilgetag, C. C., Kotter, K., & Young, M. P. (2001). Simultaneity of responses in a hierarchical visual network. *Neuroreport, 12*, 2753–2759.

Preuss, T. M. (1995). Do rats have prefrontal cortex? The Rose-Woolsey-Akert program, reconsidered. *Journal of Cognitive Neuroscience, 7*, 1–24.

Preuss, T. M., & Kaas, J. H. (1996). Parvalbumin-like immunoreactivity of layer V pyramidal cells in the motor and somatosensory cortex of adult primates. *Brain Research, 712*, 353–357.

Radonjic, N. V., Ortega, J. A., Memi, F., Dionne, K., Jakovcevski, I., & Zecevic, N. (2014). The complexity of the calretinin-expressing progenitors in the human cerebral cortex. *Frontiers in Neuroanatomy, 8* (article 82).

Reep, R. L., & Corwin, J. V. (2009). Posterior parietal cortex as part of a neural network for directed attention in rats. *Neurobiology of Learning and Memory, 91*, 104–113.

Reiner, A., Hart, N. M., Lei, W., & Deng, Y. (2010). Corticostriatal projection neurons: dichotomous types and dichotomous functions. *Frontiers in Neuroanatomy, 4* (article 142).

Rockel, A. J., Hiorns, R. W., & Powell, T. P. (1980). The basic uniformity in structure of the neocortex. *Brain: A Journal of Neurology, 103*, 221–244.

Rockland, K. S. (1994). The organization of feedback connections from area V2(18) to V1(17). In A. Peters, & K. S. Rockland (Eds.), *Primary visual cortex in primates* (pp. 261–299). New York: Plenum Press.

Rockland, K. S. (1996). Two types of cortico pulvinar terminations: round (type 2) and elongate (type 1). *Journal of Comparative Neurology, 368*, 57–87.

Rockland, K. S. (1997). Elements of cortical architecture: hierarchy revisited. In K. S. Rockland, J. H. Kaas, & A. Peters (Eds.), *Extrastriate cortex in primates* (pp. 243–293). New York: Plenum Press.

Rockland, K. S. (2004). Feedback connections: splitting the arrow. In J. H. Kaas, & C. E. Collins (Eds.), *The primate visual system* (pp. 387–406). Boca Raton, FL: CRC Press.

Rockland, K. S. (2013). Collateral branching of long-distance cortical projections in monkey. *Journal of Comparative Neurology, 521*, 4112–4123.

Rockland, K. S., & Ichinohe, N. (2004). Some thoughts on cortical minicolumns. *Experimental Brain Research, 158*, 265–277.

Rockland, K. S., & Ojima, H. (2003). Multisensory convergence in calcarine visual areas in macaque monkey. *International Journal of Psychophysiology, 50*, 19–26.

Rockland, K. S., & Van Hoesen, G. W. (1994). Direct temporal-occipital feedback connections to striate cortex (V1) in the macaque monkey. *Cerebral Cortex, 4*, 300–313.

Rosa, M. G., & Tweedale, R. (2005). Brain maps, great and small: lessons from comparative studies of primate visual cortical organization. *Philosophical Transactions of the Royal Society B: Biological Sciences, 360*, 665–691.

Rossini, L., Moroni, R. F., Tassi, L., Watakabe, A., Yamamori, T., Spreafico, R., et al. (2011). Altered layer-specific gene expression in cortical samples from patients with temporal lobe epilepsy. *Epilepsia, 52*, 1928–1937.

Rouiller, E. M., & Welker, E. (2000). A comparative analysis of the morphology of corticothalamic projections in mammals. *Brain Research Bulletin, 53*, 727–741.

Roux, L., & Buzsaki, G. (2015). Tasks for inhibitory interneurons in intact circuits. *Neuropharmacology, 88*, 10–23.

Rozzi, S., Calzavara, R., Belmalih, A., Borra, E., Gregoriou, G. G., Matelli, M., et al. (2006). Cortical connections of the inferior parietal cortical convexity of the macaque monkey. *Cerebral Cortex, 16*, 1389–1417.

Rudy, B., Fishell, G., Lee, S. H., & Hjerling-Leffler, J. (2011). Three groups of interneurons account for nearly 100% of neocortical GABAergic neurons. *Developmental Neurobiology, 71*, 45–61.

Schoonover, C. E., Tapia, J. C., Schilling, V. C., Wimmer, V., Blazeski, R., Zhang, W., et al. (2014). Comparative strength and dendritic organization of thalamocortical and corticocortical synapses onto excitatory layer 4 neurons. *The Journal of Neuroscience: The Official Journal of the Society for Neuroscience, 34*, 6746–6758.

Seeley, W. W., Merkle, F. T., Gaus, S. E., Craig, A. D., Allman, J. M., & Hof, P. R. (2012). Distinctive neurons of the anterior cingulate and frontoinsular cortex: a historical perspective. *Cerebral Cortex, 22*, 245–250.

Sensi, S. L., Paoletti, P., Koh, J. Y., Aizenman, E., Bush, A. L., & Hershfinkel, M. (2011). The neurophysiology and pathology of brain zinc. *The Journal of Neuroscience: The Official Journal of the Society for Neuroscience, 31*, 16076–16085.

Sherman, S. M., & Guillery, R. W. (2002). The role of the thalamus in the flow of information to the cortex. *Philosophical Transactions of the Royal Society B, 357*, 1695–1708.

Shipp, S. (2007). Structure and function of the cerebral cortex. *Current Biology, 17*, R44R449.

Shipp, S., Adams, R. A., & Friston, K. J. (2013). Reflections on agranular architecture: predictive coding in the motor cortex. *Trends in Neurosciences, 36*, 706–716.

Shipton, O. A., El-Gaby, M., Apergis-Schoute, J., Deisseroth, K., Bannerman, D. M., Paulsen, O., et al. (2014). Left-right dissociation of hippocampal memory processes in mice. *Proceedings of the National Academy of Sciences, 111*, 5238–5243.

Simms, M. L., Kemper, T. L., Timbie, C. M., Bauman, M. L., & Blatt, G. J. (2009). The anterior cingulate cortex in autism: heterogeneity of qualitative and quantitative cytoarchitectonic features suggests possible subgroups. *Acta Neuropathologica, 118*, 673–684.

Slomianka, L., Amrein, I., Knuesel, I., Sorensen, J. C., & Wolfer, D. P. (2011). Hippocampal pyramidal cells: the reemergence of cortical lamination. *Brain Structure & Function, 216*, 301–317.

Smit-Rigter, L. A., Wadman, W. J., & van Hooft, J. A. (2011). Alterations in apical dendritic bundling in the somatosensory cortex of 5-HT$_{3A}$ receptor knockout mice. *Frontiers in Neuroanatomy, 5* (article 64).

Sorensen, S. A., Bernard, A., Menon, V., Royall, J. J., Glattfelder, K. J., Desta, T., et al. (2015). Correlated gene expression and target specificity demonstrate excitatory projection neuron diversity. *Cerebral Cortex, 25*, 433–449.

Spocter, M. A., Hopkins, W. D., Barks, S. K., Bianchi, S., Hehmeyer, A. E., Anderson, S. M., et al. (2012). Neuropil distribution in the cerebral cortex differs between humans and chimpanzees. *Journal of Comparative Neurology, 520*, 2917–2929.

Stehberg, J., Dang, P. T., & Frostig, R. D. (2014). Unimodal primary sensory cortices are directly connected by long-range horizontal projections in rat sensory cortex. *Frontiers in Neuroanatomy, 8*, 93.

Sun, T., & Hevner, R. F. (2014). Growth and folding of the mammalian cerebral cortex: from molecules to malformations. *Nature Reviews Neuroscience, 15*, 217–232.

Suzuki, W. A., & Naya, Y. (2014). The Perirhinal cortex. *Annual Review of Neuroscience, 37*, 39–53.

Thangavel, R., Sahu, S. K., Van Hoesen, G. W., & Zaheer, A. (2009). Loss of nonphosphorylated neurofilament immunoreactivity in temporal cortical areas in Alzheimer's disease. *Neuroscience, 160*, 427–433.

Thomson, A. M. (2010). Neocortical layer 6, a review. *Frontiers in Neuroanatomy, 4* (article 13).

Tomioka, R., & Rockland, K. S. (2007). Long-distance corticocortical GABAergic neurons in the adult monkey white and gray matter. *Journal of Comparative Neurology, 505*, 526–538.

Tricoire, L., Kubota, Y., & Cauli, B. (2013). Cortical NO interneurons: from embryogenesis to functions. *Frontiers in Neural Circuits, 7* (article 105).

Uylings, H. B. M., Groenewegen, H. J., & Kolb, B. (2003). Do rats have a prefrontal cortex. *Behavioural Brain Research, 146*, 3–17.

Van Aerde, K. I., & Feldmeyer, D. (2014). Morphological and physiological characterization of pyramidal neuron subtypes in rat medial prefrontal cortex. *Cerebral Cortex, 25*, 788–805.

Vertes, R. P. (2004). Differential projections of the infralimbic and prelimbic cortex in the rat. *Synapse, 51*, 32–58.

Vogt, B. A., Hof, P. R., Zilles, K., Vogt, L. J., Herold, C., & Palomero-Gallagher, N. (2013). Cingulate area 32 homologies in mouse, rat, macaque and human: cytoarchitecture and receptor architecture. *Journal of Comparative Neurology, 521*, 4189–4204.

Vogt, B. A., & Miller, M. W. (1983). Cortical connections between rat cingulate cortex and visual, motor, and postsubicular cortices. *Journal of Comparative Neurology, 10*, 192–210.

Vogt, B. A., & Paxinos, G. (2014). Cytoarchitecture of mouse and rat cingulate cortex with human homologies. *Brain Structure & Function, 219*, 185–192.

Von Economo, C. (1927/2009). Cellular structure of the human cerebral cortex. In: L.C. Triarhou (Editor and Translator), Basel: Karger.

Wang, Q., Sporns, O., & Burkhalter, A. (2012). Network analysis of corticocortical connections reveals ventral and dorsal processing streams in mouse visual cortex. *The Journal of Neuroscience: The Official Journal of the Society for Neuroscience, 32*, 4386–4399.

Watakabe, A., Hirokawa, J., Ichinohe, N., Ohsawa, S., Kaneko, T., Rockland, K. S., et al. (2012). Area-specific substratification of deep layer neurons in the rat cortex. *Journal of Comparative Neurology, 520*, 3553–3573.

Watakabe, A., Ichinohe, N., Ohsawa, S., Hashikawa, T., Komatsu, Y., Rockland, K. S., et al. (2007). Comparative analysis of layer-specific genes in mammalian neocortex. *Cerebral Cortex, 17,* 1918–1933.

Wilber, A. A., Clark, B. J., Demecha, A. J., Mesina, L., Vos, J. M., & McNaughton, B. L. (2015). Cortical connectivity maps reveal anatomically distinct areas in the parietal cortex of the rat. *Frontiers in Neural Circuits, 8* (article 146).

Witter, M. P., Canto, C. B., Couey, J. J., Koganezawa, N., & O'Reilly, K. C. (2013). Architecture of spatial circuits in the hippocampal region. *Philosophical Transactions of the Royal Society B, 369,* 1635.

Wyss, J. M., Van Groen, T., & Sripanidkulchai, K. (1990). Dendritic bundling in layer I of granular retrosplenial cortex: intracellular labeling and selectivity of innervation. *Journal of Comparative Neurology, 295,* 33–42.

Yabuta, N. H., & Callaway, E. M. (1998). Cytochrome-oxidase blobs and intrinsic horizontal connections of layer 2/3 pyramidal neurons in primate V1. *Visual Neuroscience, 15,* 1007–1027.

Yamamori, T. (2011). Selective gene expression in regions of primate neocortex: implications for cortical specialization. *Progress in Neurobiology, 94,* 201–222.

Yamamori, T., & Rockland, K. S. (2006). Neocortical areas, layers, connections, and gene expression. *Neuroscience Research, 55,* 11–27.

Yanez, I. B., Munoz, A., Contreras, J., Gonzalez, J., Rodriguez-Veiga, E., & DeFelipe, J. (2005). Double bouquet cell in the human cerebral cortex and a comparison with other mammals. *Journal of Comparative Neurology, 486,* 344–360.

Yang, Y., Fung, S. J., Rothwell, A., Tianmei, S., & Weickert, C. S. (2011). Increased interstitial white matter neuron density in the dorsolateral prefrontal cortex of people with schizophrenia. *Biological Psychiatry, 69,* 63–70.

Zhang, L., Song, N.-N., Chen, J.-Y., Huang, Y., Li, H., & Ding, Y.-Q. (2012). Satb2 is required for dendritic arborization and soma spacing in mouse cerebral cortex. *Cerebral Cortex, 22,* 1510–1519.

Zhong, Y. M., Yukie, M., & Rockland, K. S. (2006). Distinctive morphology of hippocampal CA1 terminations in orbital and medial frontal cortex in macaque monkeys. *Experimental Brain Research, 169,* 549–553.

Zilles, K. (2004). Architecture of the human cerebral cortex. In G. Paxinos, & J. K. Mai (Eds.), *The human nervous system* (2nd ed.) (pp. 997–1060). Elsevier Academic Press.

Zilles, K., Palomero-Gallagher, N., & Amunts, K. (2013). Development of cortical folding during evolution and ontogeny. *Trends in Neurosciences, 36,* 275–284.

Zilles, K., Palomero-Gallagher, N., & Schleicher, A. (2004). Transmitter receptors and functional anatomy of the cerebral cortex. *Journal of Anatomy, 205,* 417–432.

Zilles, K., & Wree, A. (1995). Cortex: areal and laminar structure. In G. Paxinos (Ed.), *The rat nervous system* (pp. 649–685). San Diego: Academic Press.

Chapter 2

Cortical Plasticity in Response to Injury and Disease

N. Weishaupt

University of Western Ontario, London, ON, Canada

PLASTICITY: A MAJOR PLAYER IN RECOVERY FROM CENTRAL NERVOUS SYSTEM INJURY AND DISEASE

Recovery after central nervous system (CNS) injury or disease is rarely complete, leaving affected individuals with compromised brain and/or spinal cord function for the rest of their lives. This is partly because of the extremely limited ability of neurons to renew themselves. Indeed, mature cortical neurons fail to divide and are unable to undergo adult neurogenesis, a unique process characteristic to only select few brain regions. This stands in contrast to most other tissues in the body, where regeneration is a powerful repair mechanism. The process of tissue regeneration can lead to *restitutio ad integrum,* a complete restoration of the healthy tissue condition and function. Even though *restitutio ad integrum* is not part of the routine repertoire of the brain or of today's neuroscientists, we do know that the brain has a substantial ability to adapt its existing circuits to changing demands. Collectively called *plasticity,* this adaptive reorganization among nerve cells constitutes a valuable intrinsic repair mechanism for CNS injury and disease. This is most clearly evident after traumatic brain injury or postischemia, where limited functional recovery is usually observed over weeks and months. Although spontaneous plasticity may be limited in restoring compromised brain function, the real promise lies in promoting, modifying, and guiding these intrinsic rearrangements. The more understanding we gain of the complex interplay of factors involved in plasticity from a systems level to a synaptic level, the closer we move toward the goal of maximizing recovery of brain functions after injury and disease.

SYSTEMS LEVEL PLASTICITY

Experience-Based Plasticity

During development, experience within a critical window determines which neuronal connections thrive and which ones are pruned. Brain plasticity in

The Cerebral Cortex in Neurodegenerative and Neuropsychiatric Disorders.
http://dx.doi.org/10.1016/B978-0-12-801942-9.00002-1

adulthood is not fundamentally different, and is likewise driven and shaped by experience-dependent processes. At the systems level, such adaptations can be observed in the form of cortical map changes. For example, the somatosensory cortex rearranges the somatotopic representation of incoming sensory information in the absence of sensory stimuli from a distinct body part, with prevailing stimuli taking over those cortical neurons that are no longer being activated. The missing stimulus may be sensation from an amputated body part, or the lack of one entire sensory modality, such as vision. Experience-dependent rearrangements typically follow the principle of competitive occupation of free neuronal "real estate." Thus in the case of visual deprivation, cortical areas normally dedicated to processing visual information may instead respond to auditory stimuli or stimuli from other sensory modalities, a well-documented phenomenon called *cross-modal plasticity* (Kupers & Ptito, 2014). The motor cortex adheres to the same rule of activity-dependent competition. For example, the cortical areas representing motor function of the fingers is significantly expanded in professional musicians compared with individuals who do not practice such skilled finger movements in their daily routines (Elbert, Pantev, Wienbruch, Rockstroh, & Taub, 1995; Gaser & Schlaug, 2003). Motor map changes can be observed with even greater detail and spatial resolution in intracortical microstimulation experiments using animal models. For example, training rats in forelimb tasks that require different skill levels results in distinct and quantifiable motor map changes (Fig. 2.1, Nudo, 2013).

Plasticity After Brain Trauma

In patients who have lost some aspect of cortical functioning as a result of a traumatic insult or ischemia, the cortical region neighboring the lesion often accommodates the processing of information that the damaged area used to process (Carmichael, 2003). Animal experiments elegantly confirm this phenomenon in greater temporal and spatial resolution. For instance, after a focal injury to the sensory digit representation in the monkey cortex, neurons responding to incoming stimuli from this digit can be located in adjacent spared cortical areas (Jenkins & Merzenich, 1987; Nudo, Wise, SiFuentes, & Milliken, 1996). Likewise, rats with a lesion of the forelimb motor cortex develop novel forelimb representations in intact, neighboring cortical areas (Castro-Alamancos & Borrel, 1995). In cases of severe unilateral injury, the contralateral hemisphere may even take over some processing of information that was previously processed in the injured hemisphere (Takatsuru et al., 2009). In addition to these insights, animal experiments allow us to explore the mechanisms behind such reorganizations as they unfold during days, weeks, and months of recovery (Fig. 2.2, Murphy & Corbett, 2009). From studies in animals, we know that different processes are responsible for reorganizations that occur acutely versus those that occur over the course of weeks and months. Because neurite growth does not happen overnight, it has been suggested that unmasking of existing, previously silent

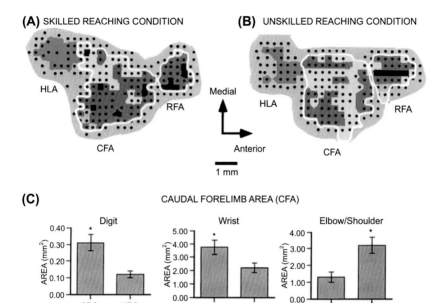

FIGURE 2.1 Analysis of forelimb motor representations in the rat motor cortex established by intracortical microstimulation. (A) Forelimb motor map after training in retrieving small pellets from a rotating platform (skilled reaching condition). (B) Forelimb motor map after training in pressing a bar (unskilled reaching condition). *CFA,* caudal forelimb area; *green,* wrist; *HLA/ dark blue,* hindlimb area; *light blue,* elbow/shoulder; *red,* digit; *RFA,* rostral forelimb area; *yellow,* head/neck. (C) Quantification of distal (digit and wrist) as well as proximal (elbow and shoulder) movement representations in the two different training paradigms. This figure demonstrates that skilled reaching training leads to an expansion of distal movement representations compared with unskilled reaching training, where instead more neurons are dedicated to elbow and shoulder movements (Nudo, 2013). *Reproduced with permission from Nudo, R.J. (2013). Recovery after brain injury: mechanisms and principles. Frontiers in Human Neuroscience, 7, 887.* http://dx.doi.org/10.3389/fnhum.2013.00887

connections in spared circuits underlies cortical changes that occur over hours and days (Jacobs & Donoghue, 1991). Taken together, these plastic changes of cortical representations are commonly recognized as substrates of recovery, because they typically go hand in hand with functional improvements. The link between cortical rearrangements and functionality is demonstrated strongly when the time course of recovery mirrors the extent of cortical changes.

Plasticity in Neurodegeneration

Though less clear-cut and less well studied than in cases of defined brain damage, plasticity can also play a role in neurodegenerative diseases. The increasingly popular expression "cognitive reserve," a measure for the ability to functionally compensate for ongoing neurodegeneration in dementia, refers to a

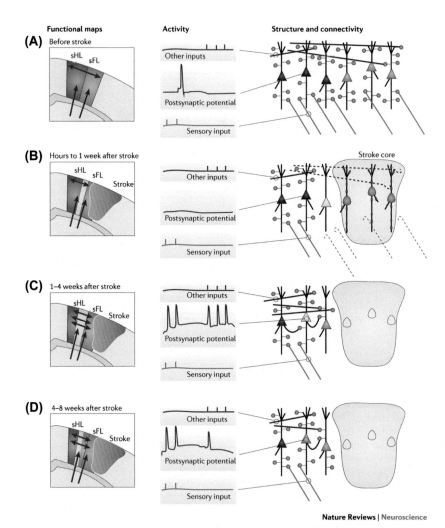

Functional maps   Activity   Structure and connectivity

(A) Before stroke

sHL sFL

Other inputs

Postsynaptic potential

Sensory input

(B) Hours to 1 week after stroke

sHL sFL
Stroke

Stroke core

Other inputs

Postsynaptic potential

Sensory input

(C) 1–4 weeks after stroke

sHL sFL Stroke

Other inputs

Postsynaptic potential

Sensory input

(D) 4–8 weeks after stroke

sHL sFL Stroke

Other inputs

Postsynaptic potential

Sensory input

Nature Reviews | Neuroscience

FIGURE 2.2 Principles of cortical plasticity in the periinfarct zone at different poststroke time points. *Left column:* Cortical somatosensory neurons selectively responding to hindlimb *(sHL, red)* or forelimb *(sFL, green)* inputs, and neurons responding to both inputs *(yellow). Middle column:* Activity of thalamic sensory inputs *(blue),* other inputs *(red),* and selected pyramidal neurons in the periinfarct zone. *Right column:* Close-up schematic of changes in neuronal connectivity and responsiveness. (A) Before stroke, somatosensory neurons are selectively responsive to specific sensory inputs, building an organized map with clear borders. (B) In the acute poststroke period, some surviving neurons in the periinfarct zone lose inputs and their activity declines. (C) During the first month after stroke, plastic processes such as axonal remodeling and synaptogenesis lead to increasing excitability in affected neurons, which become responsive to various incoming stimuli. (D) Over the course of the following weeks, some refinement in responsiveness occurs, leading to more defined somatosensory maps. In comparison with the organization before stroke, more periinfarct neurons now respond to inputs that were initially processed by cells that died in the stroke core (Murphy & Corbett, 2009). *Reproduced with permission of Nature Publishing Group from Murphy, T.H., & Corbett, D. (2009). Plasticity during stroke recovery: from synapse to behaviour.* Nature Reviews. Neuroscience, *10(12), 861–872.* http://dx.doi.org/10.1038/nrn2735

well-trained, well-used, well-experienced brain that can fall back on a multitude of established connections (Barulli & Stern, 2013). Likewise, cognitive training, which includes countless simple ways to challenge the brain with mental exercises, has been shown to be beneficial for individuals diagnosed with mild cognitive impairment or in the early stages of dementia (Hosseini, Kramer, & Kesler, 2014). There is no convincing evidence that such training can halt the degenerative processes, but it may promote compensation by establishing new connections or strengthening existing connections among spared neuronal circuits; in other words, by promoting plasticity. Unfortunately, as neurodegenerative diseases progress, we are certain to be reminded of the fact that plasticity can only work with functional neurons that are spared by pathological processes.

Systems Level Plasticity in Therapeutic Approaches

The examples mentioned above illustrate two central features of systems plasticity: it is driven by experience, and it can be molded by competition for activity. Indeed, "use it or lose it" could be termed the central dogma of plasticity. Invaluable from a therapeutic viewpoint, training is not only the most effective, but also the most accessible modifier of plasticity. Rehabilitation programs for patients with neurological disorders, including physical therapy and occupational therapy, rely heavily on the activity-dependence of neuronal plasticity. One prime example of applying the "use it or lose it" principle to rehabilitation is constraint-induced movement therapy (Sirtori, Corbetta, Moja, & Gatti, 2009). Here the patient is forced to actively use the more affected extremity by constraining the contralateral extremity or hand, a strategy that has been shown to expand the motor map in the affected motor cortex (Liepert et al., 1998). Constraint-induced movement therapy is often, though not exclusively, used in stroke patients, and works best when the cortical damage and the resulting deficits are unilateral.

Although progress can be made with these therapies, we need to keep in mind that plasticity after loss of neuronal tissue is, by nature, a rearrangement rather than a restoration. Because of the failure of neurons to regenerate within most of the CNS, definitely within cortical areas, neuronal loss is generally permanent. In other words, the original tissue organization cannot be restored. Plasticity can only work with the spared neuronal tissue and thus may create entirely new arrangements and detours where previously fine-tuned direct connections existed. Therefore with increasing severity of injury or disease, we should expect and accept successful functional rearrangements in the form of compensatory strategies rather than complete restoration of function. Plasticity can be very powerful, but it is not the complete answer for restoration of brain function after neurodegeneration or brain trauma.

Methodology: Imaging and Electrophysiology

Regional cortical activity in response to sensory stimulation or during motor or cognitive tasks can be studied noninvasively using diverse brain imaging technologies (see Chapter 1) with ever-increasing resolution. These imaging approaches are widely used to investigate cortical plasticity at the systems level in the general population and in patients. For those curious to understand processes in the top-down direction, advances in technologies such as transcranial magnetic stimulation or infrared neural stimulation now make it possible to stimulate or inhibit cortical areas of choice noninvasively (Butler & Wolf, 2007; Cayce, Friedman, Jansen, Mahavaden-Jansen, & Roe, 2011; Ziemann et al., 2014). Apart from human data, a substantial body of evidence supporting the role of plasticity in recovery stems from animal experiments. Although some sophisticated imaging methods offer a resolution high enough for use in small laboratory animals, the use of electrophysiological approaches is much more common in animal experiments for several reasons: First, electrophysiology circumvents disadvantages of imaging the brains of small laboratory animals, such as limited resolution and cost. Second, electrophysiology allows not only the recording of neuronal responses to movement or sensory stimulation, it also offers the opportunity to investigate top-down pathways most precisely (Nudo, 2013). In intracortical microstimulation experiments, cortical neurons can be electrically stimulated and evoked responses can be recorded from neuronal populations or motor nerves receiving the signal downstream (or vice versa in the sensory system). The delay between stimulation and response gives the experimenter an idea of the number of synaptic connections involved in the pathway. The threshold stimulation intensity that evokes a response serves as a measure of the strength of the neuronal connection between stimulus and response. Depending on the experimental set-up used, electrophysiology can be used to study either individual cells or field potentials, the overall activity of a population of neighboring cells (Izraeli et al., 2002). These methods are summarized in Fig. 2.4.

PLASTICITY AT THE MICROANATOMICAL LEVEL

Dendritic and Axonal Changes

Spontaneous remodeling of a neuron's cellular structure is surprisingly common, contrary to previous beliefs that neurons remained unchanged once developmental processes were finalized. Experimental evidence tells a story of constant fluidity of neuronal structures and connections, even in the healthy brain. For instance, dendritic spines, the receiving docks for synaptic signals from other cells, change their morphology and density in a matter of seconds to minutes in response to changing demands (Bhatt, Zhang, & Gan, 2009; Brown & Murphy, 2008). These changes in dendritic spine morphology are thought to correlate with strengthening, weakening, building, or pruning of functional synaptic contacts. Dendritic spine dynamics are dependent on reorganization of the actin cytoskeleton within dendrites, which is an activity-dependent process (Star, Kwiatkowski, & Murthy, 2002). Changes in dendritic arborization, such as dendritic branching patterns and dendrite lengths, are also often analyzed as a measure of plasticity (Himmler, Pellis, & Kolb, 2013).

Microanatomical plasticity, however, is by no means restricted to the receiving structures of a neuronal cell. In fact, axonal remodeling is common both after axonal injury and after loss of a postsynaptic target (Fouad, Pedersen, Schwab, & Brosamle, 2001; Weidner, Ner, Salimi, & Tuszynski, 2001). Unfortunately, true axonal regeneration, which is achievable after peripheral nerve injury (Chan, Gordon, Zochodne, & Power, 2014), is not readily achieved after CNS injury. Innovative experiments in the past have demonstrated elegantly that the local environment and immune responses differ critically between the CNS and the peripheral nervous system, two of the main reasons for exceptionally poor axonal regeneration in the brain and spinal cord (Brosius Lutz & Barres, 2014; David & Aguayo, 1981; Huebner & Strittmatter, 2009).

Axonal Plasticity of Injured Corticospinal Axons

A lot of what is known about axonal remodeling stems from researching spinal cord injury, where axons from neurons within the motor cortex that give rise to the corticospinal tract are often severed. Injured corticospinal axons consistently fail to regenerate (Fouad et al., 2001; Weidner et al., 2001), leading to permanent deficits in voluntary and fine motor control. Instead of regenerative growth originating from a growth cone at the injured axon's stump, growth cone collapse is typically observed in the injured adult CNS environment (Huebner & Strittmatter, 2009). Fortunately, it seems that compensatory axon growth, which includes sprouting of new branches from any region along an axon shaft, is more common than regeneration. Compensatory axon growth can occur in the CNS as an intrinsic, activity-dependent response to injury, even in corticospinal axons. One of the reasons for this difference in the growth behavior of corticospinal axons is that healthy, nonscarred tissue environments are more conducive to axonal plasticity, making compensatory growth a valuable option for functional improvement. Apart from spinal cord injury, axonal sprouting is also one of many adaptive changes that occur spontaneously after stroke, and is thought to be a major mechanism underlying new intrahemispheric and interhemispheric connectivity established in the aftermath of stroke (Carmichael, 2003).

Methodology: Neuronal Tracing and Histological Techniques

Visualization of the microscopic cellular structures of a neuron can be achieved with a number of methods. First, axonal pathways can be visualized in histological sections after injection of neuronal tracers in the live animal (Carmichael, Wei, Rovainen, & Woolsey, 2001). Tracers injected in the vicinity of a cell body will be taken up by the cell and travel anterogradely along the cell's projections, whereas tracers taken up by axons are transported back to the cell body retrogradely (Fig. 2.3, Vavrek, Girgis, Tetzlaff, Hiebert, & Fouad, 2006). Both approaches can be useful, depending on the question to be answered, and some tracer substances are transported better in one direction or the other. However, most tracing substances do not cross synaptic connections. If visualization of

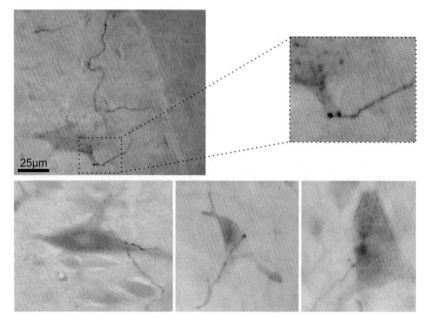

FIGURE 2.3 Visualization of contacts between two different cell populations by neuronal tracing. Retrograde tracing of propriospinal interneurons with FluoroGold (visualized with Nova Red in *red*) combined with anterograde tracing of layer V pyramidal neurons of the motor cortex with biotinylated dextran amine (visualized with diaminobenzidine in *black*) shows bouton-like contacts between corticospinal fibers *(black)* and interneuronal cell bodies *(red)* in the injured spinal cord (Vavrek et al., 2006). In this experiment, the number of such contacts was used to quantify axonal plasticity of motor cortex neurons after corticospinal tract injury. *Reproduced with permission of Oxford University Press from Vavrek, R., Girgis, J., Tetzlaff, W., Hiebert, G.W., & Fouad, K. (2006). BDNF promotes connections of corticospinal neurons onto spared descending interneurons in spinal cord injured rats.* Brain: A Journal of Neurology, 129(Pt 6), 1534–1545. http://dx.doi.org/10.1093/brain/awl087

transneuronal connectivity is crucial for testing a hypothesis, transsynaptic viral tracers are the option of choice. Second, microanatomical structures of a specific cell population can be visualized elegantly by using genetically engineered mice (Bhatt et al., 2009; Brown & Murphy, 2008). Whereas some yellow fluorescent protein (YFP)–labeled mice are commercially available, genetic YFP labeling in other rodent species is not as common. A third approach to visualizing cellular structures is using immunohistochemistry, for example, against axonal markers (eg, neurofilament, tau), dendritic markers (eg, microtubule-associated protein 2), dendritic spine markers (eg, postsynaptic density protein 95), and growth markers (eg, growth-associated protein 43). Histochemical methods such as Golgi-staining, 1,1′-Dioctadecyl-3,3,3′,3′-Tetramethylindocarbocyanine Perchlorate (DiI) staining, or the Golgi-Cox method are popular as well.

Microanatomical investigations often deal with a common challenge. Although they offer a multitude of correlational evidence, the experiments often do not provide causational proof of meaningful functional effects of the observed plasticity. Techniques to overcome the limitations of correlation become increasingly important with translation to the clinic in mind. Examples include examining the functional effects of reversible silencing of a population of neurons pharmacologically (Majchrzak & Di Scala, 2000) or by using magnetic stimulation (Radhu, Ravindran, Levinson, & Daskalakis, 2012). Novel optogenetic approaches also offer exciting opportunities for controlling firing rates of specific neuronal populations (Tsunematsu et al., 2014). Alternatively, examining the effects of irreversible severance (Krajacic, Weishaupt, Girgis, Tetzlaff, & Fouad, 2010; Weidner et al., 2001) of those structures whose reorganization is suspected to be critically implied in observed functional changes can also indicate whether functionally meaningful rewiring occurred in a given system. Finally, characterizing specific connections using electrophysiological methods can produce convincing causational evidence of new meaningful connectivity (Fouad et al., 2001). These methods are summarized in Fig. 2.4.

Synaptic Plasticity

Synaptic plasticity is one of the underlying mechanisms for many of the plastic changes observable at systems level and on dendrites. Adaptive changes at the synapse are the result of a complicated interplay of neurotransmitter release, number and variety of postsynaptic receptors, and synchronous activation of neighboring structures, which can amount to overall strengthening or weakening of synaptic connections. Functional consequences of such long-term potentiation (LTP; strengthening of a synapse) or long-term depression (LTD; weakening of a synapse) in the hippocampus, the hallmark structure for studying synaptic plasticity, have been directly linked to learning and memory (Pastalkova et al., 2006; Whitlock, Heynen, Shuler, & Bear, 2006). The region of the cerebral cortex where synaptic plasticity has received the most attention is the developing visual cortex (Berardi, Pizzorusso, Ratto, & Maffei, 2003). Experience-dependent synaptic plasticity and the intricate development of ocular dominance columns during the critical period (Hubel & Wiesel, 1963; Wiesel & Hubel, 1963) have taught us a lot about the relationship between LTP and LTD and the ability to process visual information in the cortex (Gao, Yin, Liu, Wang, & Fan, 2005; Jang et al., 2009; Smith, Heynen, & Bear, 2009). Indeed, it has been argued that the synaptic plasticity observed in visual deprivation experiments during the critical period may work in very similar ways in the adult injured brain, yet to a lesser extent (Nahmani & Turrigiano, 2014).

Many of the molecular key players thought to be universally important in LTP and LTD throughout the brain have been identified, among them different types of glutamate receptors, calcium-signaling molecules (calcium-calmodulin kinase II, calcium-response element binding protein) and the neurotrophin brain-derived neurotrophic factor (BDNF). As synaptic plasticity has been the subject of intense study for many years, the interested reader is referred to other resources for a detailed understanding of the underlying molecular processes (Bliss & Collingridge, 1993; Collingridge, Peineau, Howland, & Wang, 2010; Malenka & Bear, 2004).

Methodology: In Vitro and In Vivo Electrophysiology

The hallmark model for studying synaptic plasticity in vitro is the hippocampal slice culture. The synaptic network of the hippocampus is known in its entirety, is relatively simple in structure, and is anatomically distinct. Tissue slices harvested from the brain of a newborn animal can be kept alive in vitro for a limited time, allowing targeted electrophysiological and pharmacological experiments (Lossi, Alasia, Salio, & Merighi, 2009). Slice and cell cultures allow the experimenter to observe and quantify effects of globally applied or locally micro-injected molecules on neurotransmitter release, receptor activity, postsynaptic potentials, and molecular responses. In addition, target cells can be stimulated at various intensities and frequencies to study the effect of orchestrated cellular activity on synaptic plasticity. Apart from commonly used hippocampal slice cultures, it is also possible to study connections within the cortex in vitro using organotypic cultures (Caeser, Bonhoeffer, & Bolz, 1989; Gao et al., 2014). Even more impressive, sophisticated chronic in vivo recordings from hippocampal (Pastalkova et al., 2006; Whitlock et al., 2006) or cortical (Hengen, Lambo, Van Hooser, Katz, & Turrigiano, 2013) regions in laboratory animals have contributed greatly to our understanding of how synaptic plasticity develops, what factors it is influenced by, and how changes in synaptic transmission can impact behavior (Fig. 2.4). These methods are summarized in Fig. 2.4.

HOW CAN WE PROMOTE AND MODIFY PLASTICITY?

Any neuronal adaptation discussed in the previous sections starts at the molecular level. In order to promote plasticity in an effort to maximize functional benefit, we need to have a thorough understanding of the underlying molecular events. Such knowledge will ultimately help identify therapeutic targets to manipulate plasticity to the advantage of patients.

The two major factors that trigger intracellular signaling relevant to plasticity are cellular activity and environmental cues, including injury-related cues such as inflammatory mediators. The ensuing signaling cascades eventually drive or block the expression of genes, regulating the production of effector proteins necessary for adaptive change.

The most widely used method to promote plasticity in the wake of CNS injury or disease is to provide network activity through training. Interventions such as occupational, physical, or cognitive therapy use motor exercises, sensory stimulation, or cognitive and mental exercises to achieve the desired functional improvement through activity. More recently, direct stimulation of the neuromuscular unit (Quandt & Hummel, 2014), peripheral nerve (Sattler

Organizational Level	Examples of Plastic Changes	Commonly Used Experimental Methods	References
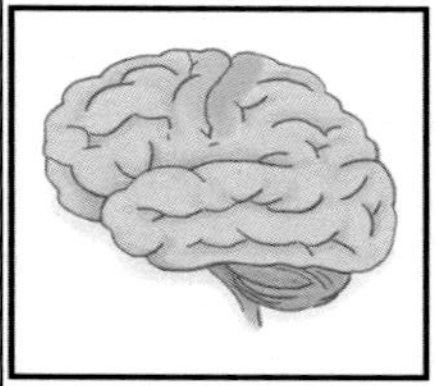	Global brain activity	Functional brain imaging	Kupers & Pito, 2014; Gaser & Schlaug, 2003
	Somatotopic representations and other regional brain maps	Transcranial magnetic stimulation	Ziemann et al., 2014; Butler & Wolf, 2007; Liepert et al., 1998
		Infrared neural stimulation	Cayce, Friedman, Jansen, Mahavaden-Jansen, & Roe, 2011
	Changes in stimulus-response patterns within circuits	Electrophysiology (incl. intracortical microstimulation)	Nudo, 2013; Izraeli et al., 2002; Nudo, Wise, SiFuentes, & Milliken, 1996; Castro-Alamancos & Borrel, 1995
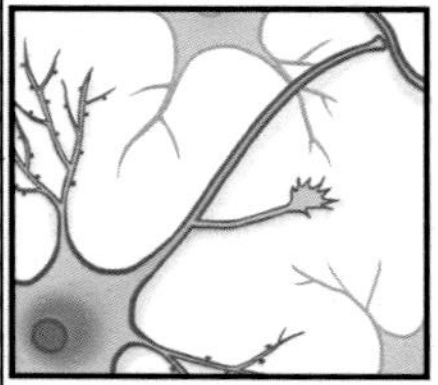	Dendritic spine density	Genetic labeling and histochemical techniques	Himmler, Pellis, & Kolb, 2013; Bhatt, Zhang, & Gan, 2009; Brown & Murphy, 2008
	Dendritic arborization	Anterograde and retrograde neuronal tracing	Vavrek, Girgis, Tetzlaff, Hiebert, & Fouad, 2006; Fouad, Pedersen, Schwab, & Brosamle, 2001; Weidner, Ner, Salimi, & Tuszynski, 2001; Carmichael, Wei, Rovainen, & Woolsey, 2001
	Axon collateral growth ("sprouting")	Electrophysiology (incl. intracortical microstimulation)	Carmichael, 2003; Fouad, Pedersen, Schwab, & Brosamle, 2001
	Genesis or pruning of synapses	In vivo electrophysiology	Hengen, Lambo, Van Hooser, Katz, & Turrigiano, 2013; Jang et al., 2009; Pastalkova et al., 2006; Whitlock, Heynen, Shuler, & Bear, 2006
	Long term potentiation		
	Long term depression	In vitro electrophysiology	Gao et al., 2014; Lossi, Alasia, Salio, & Merighi, 2009; Gao, Yin, Liu, Wang, & Fan, 2005; Caeser, Bonhoeffer, & Bolz, 1989

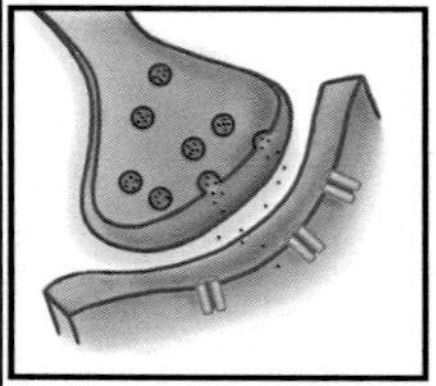

FIGURE 2.4   Overview of experimental approaches commonly used to study plasticity at different organizational levels. *Designed and created by Angela Zhang.*

et al., 2015), and even central nervous structures [eg, intraspinal microstimulation (Bamford & Mushahwar, 2011), and transcranial magnetic stimulation (Sattler et al., 2015)] have been explored as a means to drive activity-dependent recovery mechanisms. For individuals with compromised cognitive function, the principle of activity-dependent plasticity can also make an impressive impact through cognitive training (Ball et al., 2002; Willis et al., 2006). In some cases of neuropsychiatric conditions like posttraumatic stress disorder and other anxiety-disorders, cognitive therapy is aimed at rewiring the brain by expanding desired ways of thinking while trying to override detrimental associations, a process called *extinction learning* (Klumpp, Keutmann, Fitzgerald, Shankman, & Phan, 2014; Thomaes et al., 2014).

Although training is readily accessible in most settings, cues in the local tissue environment that influence microanatomical plasticity of neuronal structures are not nearly as easy to manipulate therapeutically. Neurons are exposed to a wide variety of factors relevant for plasticity, including growth-conducive (eg, laminin) or growth-aversive [eg, chondroitin-sulfate proteoglycans (CSPGs)] extracellular matrix proteins, as well as growth promoting factors (eg, neurotrophins) and growth inhibitors (eg, myelin-associated proteins). Together, these factors are thought to serve as regulators of plasticity, particularly in the adult brain. Those molecules in the CNS environment generally inhibitory to neuronal growth, such as CSPGs in perineuronal nets (Kwok, Afshari, Garcia-Alias, & Fawcett, 2008) and certain myelin proteins [eg, oligodendrocyte myelin glycoprotein, myelin-associated glycoprotein, Nogo (Akbik, Cafferty, & Strittmatter, 2012)] are produced in abundance only after the CNS has matured, and are therefore thought to protect the intricate connectivity shaped by individual experiences during development. Unfortunately, growth inhibitors also restrict the extent of microanatomical plasticity in the wake of an injury when CSPGs are produced *en masse* by activated astroglia (McKeon, Jurynec, & Buck, 1999), making the glial scar an impenetrable barrier for most growing neurons. Experimental approaches targeting these inhibitory substances have been somewhat successful by antagonizing inhibitors directly, by blocking their respective receptors on the neuronal surface (eg, protein tyrosine phosphatase σ, Nogo receptor, paired immunoglobulin-like receptor B), or by interfering with the intracellular signaling cascade they set in motion (Rho-associated protein kinase). A promising strategy to counteract growth inhibition in the glial scar with so far no reports of detrimental side effects in experimental models is the use of the bacterial enzyme chondroitinase, which effectively degrades CSPGs (Kwok et al., 2008).

Factors that promote neuronal growth are important players during neural development and during the maturation of the nervous system. Apart from non-CNS specific factors [eg, fibroblast growth factor, insulin-like growth factor, ciliary neurotrophic factor (CNTF)], glial-derived neurotrophic factor, and the classic neurotrophins stand out as growth factors with essential roles in nervous tissues. The classic neurotrophins include nerve growth factor, BDNF, and neurotrophin 3, as well as the less well characterized neurotrophin 4/5 (Skaper, 2012). Neurotrophins, especially BDNF, exert a range of impressive plasticity-promoting and neuroprotective properties through tropomyosin-related kinase receptor signaling. For example, BDNF signaling does not only promote growth of injured axons (Vavrek et al., 2006), but is directly involved in determining a cell's overall activity level (Rivera et al., 2002; Ziemlinska et al., 2014), is essential for LTP and other forms of synaptic plasticity (Gottmann, Mittmann, & Lessmann, 2009; Leal, Afonso, Salazar, & Duarte, 2014; Yamada & Nabeshima, 2003), and is probably the best known translator of cellular activity into plasticity. The latter is facilitated by one key feature of BDNF: its tightly controlled activity-dependent release (Kojima et al., 2001; Kuczewski, Porcher, Lessmann, Medina, & Gaiarsa, 2009), a characteristic other neurotrophins do not share. This unique feature makes endogenous BDNF accessible for therapeutic use, because neuronal activity will increase BDNF levels in involved circuits. This has been measured in detail in studies of physical activity such as treadmill training (Griesbach, Hovda, Molteni, Wu, & Gomez-Pinilla, 2004; Vaynman & Gomez-Pinilla, 2005). Neurotrophins have been explored for therapeutic use in virtually any condition of the CNS, often primarily with neuroprotection in mind. For example, clinical trials using neurotrophins have been conducted in patients suffering from neurodegenerative disorders such as Alzheimer's disease (Tuszynski et al., 2005), amyotrophic lateral sclerosis (Controlled, 1999; Ochs et al., 2000), and Parkinson's disease (Patel et al., 2005). The plasticity-promoting effects of neurotrophins have received more attention in studies of traumatic brain injury (Kleim, Jones, & Schallert, 2003), spinal cord injury (Boyce & Mendell, 2014; Weishaupt, Blesch, & Fouad, 2012), and stroke (Mang, Campbell, Ross, & Boyd, 2013; Ploughman et al., 2009).

Apart from neurotrophins, CNS injury itself is usually a potent stimulus for plasticity, not least because of the ensuing inflammatory response. Thus neuronal growth has been observed to be significantly more substantial in areas of ongoing inflammatory processes (Chen, Smith, & Shine, 2008). Alternatively activated (M2) macrophages, which are considered to be a central component of a reparative immune response in the CNS, are known to play an important role in promoting plasticity in the aftermath of injury and in the course of disease (Mantovani, Biswas, Galdiero, Sica, & Locati, 2013; Murray & Wynn, 2011; Sica & Mantovani, 2012). However, successfully and safely manipulating inflammation, which is an extraordinarily complex process with a fine line between benefit and harm, is an unmet challenge as of yet.

BEWARE THE DARK SIDE OF PLASTICITY

Generally speaking, plasticity has an extraordinarily good reputation for its well-acknowledged role in healthy brain performance and in the recovery from CNS illness and trauma. However, there are also good reasons why the CNS regulates plasticity so tightly. The complexity of CNS networks is enormous, and the potential for harmful reorganization or perturbation of well-tuned connectivity would be great if cellular growth and synaptic connectivity were entirely unrestricted and unregulated. Some undesired effects of plasticity occur despite the many safeguards that the CNS has in place to control adaptive changes. Examples of such maladaptive changes include phantom pain, some forms of neuropathic pain, and spasticity. To make things more complicated, many of the plasticity-promoting factors mentioned, the prime example being BDNF, can be involved in the development of these maladaptive reorganizations. Thus undesired BDNF signaling can lead to hyperexcitability in brain circuits, causing seizures (Scharfman, 2005).

Another example of plasticity potentially causing harm is task-specific training. Task-specific training is widely accepted as one of most straightforward and safe strategies to promote recovery of function by enhancing plasticity. However, observations in experimental animals and human subjects living with a disruption of the corticospinal tract indicate that whereas performance in the trained activity improves, the function gained will remain specific to the trained task, and will often not even translate into related tasks (Grasso et al., 2004; Magnuson et al., 2009). Furthermore, some experimental evidence indicates that performance in nontrained tasks may even be worse after task-specific training (Garcia-Alias, Barkhuysen, Buckle, & Fawcett, 2009; Girgis et al., 2007). Whatever we do to manipulate plasticity, we should always be aware of the potential to cause harm in a system as complex as the mature CNS.

CHALLENGES AND HOPES FOR THE INVESTIGATION OF CENTRAL NERVOUS SYSTEM PLASTICITY

There is no doubt that plasticity can be a game changer when the brain has suffered irreversible damage. The better our understanding of how we can mold plasticity to our advantage, the greater the potential impact plasticity may have on recovery from virtually any pathological condition of the CNS. Investigations so far have taught us that there is no single "knob" to be turned to control plasticity. Instead, research results inspire a humble but very hopeful view on the future of the field, as we are constantly reminded of the complexity of the systems that we are trying to understand. An effective approach to promote and direct plasticity will most likely rely on combinatory strategies targeting various aspects of the interplay between tissue environment, receptors, signaling molecules, gene expression, and neuronal activity. The prospect of maximizing meaningful and beneficial plasticity promises exciting new routes for promoting recovery from a variety of CNS conditions. Certainly, future discoveries will greatly impact not only how we improve the lives of patients, but also how we think about the healthy brain and its potential.

REFERENCES

Akbik, F., Cafferty, W. B., & Strittmatter, S. M. (2012). Myelin associated inhibitors: a link between injury-induced and experience-dependent plasticity. *Experimental Neurology, 235*(1), 43–52. http://dx.doi.org/10.1016/j.expneurol.2011.06.006.

Ball, K., Berch, D. B., Helmers, K. F., Jobe, J. B., Leveck, M. D., Marsiske, M., et al. (2002). Effects of cognitive training interventions with older adults: a randomized controlled trial. *JAMA, 288*(18), 2271–2281.

Bamford, J. A., & Mushahwar, V. K. (2011). Intraspinal microstimulation for the recovery of function following spinal cord injury. *Progress in Brain Research, 194*, 227–239. http://dx.doi.org/10.1016/B978-0-444-53815-4.00004-2.

Barulli, D., & Stern, Y. (2013). Efficiency, capacity, compensation, maintenance, plasticity: emerging concepts in cognitive reserve. *Trends in Cognitive Sciences, 17*(10), 502–509. http://dx.doi.org/10.1016/j.tics.2013.08.012.

Berardi, N., Pizzorusso, T., Ratto, G. M., & Maffei, L. (2003). Molecular basis of plasticity in the visual cortex. *Trends in Neurosciences, 26*(7), 369–378. http://dx.doi.org/10.1016/S0166-2236(03)00168-1.

Bhatt, D. H., Zhang, S., & Gan, W. B. (2009). Dendritic spine dynamics. *Annual Review of Physiology, 71*, 261–282. http://dx.doi.org/10.1146/annurev.physiol.010908.163140.

Bliss, T. V., & Collingridge, G. L. (1993). A synaptic model of memory: long-term potentiation in the hippocampus. *Nature, 361*(6407), 31–39. http://dx.doi.org/10.1038/361031a0.

Boyce, V. S., & Mendell, L. M. (2014). Neurotrophic factors in spinal cord injury. *Handbook of Experimental Pharmacology, 220*, 443–460. http://dx.doi.org/10.1007/978-3-642-45106-5-16.

Brosius Lutz, A., & Barres, B. A. (2014). Contrasting the glial response to axon injury in the central and peripheral nervous systems. *Developmental Cell, 28*(1), 7–17. http://dx.doi.org/10.1016/j.devcel.2013.12.002.

Brown, C. E., & Murphy, T. H. (2008). Livin' on the edge: imaging dendritic spine turnover in the peri-infarct zone during ischemic stroke and recovery. *Neuroscientist, 14*(2), 139–146. http://dx.doi.org/10.1177/1073858407309854.

Butler, A. J., & Wolf, S. L. (2007). Putting the brain on the map: use of transcranial magnetic stimulation to assess and induce cortical plasticity of upper-extremity movement. *Physical Therapy, 87*(6), 719–736. http://dx.doi.org/10.2522/ptj.20060274.

Caeser, M., Bonhoeffer, T., & Bolz, J. (1989). Cellular organization and development of slice cultures from rat visual cortex. *Experimental Brain Research, 77*(2), 234–244.

Carmichael, S. T. (2003). Plasticity of cortical projections after stroke. *Neuroscientist, 9*(1), 64–75.

Carmichael, S. T., Wei, L., Rovainen, C. M., & Woolsey, T. A. (2001). New patterns of intracortical projections after focal cortical stroke. *Neurobiology of Disease, 8*(5), 910–922. http://dx.doi.org/10.1006/nbdi.2001.0425.

Castro-Alamancos, M. A., & Borrel, J. (1995). Functional recovery of forelimb response capacity after forelimb primary motor cortex damage in the rat is due to the reorganization of adjacent areas of cortex. *Neuroscience, 68*(3), 793–805.

Cayce, J. M., Friedman, R. M., Jansen, E. D., Mahavaden-Jansen, A., & Roe, A. W. (2011). Pulsed infrared light alters neural activity in rat somatosensory cortex in vivo. *Neuroimage, 57*(1), 155–166. http://dx.doi.org/10.1016/j.neuroimage.2011.03.084.

Chan, K. M., Gordon, T., Zochodne, D. W., & Power, H. A. (2014). Improving peripheral nerve regeneration: from molecular mechanisms to potential therapeutic targets. *Experimental Neurology, 261*, 826–835. http://dx.doi.org/10.1016/j.expneurol.2014.09.006.

Chen, Q., Smith, G. M., & Shine, H. D. (2008). Immune activation is required for NT-3-induced axonal plasticity in chronic spinal cord injury. *Experimental Neurology, 209*(2), 497–509. http://dx.doi.org/10.1016/j.expneurol.2007.11.025.

Collingridge, G. L., Peineau, S., Howland, J. G., & Wang, Y. T. (2010). Long-term depression in the CNS. *Nature Reviews. Neuroscience, 11*(7), 459–473. http://dx.doi.org/10.1038/nrn2867.

A controlled trial of recombinant methionyl human BDNF in ALS: the BDNF Study Group (Phase III). *Neurology, 52*(7), (1999), 1427–1433.

David, S., & Aguayo, A. J. (1981). Axonal elongation into peripheral nervous system "bridges" after central nervous system injury in adult rats. *Science, 214*(4523), 931–933.

Elbert, T., Pantev, C., Wienbruch, C., Rockstroh, B., & Taub, E. (1995). Increased cortical representation of the fingers of the left hand in string players. *Science, 270*(5234), 305–307.

Fouad, K., Pedersen, V., Schwab, M. E., & Brosamle, C. (2001). Cervical sprouting of corticospinal fibers after thoracic spinal cord injury accompanies shifts in evoked motor responses. *Current Biology: CB, 11*(22), 1766–1770.

Gao, M., Maynard, K. R., Chokshi, V., Song, L., Jacobs, C., Wang, H., et al. (2014). Rebound potentiation of inhibition in juvenile visual cortex requires vision-induced BDNF expression. *The Journal of Neuroscience: The Official Journal of the Society for Neuroscience, 34*(32), 10770–10779. http://dx.doi.org/10.1523/JNEUROSCI.5454-13.2014.

Gao, P., Yin, Z., Liu, Y., Wang, S., & Fan, H. (2005). Study on long-term potentiation in developing rat visual cortex during the critical period of plasticity. *Yan Ke Xue Bao, 21*(1), 38–43.

Garcia-Alias, G., Barkhuysen, S., Buckle, M., & Fawcett, J. W. (2009). Chondroitinase ABC treatment opens a window of opportunity for task-specific rehabilitation. *Nature Neuroscience, 12*(9), 1145–1151. http://dx.doi.org/10.1038/nn.2377.

Gaser, C., & Schlaug, G. (2003). Brain structures differ between musicians and non-musicians. *The Journal of Neuroscience: The Official Journal of the Society for Neuroscience, 23*(27), 9240–9245.

Girgis, J., Merrett, D., Kirkland, S., Metz, G. A., Verge, V., & Fouad, K. (2007). Reaching training in rats with spinal cord injury promotes plasticity and task specific recovery. *Brain: A Journal of Neurology, 130*(Pt 11), 2993–3003. http://dx.doi.org/10.1093/brain/awm245.

Gottmann, K., Mittmann, T., & Lessmann, V. (2009). BDNF signaling in the formation, maturation and plasticity of glutamatergic and GABAergic synapses. *Experimental Brain Research, 199*(3–4), 203–234. http://dx.doi.org/10.1007/s00221-009-1994-z.

Grasso, R., Ivanenko, Y. P., Zago, M., Molinari, M., Scivoletto, G., & Lacquaniti, F. (2004). Recovery of forward stepping in spinal cord injured patients does not transfer to untrained backward stepping. *Experimental Brain Research, 157*(3), 377–382. http://dx.doi.org/10.1007/s00221-004-1973-3.

Griesbach, G. S., Hovda, D. A., Molteni, R., Wu, A., & Gomez-Pinilla, F. (2004). Voluntary exercise following traumatic brain injury: brain-derived neurotrophic factor upregulation and recovery of function. *Neuroscience, 125*(1), 129–139. http://dx.doi.org/10.1016/j.neuroscience.2004.01.030.

Hengen, K. B., Lambo, M. E., Van Hooser, S. D., Katz, D. B., & Turrigiano, G. G. (2013). Firing rate homeostasis in visual cortex of freely behaving rodents. *Neuron, 80*(2), 335–342. http://dx.doi.org/10.1016/j.neuron.2013.08.038.

Himmler, B. T., Pellis, S. M., & Kolb, B. (2013). Juvenile play experience primes neurons in the medial prefrontal cortex to be more responsive to later experiences. *Neuroscience Letters, 556*, 42–45. http://dx.doi.org/10.1016/j.neulet.2013.09.061.

Hosseini, S. M., Kramer, J. H., & Kesler, S. R. (2014). Neural correlates of cognitive intervention in persons at risk of developing Alzheimer's disease. *Front Aging Neurosci, 6*, 231. http://dx.doi.org/10.3389/fnagi.2014.00231.

Hubel, D. H., & Wiesel, T. N. (1963). Shape and arrangement of columns in cat's striate cortex. *The Journal of Physiology*, *165*, 559–568.

Huebner, E. A., & Strittmatter, S. M. (2009). Axon regeneration in the peripheral and central nervous systems. *Results and Problems in Cell Differentiation*, *48*, 339–351. http://dx.doi.org/10.1007/400-2009-19.

Izraeli, R., Koay, G., Lamish, M., Heicklen-Klein, A. J., Heffner, H. E., Heffner, R. S., et al. (2002). Cross-modal neuroplasticity in neonatally enucleated hamsters: structure, electrophysiology and behaviour. *The European Journal of Neuroscience*, *15*(4), 693–712.

Jacobs, K. M., & Donoghue, J. P. (1991). Reshaping the cortical motor map by unmasking latent intracortical connections. *Science*, *251*(4996), 944–947.

Jang, H. J., Cho, K. H., Kim, H. S., Hahn, S. J., Kim, M. S., & Rhie, D. J. (2009). Age-dependent decline in supragranular long-term synaptic plasticity by increased inhibition during the critical period in the rat primary visual cortex. *Journal of Neurophysiology*, *101*(1), 269–275. http://dx.doi.org/10.1152/jn.90900.2008.

Jenkins, W. M., & Merzenich, M. M. (1987). Reorganization of neocortical representations after brain injury: a neurophysiological model of the bases of recovery from stroke. *Progress in Brain Research*, *71*, 249–266.

Kleim, J. A., Jones, T. A., & Schallert, T. (2003). Motor enrichment and the induction of plasticity before or after brain injury. *Neurochemical Research*, *28*(11), 1757–1769.

Klumpp, H., Keutmann, M. K., Fitzgerald, D. A., Shankman, S. A., & Phan, K. L. (2014). Resting state amygdala-prefrontal connectivity predicts symptom change after cognitive behavioral therapy in generalized social anxiety disorder. *Biology of Mood & Anxiety Disorders*, *4*(1), 14. http://dx.doi.org/10.1186/s13587-014-0014-5.

Kojima, M., Takei, N., Numakawa, T., Ishikawa, Y., Suzuki, S., Matsumoto, T., et al. (2001). Biological characterization and optical imaging of brain-derived neurotrophic factor-green fluorescent protein suggest an activity-dependent local release of brain-derived neurotrophic factor in neurites of cultured hippocampal neurons. *Journal of Neuroscience Research*, *64*(1), 1–10.

Krajacic, A., Weishaupt, N., Girgis, J., Tetzlaff, W., & Fouad, K. (2010). Training-induced plasticity in rats with cervical spinal cord injury: effects and side effects. *Behavioural Brain Research*, *214*(2), 323–331. http://dx.doi.org/10.1016/j.bbr.2010.05.053.

Kuczewski, N., Porcher, C., Lessmann, V., Medina, I., & Gaiarsa, J. L. (2009). Activity-dependent dendritic release of BDNF and biological consequences. *Molecular Neurobiology*, *39*(1), 37–49. http://dx.doi.org/10.1007/s12035-009-8050-7.

Kupers, R., & Ptito, M. (2014). Compensatory plasticity and cross-modal reorganization following early visual deprivation. *Neuroscience and Biobehavioral Reviews*, *41*, 36–52. http://dx.doi.org/10.1016/j.neubiorev.2013.08.001.

Kwok, J. C., Afshari, F., Garcia-Alias, G., & Fawcett, J. W. (2008). Proteoglycans in the central nervous system: plasticity, regeneration and their stimulation with chondroitinase ABC. *Restorative Neurology and Neuroscience*, *26*(2–3), 131–145.

Leal, G., Afonso, P. M., Salazar, I. L., & Duarte, C. B. (2014). Regulation of hippocampal synaptic plasticity by BDNF. *Brain Research*. http://dx.doi.org/10.1016/j.brainres.2014.10.019.

Liepert, J., Miltner, W. H., Bauder, H., Sommer, M., Dettmers, C., Taub, E., et al. (1998). Motor cortex plasticity during constraint-induced movement therapy in stroke patients. *Neuroscience Letters*, *250*(1), 5–8.

Lossi, L., Alasia, S., Salio, C., & Merighi, A. (2009). Cell death and proliferation in acute slices and organotypic cultures of mammalian CNS. *Progress in Neurobiology*, *88*(4), 221–245. http://dx.doi.org/10.1016/j.pneurobio.2009.01.002.

Magnuson, D. S., Smith, R. R., Brown, E. H., Enzmann, G., Angeli, C., Quesada, P. M., et al. (2009). Swimming as a model of task-specific locomotor retraining after spinal cord injury in the rat. *Neurorehabilitation and Neural Repair, 23*(6), 535–545. http://dx.doi.org/ 10.1177/1545968308331147.

Majchrzak, M., & Di Scala, G. (2000). GABA and muscimol as reversible inactivation tools in learning and memory. *Neural Plasticity, 7*(1–2), 19–29. http://dx.doi.org/10.1155/NP.2000.19.

Malenka, R. C., & Bear, M. F. (2004). LTP and LTD: an embarrassment of riches. *Neuron, 44*(1), 5–21. http://dx.doi.org/10.1016/j.neuron.2004.09.012.

Mang, C. S., Campbell, K. L., Ross, C. J., & Boyd, L. A. (2013). Promoting neuroplasticity for motor rehabilitation after stroke: considering the effects of aerobic exercise and genetic variation on brain-derived neurotrophic factor. *Physical Therapy, 93*(12), 1707–1716. http://dx.doi.org/10.2522/ptj.20130053.

Mantovani, A., Biswas, S. K., Galdiero, M. R., Sica, A., & Locati, M. (2013). Macrophage plasticity and polarization in tissue repair and remodelling. *The Journal of Pathology, 229*(2), 176–185. http://dx.doi.org/10.1002/path.4133.

McKeon, R. J., Jurynec, M. J., & Buck, C. R. (1999). The chondroitin sulfate proteoglycans neurocan and phosphacan are expressed by reactive astrocytes in the chronic CNS glial scar. *The Journal of Neuroscience: The Official Journal of the Society for Neuroscience, 19*(24), 10778–10788.

Murphy, T. H., & Corbett, D. (2009). Plasticity during stroke recovery: from synapse to behaviour. *Nature Reviews. Neuroscience, 10*(12), 861–872. http://dx.doi.org/10.1038/nrn2735.

Murray, P. J., & Wynn, T. A. (2011). Protective and pathogenic functions of macrophage subsets. *Nature Reviews. Immunology, 11*(11), 723–737. http://dx.doi.org/10.1038/nri3073.

Nahmani, M., & Turrigiano, G. G. (2014). Adult cortical plasticity following injury: recapitulation of critical period mechanisms? *Neuroscience, 283,* 4–16. http://dx.doi.org/10.1016/ j.neuroscience.2014.04.029.

Nudo, R. J. (2013). Recovery after brain injury: mechanisms and principles. *Frontiers in Human Neuroscience, 7,* 887. http://dx.doi.org/10.3389/fnhum.2013.00887.

Nudo, R. J., Wise, B. M., SiFuentes, F., & Milliken, G. W. (1996). Neural substrates for the effects of rehabilitative training on motor recovery after ischemic infarct. *Science, 272*(5269), 1791–1794.

Ochs, G., Penn, R. D., York, M., Giess, R., Beck, M., Tonn, J., et al. (2000). A phase I/II trial of recombinant methionyl human brain derived neurotrophic factor administered by intrathecal infusion to patients with amyotrophic lateral sclerosis. *Amyotrophic Lateral Sclerosis and Frontotemporal Degeneration, 1*(3), 201–206.

Pastalkova, E., Serrano, P., Pinkhasova, D., Wallace, E., Fenton, A. A., & Sacktor, T. C. (2006). Storage of spatial information by the maintenance mechanism of LTP. *Science, 313*(5790), 1141–1144. http://dx.doi.org/10.1126/science.1128657.

Patel, N. K., Bunnage, M., Plaha, P., Svendsen, C. N., Heywood, P., & Gill, S. S. (2005). Intraputamenal infusion of glial cell line-derived neurotrophic factor in PD: a two-year outcome study. *Annals of Neurology, 57*(2), 298–302. http://dx.doi.org/10.1002/ana.20374.

Ploughman, M., Windle, V., MacLellan, C. L., White, N., Dore, J. J., & Corbett, D. (2009). Brain-derived neurotrophic factor contributes to recovery of skilled reaching after focal ischemia in rats. *Stroke: A Journal of Cerebral Circulation, 40*(4), 1490–1495. http://dx.doi.org/10.1161/STROKEAHA.108.531806.

Quandt, F., & Hummel, F. C. (2014). The influence of functional electrical stimulation on hand motor recovery in stroke patients: a review. *Experimental & Translational Stroke Medicine, 6,* 9. http://dx.doi.org/10.1186/2040-7378-6-9.

Radhu, N., Ravindran, L. N., Levinson, A. J., & Daskalakis, Z. J. (2012). Inhibition of the cortex using transcranial magnetic stimulation in psychiatric populations: current and future directions. *Journal of Psychiatry & Neuroscience: JPN, 37*(6), 369–378. http://dx.doi.org/10.1503/jpn.120003.

Rivera, C., Li, H., Thomas-Crusells, J., Lahtinen, H., Viitanen, T., Nanobashvili, A., et al. (2002). BDNF-induced TrkB activation down-regulates the K^+–Cl^- cotransporter KCC2 and impairs neuronal Cl^- extrusion. *The Journal of Cell Biology, 159*(5), 747–752. http://dx.doi.org/10.1083/jcb.200209011.

Sattler, V., Acket, B., Raposo, N., Albucher, J. F., Thalamas, C., Loubinoux, I., et al. (2015). Anodal tDCS combined with radial nerve stimulation promotes hand motor recovery in the acute phase after ischemic stroke. *Neurorehabilitation and Neural Repair.* http://dx.doi.org/10.1177/1545968314565465.

Scharfman, H. E. (2005). Brain-derived neurotrophic factor and epilepsy: a missing link? *Epilepsy Currents, 5*(3), 83–88. http://dx.doi.org/10.1111/j.1535-7511.2005.05312.x.

Sica, A., & Mantovani, A. (2012). Macrophage plasticity and polarization: in vivo veritas. *The Journal of Clinical Investigation, 122*(3), 787–795. http://dx.doi.org/10.1172/JCI59643.

Sirtori, V., Corbetta, D., Moja, L., & Gatti, R. (2009). Constraint-induced movement therapy for upper extremities in stroke patients. *The Cochrane Database of Systematic Reviews, 4,* CD004433. http://dx.doi.org/10.1002/14651858.CD004433.pub2.

Skaper, S. D. (2012). The neurotrophin family of neurotrophic factors: an overview. *Methods in Molecular Biology, 846,* 1–12. http://dx.doi.org/10.1007/978-1-61779-536-7_1.

Smith, G. B., Heynen, A. J., & Bear, M. F. (2009). Bidirectional synaptic mechanisms of ocular dominance plasticity in visual cortex. *Philosophical Transactions of the Royal Society of London. Series B, Biological Sciences, 364*(1515), 357–367. http://dx.doi.org/10.1098/rstb.2008.0198.

Star, E. N., Kwiatkowski, D. J., & Murthy, V. N. (2002). Rapid turnover of actin in dendritic spines and its regulation by activity. *Nature Neuroscience, 5*(3), 239–246. http://dx.doi.org/10.1038/nn811.

Takatsuru, Y., Fukumoto, D., Yoshitomo, M., Nemoto, T., Tsukada, H., & Nabekura, J. (2009). Neuronal circuit remodeling in the contralateral cortical hemisphere during functional recovery from cerebral infarction. *The Journal of Neuroscience: The Official Journal of the Society for Neuroscience, 29*(32), 10081–10086. http://dx.doi.org/10.1523/JNEUROSCI.1638-09.2009.

Thomaes, K., Dorrepaal, E., Draijer, N., Jansma, E. P., Veltman, D. J., & van Balkom, A. J. (2014). Can pharmacological and psychological treatment change brain structure and function in PTSD? A systematic review. *Journal of Psychiatric Research, 50,* 1–15. http://dx.doi.org/10.1016/j.jpsychires.2013.11.002.

Tsunematsu, T., Ueno, T., Tabuchi, S., Inutsuka, A., Tanaka, K. F., Hasuwa, H., et al. (2014). Optogenetic manipulation of activity and temporally controlled cell-specific ablation reveal a role for MCH neurons in sleep/wake regulation. *The Journal of Neuroscience: The Official Journal of the Society for Neuroscience, 34*(20), 6896–6909. http://dx.doi.org/10.1523/JNEUROSCI.5344-13.2014.

Tuszynski, M. H., Thal, L., Pay, M., Salmon, D. P., Hoi Sang, U., Bakay, R., et al. (2005). A phase 1 clinical trial of nerve growth factor gene therapy for Alzheimer disease. *Nature Medicine, 11*(5), 551–555. http://dx.doi.org/10.1038/nm1239.

Vavrek, R., Girgis, J., Tetzlaff, W., Hiebert, G. W., & Fouad, K. (2006). BDNF promotes connections of corticospinal neurons onto spared descending interneurons in spinal cord injured rats. *Brain: A Journal of Neurology, 129*(Pt 6), 1534–1545. http://dx.doi.org/10.1093/brain/awl087.

Vaynman, S., & Gomez-Pinilla, F. (2005). License to run: exercise impacts functional plasticity in the intact and injured central nervous system by using neurotrophins. *Neurorehabilitation and Neural Repair, 19*(4), 283–295. http://dx.doi.org/10.1177/1545968305280753.

Weidner, N., Ner, A., Salimi, N., & Tuszynski, M. H. (2001). Spontaneous corticospinal axonal plasticity and functional recovery after adult central nervous system injury. *Proceedings of the National Academy of Sciences USA*, *98*(6), 3513–3518. http://dx.doi.org/10.1073/pnas.051626798.

Weishaupt, N., Blesch, A., & Fouad, K. (2012). BDNF: the career of a multifaceted neurotrophin in spinal cord injury. *Experimental Neurology*, *238*(2), 254–264. http://dx.doi.org/10.1016/j.expneurol.2012.09.001.

Whitlock, J. R., Heynen, A. J., Shuler, M. G., & Bear, M. F. (2006). Learning induces long-term potentiation in the hippocampus. *Science*, *313*(5790), 1093–1097. http://dx.doi.org/10.1126/science.1128134.

Wiesel, T. N., & Hubel, D. H. (1963). Single-cell responses in striate cortex of kittens deprived of vision in one eye. *Journal of Neurophysiology*, *26*, 1003–1017.

Willis, S. L., Tennstedt, S. L., Marsiske, M., Ball, K., Elias, J., Koepke, K. M., et al. (2006). Long-term effects of cognitive training on everyday functional outcomes in older adults. *JAMA*, *296*(23), 2805–2814. http://dx.doi.org/10.1001/jama.296.23.2805.

Yamada, K., & Nabeshima, T. (2003). Brain-derived neurotrophic factor/TrkB signaling in memory processes. *Journal of Pharmacological Sciences*, *91*(4), 267–270.

Ziemann, U., Reis, J., Schwenkreis, P., Rosanova, M., Strafella, A., Badawy, R., et al. (2014). TMS and drugs revisited 2014. *Clinical Neurophysiology: Official Journal of the International Federation of Clinical Neurophysiology*. http://dx.doi.org/10.1016/j.clinph.2014.08.028.

Ziemlinska, E., Kugler, S., Schachner, M., Wewior, I., Czarkowska-Bauch, J., & Skup, M. (2014). Overexpression of BDNF increases excitability of the lumbar spinal network and leads to robust early locomotor recovery in completely spinalized rats. *PLoS One*, *9*(2), e88833. http://dx.doi.org/10.1371/journal.pone.0088833.

Chapter 3

Imaging Approaches to Cerebral Cortex Pathology

R. Bartha[1], T.-Y. Lee[1,2]
[1]University of Western Ontario, London, ON, Canada; [2]St. Joseph's Health Centre, London, ON, Canada

INTRODUCTION

Brain imaging in neurodegenerative and neuropsychiatric conditions can aid in diagnostic accuracy and in treatment management. However, in many such diseases, cortical changes are subtle, particularly early in the disease course. Development of imaging biomarkers of disease progression is a major ongoing research focus whose main imperatives include the improvement of diagnostic accuracy and the acceleration of drug development. In recent years, major imaging initiatives have been undertaken particularly in neurodegenerative diseases like Alzheimer's disease (AD) and Parkinson's disease to define imaging biomarkers of disease progression. Of particular note is the Alzheimer's Disease Neuroimaging Initiative, which has set the bar for international large-scale, multisite research efforts. Such large-scale initiatives have provided a wealth of information about disease course in some of the more common neurodegenerative conditions. However, further research is needed to advance knowledge in less common diseases and to develop novel imaging metrics. Recently, imaging has taken a greater role in the management of patients with neurodegenerative disease. For example in cases of suspected AD, imaging can be used after diagnosis to increase the certainty that AD pathology underlies dementia (Jack et al., 2011; McKhann et al., 2011). Before diagnosis in the prodromal phase, imaging can be used to establish the etiology of disease and may help predict progression to dementia (Albert et al., 2011). Finally, in the presymptomatic phase, imaging markers of amyloid accumulation and neurodegeneration can be used to establish pathophysiological changes in the brain (Sperling et al., 2011). The focus of this chapter is to introduce the main imaging modalities used in large-scale, multisite studies in neurodegenerative and neuropsychiatric disease. There is a particular emphasis on AD because it is the most common neurodegenerative disease and cause of dementia in adults (Amin, Morrow, Lake, & Churchill, 1994; Cummings, 2004).

The Cerebral Cortex in Neurodegenerative and Neuropsychiatric Disorders.
http://dx.doi.org/10.1016/B978-0-12-801942-9.00003-3

MAGNETIC RESONANCE IMAGING

Magnetic resonance imaging (MRI) has become one of the most important and accessible tools of modern medicine and has made significant contributions to the understanding of neurodegenerative and neuropsychiatric diseases showing changes in metabolism (Kantarci et al., 2003; Miller et al., 1993; Rapoport, 2002; Shonk et al., 1995), function (Lind et al., 2006), tissue diffusion (Rose, Janke, & Chalk, 2008; de la Torre, Butler, Kozlowski, Fortin, & Saunders, 1995;), and brain tissue atrophy (Fox, Freeborough, & Rossor, 1996; Fox & Schott, 2004; Jack et al., 1997). With disease-modifying treatments on the horizon for some conditions, the detection of subtle early signs of disease before gross structural changes are evident has become a major research focus, as well as the development of sensitive measures to predict treatment response. For example, brain tissue atrophy is now easily observed in subjects with AD; however, this gross measure of cell death represents the end stage of the disease process and is known to be preceded by metabolic impairment, increased amyloid deposition, altered perfusion, loss of synapses, and decreased neuronal function. Such changes are most commonly detected by MRI and positron emission tomography (PET) and are described in the following sections.

Brain Volumetry (T_1-Weighted Magnetic Resonance Imaging)

Serial magnetic resonance (MR) volumetric imaging studies (Freeborough & Fox, 1997) have shown volumetric changes indicative of neurodegeneration in the hippocampus (Barnes et al., 2007; Nestor, Gibson, Gao, Kiss, & Black, 2013; Thompson et al., 2004), ventricles (Nestor et al., 2008), and whole brain in the early stages of AD (Fox & Freeborough, 1997; Leinsinger et al., 2003; Leung, Ridgway, Ourselin, & Fox, 2012; Schott et al., 2005). These change may be evident years before the actual clinical diagnosis of dementia (Gosche, Mortimer, Smith, Markesbery, & Snowdon, 2002; Kantarci et al., 2004). Using such techniques, the rate of global atrophy in AD has been estimated at 3–6% annually (Fox et al., 1996). Similar volumetric results have also been found for patients with mild cognitive impairment (MCI) (Devanand et al., 2007). Ventricle volume is a particularly attractive biomarker because the boundaries of the ventricle are well defined in T_1-weighted MR images, allowing rapid and precise segmentation of this structure (Nestor et al., 2008). Recent efforts have focused on standardization (Boccardi et al., 2015; Duchesne et al., 2015; Frisoni et al., 2015) and automation of volumetric measurements, particularly within the hippocampus, including the quantification of hippocampal subfields (Marizzoni et al., 2015). All such imaging biomarkers are capable of assessing longitudinal changes that correlate with cognitive measurements, and it has been shown that the use of structural imaging can reduce sample sizes in clinical trials studying therapeutic drugs (Jack et al., 2004).

Brain Metabolite Levels (^{1}H Magnetic Resonance Spectroscopy)

The molecular neuropathology of AD is thought to precede structural brain alteration by many years. Hence metabolite measurements are sensitive indicators of very early disease processes. ^{1}H MR spectroscopy (MRS) is a noninvasive technique used to measure the concentration of low–molecular-weight metabolites in vivo, with a detection threshold of approximately 1 mmol/L (mM) from a volume of interest between 1 and 8 cm^3. Detectable in vivo brain metabolites including *N*-acetylaspartate (NAA; a putative marker of neuronal integrity and function), glutamate, glutamine, choline-containing compounds, creatine compounds, and myoinositol have a typical concentration between 1 and 12 mM. Previous studies have shown altered tissue metabolite levels in the brain between subjects aging normally, subjects with MCI, and subjects with AD (Ackl et al., 2005; Adalsteinsson, Sullivan, Kleinhans, Spielman, & Pfefferbaum, 2000; Frederick et al., 2004; Hattori, Abe, Sakoda, & Sawada, 2002; Jessen et al., 2001; Kantarci, 2007; Kantarci et al., 2003; Metastasio et al., 2006; Modrego, Fayed, & Pina, 2005; Parnetti et al., 1997). Measurement of metabolite levels can also improve the differential diagnosis between AD, vascular dementia, or Parkinson's disease dementia (Hsu, Du, Schuff, & Weiner, 2001; Schuff et al., 2003), and are sensitive to changes induced by drug interventions (Bartha et al., 2008; Frederick et al., 2002; Glodzik et al., 2008; Krishnan et al., 2003; Penner et al., 2010). Therefore metabolic impairment is potentially a highly sensitive diagnostic measure and indicator of treatment response. Recent reviews of MRS in neurodegenerative conditions provide excellent summaries of the field (Oz et al., 2014).

The most commonly reported finding in neurodegenerative conditions is the reduction of NAA. NAA is an amino acid found primarily within neurons in the central nervous system. The concentration of NAA is approximately 8–10 mM in brain tissue, resulting in a large peak in the in-vivo ^{1}H spectrum at 2.01 ppm (Pouwels & Frahm, 1998; Valenzuela & Sachdev, 2001). Inside the neuron, NAA is found mostly in the cytosol (75%), but also in the mitochondria (Birken & Oldendorf, 1989). Because it is found mostly in neuronal cells, many MRS studies in psychiatric and neurological disease have focused on NAA. Reduced NAA levels have been found in diseases such as Huntington disease (Davie, Barker, Quinn, Tofts, & Miller, 1994; Harms, Meierkord, Timm, Pfeiffer, & Ludolph, 1997; Hoang et al., 1998; Jenkins, Koroshetz, Beal, & Rosen, 1993, Jenkins et al., 1998; Reynolds & Pearson, 1994; Sanchez-Pernaute, Garcia-Segura, del Barrio Alba, Viano, & de Yebenes, 1999; Taylor-Robinson et al., 1994, 1996) and Parkinson's disease (Axelson et al., 2002; Bowen et al., 1995; Clarke & Lowry, 2001; Griffith et al., 2008; Hoang et al., 1998; Summerfield et al., 2002), as well as AD (Chen, Charles, Barboriak, & Doraiswamy, 2000; Dixon, Bradley, Budge, Styles, & Smith, 2002; Parnetti et al., 1997; Rapoport, 2002; Shonk et al., 1995; Stoppe, Bruhn, Pouwels, Hanicke, & Frahm, 2000). Additional support for the functional significance of NAA comes from studies that show that NAA levels covary with cognitive performance (Jung et al., 1999).

Interpretation of NAA changes is dependent on the context of the measurement. The rate of mitochondrial activity has been associated with NAA synthesis in vitro (Bates et al., 1996). Therefore declining levels of NAA may indicate neurometabolic impairment or, in the case of severe injury, may indicate neuronal death and reduced neuronal density. Additional support for the use of NAA to indicate the viability of neurons comes from studies that show that NAA declines can be reversed after treatment, for example, in disorders such as epilepsy (Hugg et al., 1996), head trauma (Brooks et al., 2000), and multiple sclerosis (Khan et al., 2005). The fact that NAA decline has been found in both the gray matter and white matter of AD patients suggests that both neuronal cell bodies and axons may be affected. The link between NAA and neuronal viability may make NAA an important indicator of the efficacy of drug treatments. Other metabolites including myoinositol, a putative marker of gliosis, and glutamate, the major excitatory neurotransmitter in the brain have also been reported to change in neurodegenerative disease (Rupsingh, Borrie, Smith, Wells, & Bartha, 2011; Siger, Schuff, Zhu, Miller, & Weiner, 2009). Recent reviews of spectroscopy changes in neurodegenerative conditions provide excellent summaries (Burhan et al., 2013; Griffith, Stewart, & den Hollander, 2009).

White Matter Lesions (T_2-Weighted Imaging and Fluid-Attenuated Inversion Recovery)

White matter hyperintensities on T_2-weighted or fluid-attenuated inversion recovery MRI scans are prevalent in elderly subjects and have received increased attention because of the emergence of automated methods to identify and quantify the extent of such tissue (Maniega et al., 2015; Ramirez et al., 2014). Although often clinically silent until the white matter burden becomes large, the relevance of these hyperintense regions has been the subject of considerable interest and debate. It is generally believed that these hyperintensities are related to vascular pathology, particularly small vessel disease. Periventricular hyperintensities may be related to blood–brain barrier (BBB) disruption or intraparenchymal venular disease (Black, Gao, & Bilbao, 2009). Regardless of the underlying pathology, the result is likely hypoperfusion, resulting in white matter injury (Black et al., 2009). Periventricular hyperintensities have been shown to correlate with executive function, potentially by interrupting white matter tracks. However, in assessing the influence of such changes, one must consider not only the volume, but also the location of the lesion.

Cerebral Microbleeds (T_2*-Weighted Imaging and Susceptibility Weighted Imaging)

Relatively little is known about the relationship between microbleeds and cognitive function. Cerebral microbleeds are best visualized using gradient echo T_2*-weighted MRI pulse sequences followed by susceptibility weighted image processing (Yates et al., 2014). The small amounts of iron (hemosiderin) deposited in the tissue from the bleeds can be detected by such gradient-echo imaging methods. Typically microbleeds are round hypointensities 2–10 mm in diameter located away from sulcal regions (Koennecke, 2006). Previous studies have shown that roughly 6% of subjects without cerebrovascular disease have cerebral microbleeds, whereas that number increases significantly in subjects with cerebrovascular disease, including intracerebral hemorrhage and stroke (Koennecke, 2006). They are often found in older individuals but may have little clinical relevance. In AD, microbleeds may be caused by cerebral amyloid angiopathy or by vascular risk factors (eg, hypertension, atherosclerosis). Recently the role of microbleeds in exacerbating AD pathology has been more intensely studied (Yates et al., 2014). The number and location of microbleeds may play a part in the onset of dementia. The prevalence of microbleeds ranges from approximately 15% in people with MCI to more than 20% in people with AD. Because hemosiderin distorts local magnetic fields, high-field (3 T and above) MRI is ideally suited to visualize such lesions. In fact, susceptibility weighted imaging is an MRI technique that exploits the effect of variations in magnetic susceptibility in gradient-echo images to enhanced the contrast produced by microbleeds, which appear as hypointense dots on the MRI image.

Diffusion Tensor Imaging

Diffusion tensor imaging is sensitive to the diffusion of water molecules within tissue (Basser, Mattiello, & LeBihan, 1994). The diffusion of water can be impeded by tissue microstructure (Basser, 1995) and therefore diffusion tensor imaging is sensitive to changes in tissue microstructure induced by disease (Fellgiebel & Yakushev, 2011; Travers et al., 2012). There are two common parameters that are measured: the mean diffusivity and the fractional anisotropy (Basser, 1995). The mean diffusivity is an indicator of the overall mean squared distance a water molecule diffuses through the tissue (Alexander, Lee, Lazar, & Field, 2007; Le Bihan et al., 2001). The fractional anisotropy measures the proportion of diffusion that is attributed to anisotropic diffusion processes (Le Bihan et al., 2001). Often fractional anisotropy declines and mean diffusivity increases in structural lesions, demyelination, and axonal loss (Poloni, Minagar, Haacke, & Zivadinov, 2011). Diffusion tensor imaging has shown changes in connectivity in AD (Rose et al., 2000).

Resting State Brain Network Function

The predominant use of blood oxygenation level–dependent (BOLD) functional MRI (fMRI) is to identify brain regions that are active during a task. An event-related or block design is implemented to allow the comparison of signal intensities between task and no-task states. The BOLD signal recorded in the absence of specific thoughts or tasks is referred to as *resting state fMRI (rs-fMRI)*

(Gusnard, Raichle, & Raichle, 2001). The rs-fMRI signal shows spatiotemporal correlations between different regions of the mammalian brain (Auer, 2008). These correlations are indicative of functional connectivity. Consistent patterns of spatial connectivity are found in healthy subjects (Damoiseaux et al., 2006; Smith et al., 2009) and are referred to as *resting state networks*. Although there have been some inconsistent results between studies, simultaneous local field potential and BOLD recordings in animal models are highly correlated, providing strong evidence of the neural basis of these signals (Logothetis, 2003; Pan, Alagapan, Franca, Brewer, & Wheeler, 2011). Along with synaptic loss, it has been shown that brain network function is affected in AD. When considering the different resting state networks, the default mode network is the most relevant in AD because it is involved in episodic memory formation and attention (Beason-Held, 2011; Buckner, Andrews-Hanna, & Schacter, 2008; Wermke, Sorg, Wohlschlager, & Drzezga, 2008). The default mode network includes the posterior cingulate cortex and hippocampus as well as the precuneus, inferior parietal cortex, and medial prefrontal cortex. Brain connectivity studies have found reduced connectivity between the hippocampus and the posterior cingulate, among other regions in people with AD (Allen et al., 2007; Wang et al., 2007; Zhang et al., 2009) as well as people with MCI (Bai et al., 2009).

POSITRON EMISSION TOMOGRAPHY

PET can be used to study the functional, metabolic, cellular, and molecular bases of neurodegenerative diseases because of its ability to image the biomolecules/ligands that participate in either normal or aberrant processes in the brain. In this section, we will discuss PET studies in each of these four categories: functional (blood flow/perfusion, BBB permeability surface), metabolic (glucose metabolism, oxidative stress), cellular (inflammatory cells), and molecular (β-amyloidosis, tauopathy).

Cerebral Perfusion, Glucose Metabolism and Oxidative Stress

Hypoperfusion and hypometabolism are hallmarks of AD (Mosconi, 2005). These reductions are regional in nature rather than global. The posterior cingulate gyrus and precuneus are the first to be affected in very early AD, followed by the medial temporal structures and parietotemporal association cortex as disease progresses (Matsuda, 2001). Both effects on perfusion and glucose metabolism are associated with brain amyloid-β burden and apolipoprotein E ε4 genotype (Carbonell, Charil, Zijdenbos, Evans, & Bedell, 2014; Matsuda, 2001; Mattsson et al., 2014). As an example, Fig. 3.1 shows hippocampal hypometabolism as visualized with ^{18}F-fluorodeoxyglucose (^{18}F-FDG) PET in a mildly cognitively impaired subject and an AD subject. ^{18}F-FDG is a glucose analog, which when phosphorylated by hexokinase accumulates in the brain. As such, ^{18}F-FDG uptake imaged by PET is a surrogate marker for brain glucose metabolism (Phelps et al., 1979).

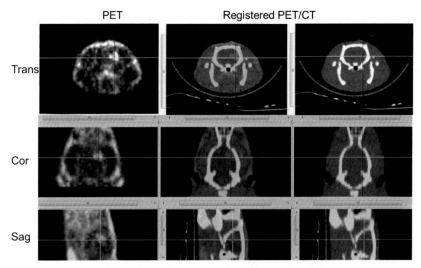

FIGURE 3.1   **Hypometabolism in mild cognitive impairment (MCI) and Alzheimer's disease (AD).** Left to right are the ^{18}F-fluorodeoxyglucose (^{18}F-FDG) positron emission tomography (PET) scans of a normal subject and subjects with, MCI and AD subject. Top and bottom rows are coronal and axial scans of the same subject. The intersection of the *red lines* indicates the hippocampal region. The PET ^{18}F-FDG scans of all three subjects were coregistered. Glucose metabolism in the hippocampus showed a gradation from normal in the normal subject to mild decrease in MCI to severe suppression in AD. In addition, hippocampal hypometabolism was more severe in the left hemisphere in the MCI subject and became more bilateral in the AD subject. *PET-CT,* Positron emission tomography–computed tomography. *From Mosconi, L. (2005). Brain glucose metabolism in the early and specific diagnosis of Alzheimer's disease: FDG-PET studies in MCI and AD. European Journal of Nuclear Medicine and Molecular Imaging, 32(4), 486–510.*

The cause of hypoperfusion was elucidated by Maier et al. (2014) in longitudinal studies of the time profile of β-amyloid (Aβ) deposition and the decline of cerebral perfusion in amyloid precursor protein transgenic mouse models of AD. Only in the presence of cerebral Ao angiopathy (CAA) would parenchymal β-amyloidosis lead to decline of cerebral perfusion, which additionally correlates with the growth of Aβ plaque burden but not with the number of CAA-induced microhemorrhages (microbleeds). This new result lends support to the vascular hypothesis of AD (Zlokovic, 2011).

Other metabolic factors that have been associated with neurodegeneration are insulin resistance (Willette et al., 2015) and oxidative stress (Yoshii et al., 2012). Specifically, in a population of late middle-aged adults with parental history of AD, insulin resistance is not only associated with lower global glucose metabolism but also regional hypometabolism in frontal, lateral parietal, lateral temporal, and medial temporal lobes. Additionally, lower glucose metabolism in the left medial temporal lobe is associated with mildly impaired immediate and delayed memory (Willette et al., 2015). One candidate mechanism linking insulin resistance to neurodegeneration is oxidative stress from mitochondrial dysfunction (Chen & Zhong, 2013; Craft, Cholerton, & Baker, 2013). One consequence of mitochondria-induced oxidative stress is the excessive accumulation of electrons, leading to an overreductive state in the mitochondria (Chen & Zhong, 2013). Existing PET hypoxia imaging agents, eg, ^{62}Cu-ATSM, which binds to cellular components after being reduced in the electron-rich environment of dysfunctioning mitochondria, can be used to examine oxidative stress in neurodegenerative disease (Okazawa, Ikawa, Tsujikawa, Kiyono, & Yoneda, 2014). In normal brain, there is a tight coupling of blood flow and metabolism (oxygen, hence by inference, glucose; see Fig. 3.1) (Peterson, Wang, & Britz, 2011). Increased metabolism coupled with diminished perfusion (oxygen supply) has been used as an imaging biomarker for tumor hypoxia (Mankoff et al., 2002; Miles & Williams, 2008). As such, measurement of glucose metabolic rate and perfusion could be an alternative to hypoxic ligands to image oxidative stress; namely, a high ratio would suggest hypoxia or oxidative stress.

Blood–Brain Barrier Dysfunction

The BBB arising from the tight junctions of endothelial cells (Reese & Karnovsky, 1967) serves to tightly regulate the homeostasis of the brain by restricting entry of molecules to either passive diffusion or active transport. Evidence for involvement of the BBB in neurodegeneration has been the observation of elevated level of albumin, a high–molecular-weight protein that does not cross an intact BBB in cerebrospinal fluid of AD patients (Farrall & Wardlaw, 2009). Imaging of BBB dysfunction has been attempted with PET (Schlageter, Carson, & Rapoport, 1987), dynamic contrast enhanced MRI (Wang, Golob, & Su, 2006), and dynamic contrast enhanced computed tomography (Caserta, Caccioppo, Lapin, Ragin, & Groothuis, 1998; Dysken, Nelson, Hoover, Kuskowski, & McGeachie, 1990). However, the results are conflicting; whereas some studies show BBB dysfunction (Dysken et al., 1990; Wang et al., 2006), others do not (Caserta et al., 1998; Schlageter et al., 1987). A possible explanation could be inclusion of silent cerebrovascular disease (eg, CAA) to different extents in the study populations.

Inflammatory Cells

PET with the benzodiazepine receptor ligand (^{11}C-PK11195) can be used to image activated microglia in the brain (Cagnin, Kassiou, Meikle, & Banati, 2006). They are recognized as the resident macrophages in the brain and play important roles in innate immune/inflammatory responses in different neurodegenerative disorders, including AD (Mandrekar-Colucci & Landreth, 2010). There are likely to be multiple stimuli for the activation of microglia in the AD brain, but Aβ deposits appear to be especially potent, as indicated by the dense accumulations of activated microglia within and around such deposits (Rogers, Luber-Narod, Styren, & Civin, 1988). PET using benzodiazepine ligand (^{11}C-PK11195) for activated microglia has shown increased uptake by these cells in living AD versus control subjects (Cagnin et al., 2001; Edison et al., 2008) and an inverse correlation between benzodiazepine uptake and cognitive status scores (Edison et al., 2008), but such uptake did not correlate with amyloid-β burden in the same subjects (Edison et al., 2008). Another study was unable to confirm benzodiazepine associated activated microglia in AD subjects even in the presence of Aβ deposits (Wiley et al., 2009). It is possible that benzodiazepine uptake is mediated by microglia that is less activated by amyloid-β.

In vivo PET imaging of activated microglia with ^{11}C-PK11195 is limited by the low affinity and low extraction in the brain, resulting in poor signal-to-noise ratio (Banati et al., 2000). Search for second-generation benzodiazepine ligands with better in vivo and physical characteristics, such as ^{11}C-PBR28 (Owen et al., 2011) and ^{18}F-FEPPA (Mizrahi et al., 2012), have revealed, surprisingly, that these new radioligands have large interindividual variability in binding affinity that can be broadly classified into high, low, and mixed (Owen et al., 2011). The existence of these different binding affinities means that varying uptakes of these radioligands cannot be interpreted as more or less activated microglia across individuals. Fortunately, the high, low, and mixed binding affinity of ^{18}F-FEPPA can be predicted by a polymorphism (rs6971) located in exon 4 of the benzodiazepine [translocator protein *(TSPO)*] gene. Thus quantitative evaluation of microglial activation with ^{18}F-FEPPA PET will mandate testing for the rs6971 polymorphism status (Mizrahi et al., 2012).

β-Amyloidosis

AD, characterized by the progressive deterioration of the cognitive and memory functions of the brain, is associated with extracellular deposition of Aβ peptide aggregates and fibrillary tangles of hyperphosphorylated tau protein within neurons in the brain (Braak & Braak, 1994; Corder et al., 2000). According to the amyloid hypothesis, amyloid deposition causes severe damage to neurons many years before onset of dementia via a cascade of several downstream effects (Haass & Selkoe, 2007). One treatment strategy would be to target Aβ, including immunotherapy (Panza et al., 2011) and inhibition of secretase (Panza et al., 2009). For such treatments to be effective, patients at an early stage of disease (MCI) who will progress to AD need to be identified and treatment effect, which can be slow and not easily detectable by cognitive testing, needs to be sensitively and accurately evaluated. For these reasons, markers of Aβ have long been sought after. Table 3.1 lists the available PET radiolabeled ligands that have been used for Aβ imaging, and Fig. 3.2 shows the patterns of uptake of these ligands in AD. As reviewed by Villemagne and Rowe (2013), these imaging agents provide highly accurate (better than glucose metabolism with ^{18}F-FDG), reliable, and reproducible quantitative estimates of regional or global Aβ burden in the brain, essential for therapeutic trial recruitment and for the evaluation of anti-Aβ treatment effects over time. Instead of correlating with cognitive

TABLE 3.1 Positron Emission Tomography Radiolabeled Ligands for Imaging β-Amyloid

	Pittsburgh Compound B	Flutemetamol	Florbetapir	Florbetaben
Synonyms	PiB	GE-067, 3'-fluoro-PIB	AV-45	BAY-94-9172, AV-1
Chemical group	Benzothiazole	Benzothiazole	Styrylpyridine	Stilbene
Isotope label	Carbon-11	Fluorine-18	Fluorine-18	Fluorine-18
Amyloid affinity (Ki, nM)	0.9	0.7	2.2	2.4
Plasma metabolites	Polar	Polar	Polar and nonpolar	Polar and nonpolar
Typical injected dose (MBq)	250–450	185	300	300
Typical imaging time (min)	40–90	80–100	50–70	90–130
Effective radiation dose (mSv; µSv/MBq)	1.3–2.4 (5.3)	6.3 (33.8)	5.8 (19.3)	4.4 (14.7)

From Herholz, K., & Ebmeier, K. (2011). Clinical amyloid imaging in Alzheimer's disease. *Lancet Neurology, 10*(7), 667–670.

impairment in AD, PET assessed Aβ burden is more associated with memory impairment and a higher risk for cognitive decline in the aging population and MCI subjects. As memory impairment is one of the earliest symptoms of AD, this result suggests that β-amyloidosis in the brain likely represents preclinical AD in asymptomatic individuals and prodromal AD in MCI.

Tau Protein Aggregation

Besides extracellular neuritic plaques composed of aggregated Aβ, intracellular neurofibrillary tangles (NFTs) composed of the aggregated tau protein coexist in the AD brain (Braak & Braak, 1994; Corder et al., 2000). The development of tau imaging agent was spurred on by the well-known clinical conundrum that Aβ burden as assessed by PET does not strongly correlate with cognitive

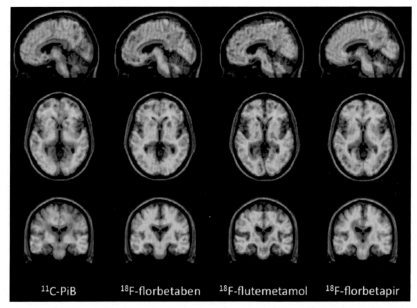

FIGURE 3.2 β-Amyloidosis. Representative sagittal (top row), transaxial (middle row), and coronal (bottom row) positron emission tomography (PET) images overlaid on magnetic resonance imaging (MRI) from patients with Alzheimer's disease (AD) obtained with different Aβ radiolabeled ligands. From left to right, ^{11}C-Pittsburgh compound B (^{11}C-PiB), ^{18}F-florbetaben, ^{18}F-flutemetamol, and ^{18}F-florbetapir. The images show the typical pattern of tracer retention in AD, with the highest retention in frontal, temporal, and posterior cingulate cortices, reflecting Aβ plaque burden. *From Villemagne, V.L., Rowe, C.C. (2013). Long night's journey into the day: amyloid-beta imaging in Alzheimer's disease. Journal of Alzheimer's Disease, 33(Suppl. 1), S349–S359.*

impairment in AD patients (Villemagne et al., 2011). Additionally, there is Aβ deposition in a high percentage of asymptomatic subjects (Katzman et al., 1988), and human postmortem results indicate that it is the density of NFTs and not of Aβ insoluble plaques that strongly correlates with neurodegeneration and cognitive deficits (Arriagada, Growdon, Hedley-Whyte, & Hyman, 1992). Taken together, this evidence suggests Aβ deposition is an early and necessary, though not sufficient, cause for cognitive impairment in AD and points to the involvement of other downstream mechanisms, such as tau aggregation and NFT formation, leading to synaptic failure and eventually neuronal loss (Villemagne et al., 2008).

Tau protein stabilizes microtubules within neurons so that the latter can give structural support and guide nutritional supply to neurons. Hyperphosphorylation causes tau proteins to pair up as paired helical filaments (PHFs) and to form tangles, which become extremely insoluble aggregates in neurons. These changes disrupt a neuron's transport and communication system and eventually lead to cell death (Iqbal, Liu, Gong, & Grundke-Iqbal, 2010). Tau aggregation is a pathological feature of not only AD but also of other neurodegenerative conditions such as frontotemporal dementia (FTD), progressive supranuclear palsy (PSP), and Pick disease (PiD). Additionally, the spatial distributions of the tau aggregates in these tauopathies are different in the mesial temporal cortex and cortical gray-matter areas for AD (Braak & Braak, 1994); in the frontal and striatal brain regions for FTD; in the brainstem, cerebellar white matter, and basal ganglia for PSP (Dickson, 1999); and in the frontal and temporal neocortex for PiD (Dickson, 2001). These different brain distributions can be used as differential tauopathy diagnoses, assuming the same tau imaging agent binds to all different forms of tau aggregates with similar affinity.

A number of PET tau imaging agents have been synthesized and reported in the literature, including ^{11}C-PBB3 (Maruyama et al., 2013), ^{18}F-THK5105 and ^{18}F-THK5117 (Okamura et al., 2013), and ^{18}F-T807 (^{18}F-AV-1451) (Chien et al., 2013). ^{18}F-TKH5105 has been shown to selectively bind to pathological tau PHF in living patients with AD in the temporal cortex, an area that is known to have high densities of NFTs in the AD population as compared with the cerebellum. In contrast, healthy controls' uptake in the inferior temporal cortex was identical to that in the cerebellum. Notably, unlike ^{11}C-Pittsburgh compound B (^{11}C-PiB) used to image Aβ deposits, ^{18}F-THK5105 uptake was significantly correlated with cognitive impairment and reduction in hippocampal and whole brain gray-matter volumes, which was consistent with findings from previous postmortem studies showing significant correlations of NFT density with dementia severity or neuronal loss (Okamura et al., 2014).

^{18}F-AV-1451 demonstrates high selective binding to tau PHF but not normal monomeric tau proteins in the postmortem brain with tau pathologies (Marquie et al., 2015). One preclinical investigation of ^{18}F-AV-1451 showed that brains with significant tau tangle burden or in combination with Aβ had increased uptake of the agent in the gray matter. Healthy controls and brains containing mostly Aβ did not demonstrate such findings (Xia et al., 2013). These results suggested that ^{18}F-AV-1451 is selectively bound to PHFs and has very weak or no affinity to the Aβ accumulation. Early clinical PET imaging with ^{18}F-AV-1451 has confirmed the findings, showing a low diffuse background activity in healthy controls but regional distinct uptakes in areas involved in cognitive dysfunction (eg, entorhinal cortex) in patients with high probability of AD (Chien et al., 2013). Fig. 3.3 compares the uptake of ^{18}F-AV-1451 in a normal subject and a subject with mild cognitive impairment.

The latest entry in the list of tau imaging agents is ^{11}C-PBB3 (Maruyama et al., 2013). Preliminary clinical studies in three healthy control volunteers and three AD patients assessed with both ^{11}C-PBB3 and ^{11}C-PiB showed a different pattern of brain retention between the two tracers, suggesting that ^{11}C-PBB3 binds selectively to tau but not Aβ. An ^{11}C-PBB3 PET study in a patient diagnosed with corticobasal degeneration showed tracer retention in the basal ganglia region, suggesting ^{11}C-PBB3 might bind other non-AD tau conformations (Maruyama et al., 2013).

(A)

(B)

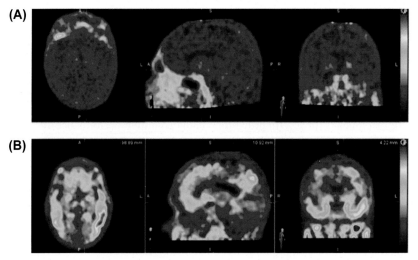

FIGURE 3.3   **Abnormal hyperphosphorylated tau aggregates.** (A) ^{18}F-AV-1451 positron emission tomography (PET) study of an elderly, cognitively normal subject showing no abnormal uptake of the tau agent above the diffuse background. (B) Study of a subject with mild Alzheimer's disease (AD) showing abnormal ^{18}F-AV-1451 accumulation in bilateral temporal lobes. *From James, O. G., Doraiswamy, P. M., & Borges-Neto, S. (2015). PET Imaging of Tau Pathology in Alzheimer's Disease and Tauopathies. Frontiers in Neurology, 6, 38. http://dx.doi.org/10.3389/fneur.2015.00038.*

FUTURE DIRECTION AND EXPERT OPINION

The use of imaging biomarkers of neurodegenerative and neuropsychiatric disease could substantially accelerate the development of novel therapeutics by providing quantitative metrics of disease progression that relate directly to the underlying pathology. For example, in AD, the loss of synapses may be one of the earliest pathological changes (Scheff, Price, Schmitt, DeKosky, Mufson, 2007; Scheff, Price, Schmitt, & Mufson, 2006) and could produce subtle change in brain function. In addition, development of ligands for visualization of amyloid deposition and hyperphosphorylated tau aggregation by PET will lead to a greater understanding of the consequences of these pathological changes in relation to neurodegeneration. The use of high–field-strength MRI (3 T and above) along with advancements in image acquisition and processing technology is ever improving image quality and contrast in our attempts to better visualize structural and metabolic features of disease.

A number of clinical trials involving antiinflammatory drugs, secretase inhibitors and modulators, statins, and monoclonal antibodies against Aβ have failed to show efficacy against the relentless progression of AD (Aisen, Vellas, & Hampel, 2013). This is partly because these clinical trials have used the amelioration of cognitive deficits as the outcome measure of clinical efficacy (Becker, Greig, Giacobini, Schneider, & Ferrucci, 2014). However, emerging evidence suggests that "clinically silent" AD neuropathologies (eg, Aβ deposits and NFTs composed of the aggregated tau protein) accumulate for a decade or more before clinically observable cognitive deficits appear (Buchhave et al., 2012). If the paradigm for clinical efficacy remains to be cognitive improvement, then unless enrolled patients are monitored for 10 years or more, it is unlikely that clinical efficacy of anti-Aβ or tau-based drugs being tested in proposed clinical trials will be observed. It is in this context that imaging biomarkers, particularly the PET ligands for Aβ deposits and NFTs, are especially helpful to prevent a potentially useful drug being abandoned for lack of clinical efficacy (improves/maintains cognitive performance). Related to this consideration, it is also important to recognize that quantitative PET imaging to document abnormal Aβ and NFT accumulation is less than optimal. Specifically, in the standard quantification procedure, the regional radioactivity concentration is first converted to standardized uptake values (SUVs) by normalizing against total injected radioactivity and body weight. Then the ratio between target and reference region (cerebellum or brain stem) is calculated to obtain a regional SUV, which is accepted as a surrogate for Aβ and aggregated tau protein load in the target. For Aβ ligands, the overestimation was estimated to be approximately 18% (Wong et al., 2010). More recently, van Berckel et al. (2013) further showed that the overestimation with a regional SUV is larger when the blood flow in the target region is reduced compared with the reference region. This effect is a concern because reduced blood flow is a core feature of AD pathology. Taken together, although PET imaging of Aβ and NFT is essential for understanding the mechanisms of neurodegeneration and as biomarkers of treatment effects, to guarantee its continuing relevance to these applications, semiquantitative regional SUVs have to be replaced by fully quantitative methods based on kinetics modeling (van Berckel et al., 2013).

REFERENCES

Ackl, N., Ising, M., Schreiber, Y. A., Atiya, M., Sonntag, A., & Auer, D. P. (2005). Hippocampal metabolic abnormalities in mild cognitive impairment and Alzheimer's disease. *Neuroscience Letters, 384*(1–2), 23–28.

Adalsteinsson, E., Sullivan, E. V., Kleinhans, N., Spielman, D. M., & Pfefferbaum, A. (2000). Longitudinal decline of the neuronal marker *N*-acetylaspartate in Alzheimer's disease. *Lancet, 355*(9216), 1696–1697.

Aisen, P. S., Vellas, B., & Hampel, H. (2013). Moving towards early clinical trials for amyloid-targeted therapy in Alzheimer's disease. *Nature Reviews. Drug Discovery, 12*(4), 324.

Albert, M. S., DeKosky, S. T., Dickson, D., Dubois, B., Feldman, H. H., Fox, N. C., et al. (2011). The diagnosis of mild cognitive impairment due to Alzheimer's disease: recommendations from the National Institute on Aging-Alzheimer's Association Workgroups on Diagnostic Guidelines for Alzheimer's Disease. *Alzheimer's & Dementia: The Journal of the Alzheimer's Association, 7*(3), 270–279.

Alexander, A. L., Lee, J. E., Lazar, M., & Field, A. S. (2007). Diffusion tensor imaging of the brain. *Neurotherapeutics: The Journal of the American Society for Experimental Neurotherapeutics, 4*(3), 316–329.

Allen, G., Barnard, H., McColl, R., Hester, A. L., Fields, J. A., Weiner, M. F., et al. (2007). Reduced hippocampal functional connectivity in Alzheimer disease. *Archives of Neurology, 64*(10), 1482–1487.

Amin, S., Morrow, J. R., Lake, C. H., & Churchill, M. R. (1994). Lanthanide(III) tetraamide macrocyclic complexes as synthetic robonucleases: structure and catalytic properties of [La(tcmc) $(CF_3SO_3)(EtOH)](CF_3SO_3)_2$. *Angewandte Chemie, 33*(7), 773–775.

Arriagada, P. V., Growdon, J. H., Hedley-Whyte, E. T., & Hyman, B. T. (1992). Neurofibrillary tangles but not senile plaques parallel duration and severity of Alzheimer's disease. *Neurology, 42*(3 Pt 1), 631–639.

Auer, D. P. (2008). Spontaneous low-frequency blood oxygenation level-dependent fluctuations and functional connectivity analysis of the 'resting' brain. *Magnetic Resonance Imaging, 26*(7), 1055–1064.

Axelson, D., Bakken, I. J., Susann Gribbestad, I., Ehrnholm, B., Nilsen, G., & Aasly, J. (2002). Applications of neural network analyses to in vivo ^{1}H magnetic resonance spectroscopy of Parkinson disease patients. *Journal of Magnetic Resonance Imaging: JMRI, 16*(1), 13–20.

Bai, F., Watson, D. R., Yu, H., Shi, Y., Yuan, Y., & Zhang, Z. (2009). Abnormal resting-state functional connectivity of posterior cingulate cortex in amnestic type mild cognitive impairment. *Brain Research, 1302*, 167–174.

Banati, R. B., Newcombe, J., Gunn, R. N., Cagnin, A., Turkheimer, F., Heppner, F., et al. (2000). The peripheral benzodiazepine binding site in the brain in multiple sclerosis: quantitative in vivo imaging of microglia as a measure of disease activity. *Brain: A Journal of Neurology, 123*(Pt 11), 2321–2337.

Barnes, J., Boyes, R. G., Lewis, E. B., Schott, J. M., Frost, C., Scahill, R. I., et al. (2007). Automatic calculation of hippocampal atrophy rates using a hippocampal template and the boundary shift integral. *Neurobiology of Aging, 28*(11), 1657–1663.

Bartha, R., Smith, M., Rupsingh, R., Rylett, J., Wells, J. L., & Borrie, M. J. (2008). High field (1)H MRS of the hippocampus after donepezil treatment in Alzheimer disease. *Progress in Neuro-Psychopharmacology & Biological Psychiatry, 32*(3), 786–793.

Basser, P. J. (1995). Inferring microstructural features and the physiological state of tissues from diffusion-weighted images. *NMR in Biomedicine, 8*(7–8), 333–344.

Basser, P. J., Mattiello, J., & LeBihan, D. (1994). MR diffusion tensor spectroscopy and imaging. *Biophysical Journal, 66*(1), 259–267.

Bates, T. E., Strangward, M., Keelan, J., Davey, G. P., Munro, P. M., & Clark, J. B. (1996). Inhibition of *N*-acetylaspartate production: implications for ^{1}H MRS studies in vivo. *Neuroreport, 7*(8), 1397–1400.

Beason-Held, L. L. (2011). Dementia and the default mode. *Current Alzheimer Research, 8*(4), 361–365.

Becker, R. E., Greig, N. H., Giacobini, E., Schneider, L. S., & Ferrucci, L. (2014). A new roadmap for drug development for Alzheimer's disease. *Nature Reviews. Drug Discovery, 13*(2), 156.

Birken, D. L., & Oldendorf, W. H. (1989). *N*-acetyl-L-aspartic acid: a literature review of a compound prominent in ^{1}H-NMR spectroscopic studies of brain. *Neuroscience and Biobehavioral Reviews, 13*(1), 23–31.

Black, S., Gao, F., & Bilbao, J. (2009). Understanding white matter disease: imaging–pathological correlations in vascular cognitive impairment. *Stroke: A Journal of Cerebral Circulation, 40*(Suppl. 3), S48–S52.

Boccardi, M., Bocchetta, M., Apostolova, L. G., Barnes, J., Bartzokis, G., Corbetta, G., et al. (2015). Delphi definition of the EADC-ADNI Harmonized Protocol for hippocampal segmentation on magnetic resonance. *Alzheimer's & Dementia: The Journal of the Alzheimer's Association, 11*(2), 126–138.

Bowen, B. C., Block, R. E., Sanchez-Ramos, J., Pattany, P. M., Lampman, D. A., Murdoch, J. B., et al. (1995). Proton MR spectroscopy of the brain in 14 patients with Parkinson disease. *AJNR. American Journal of Neuroradiology, 16*(1), 61–68.

Braak, H., & Braak, E. (1994). Morphological criteria for the recognition of Alzheimer's disease and the distribution pattern of cortical changes related to this disorder. *Neurobiology of Aging, 15*(3), 355–356 discussion 379–380.

Brooks, W. M., Stidley, C. A., Petropoulos, H., Jung, R. E., Weers, D. C., Friedman, S. D., et al. (2000). Metabolic and cognitive response to human traumatic brain injury: a quantitative proton magnetic resonance study. *Journal of Neurotrauma, 17*(8), 629–640.

Buchhave, P., Minthon, L., Zetterberg, H., Wallin, A. K., Blennow, K., & Hansson, O. (2012). Cerebrospinal fluid levels of beta-amyloid 1-42, but not of tau, are fully changed already 5 to 10 years before the onset of Alzheimer dementia. *Archives of General Psychiatry, 69*(1), 98–106.

Buckner, R. L., Andrews-Hanna, J. R., & Schacter, D. L. (2008). The brain's default network: anatomy, function, and relevance to disease. *Annals of the New York Academy of Sciences, 1124*, 1–38.

Burhan, A. M., Bartha, R., Bocti, C., Borrie, M., Laforce, R., Rosa-Neto, P., et al. (2013). Role of emerging neuroimaging modalities in patients with cognitive impairment: a review from the Canadian Consensus Conference on the Diagnosis and Treatment of Dementia 2012. *Alzheimer's Research & Therapy, 5*(Suppl. 1), S4.

Cagnin, A., Brooks, D. J., Kennedy, A. M., Gunn, R. N., Myers, R., Turkheimer, F. E., et al. (2001). In-vivo measurement of activated microglia in dementia. *Lancet, 358*(9280), 461–467.

Cagnin, A., Kassiou, M., Meikle, S. R., & Banati, R. B. (2006). In vivo evidence for microglial activation in neurodegenerative dementia. *Acta Neurologica Scandinavica. Supplementum, 185*, 107–114.

Carbonell, F., Charil, A., Zijdenbos, A. P., Evans, A. C., & Bedell, B. J. (2014). Beta-amyloid is associated with aberrant metabolic connectivity in subjects with mild cognitive impairment. *Journal of Cerebral Blood Flow & Metabolism, 34*(7), 1169–1179.

Caserta, M. T., Caccioppo, D., Lapin, G. D., Ragin, A., & Groothuis, D. R. (1998). Blood–brain barrier integrity in Alzheimer's disease patients and elderly control subjects. *The Journal of Neuropsychiatry and Clinical Neurosciences, 10*(1), 78–84.

Chen, J. G., Charles, H. C., Barboriak, D. P., & Doraiswamy, P. M. (2000). Magnetic resonance spectroscopy in Alzheimer's disease: focus on *N*-acetylaspartate. *Acta Neurologica Scandinavica. Supplementum, 176*, 20–26.

Chen, Z., & Zhong, C. (2013). Decoding Alzheimer's disease from perturbed cerebral glucose metabolism: implications for diagnostic and therapeutic strategies. *Progress in Neurobiology, 108*, 21–43.

Chien, D. T., Bahri, S., Szardenings, A. K., Walsh, J. C., Mu, F., Su, M. Y., et al. (2013). Early clinical PET imaging results with the novel PHF-tau radioligand [F-18]-T807. *Journal of Alzheimer's Disease, 34*(2), 457–468.

Clarke, C. E., & Lowry, M. (2001). Systematic review of proton magnetic resonance spectroscopy of the striatum in parkinsonian syndromes. *European Journal of Neurology: The Official Journal of the European Federation of Neurological Societies, 8*(6), 573–577.

Corder, E. H., Woodbury, M. A., Volkmann, I., Madsen, D. K., Bogdanovic, N., & Winblad, B. (2000). Density profiles of Alzheimer disease regional brain pathology for the Huddinge brain bank: pattern recognition emulates and expands upon Braak staging. *Experimental Gerontology, 35*(6–7), 851–864.

Craft, S., Cholerton, B., & Baker, L. D. (2013). Insulin and Alzheimer's disease: untangling the web. *Journal of Alzheimer's Disease, 33*(Suppl. 1), S263–S275.

Cummings, J. L. (2004). Alzheimer's disease. *The New England Journal of Medicine, 351*(1), 56–67.

Damoiseaux, J. S., Rombouts, S. A., Barkhof, F., Scheltens, P., Stam, C. J., Smith, S. M., et al. (2006). Consistent resting-state networks across healthy subjects. *Proceedings of the National Academy of Sciences USA, 103*(37), 13848–13853.

Davie, C. A., Barker, G. J., Quinn, N., Tofts, P. S., & Miller, D. H. (1994). Proton MRS in Huntington's disease. *Lancet, 343*(8912), 1580.

Devanand, D. P., Pradhaban, G., Liu, X., Khandji, A., De Santi, S., Segal, S., et al. (2007). Hippocampal and entorhinal atrophy in mild cognitive impairment: prediction of Alzheimer disease. *Neurology, 68*(11), 828–836.

Dickson, D. W. (1999). Neuropathologic differentiation of progressive supranuclear palsy and corticobasal degeneration. *Journal of Neurology, 246*(Suppl. 2), II6–15.

Dickson, D. W. (2001). Neuropathology of Pick's disease. *Neurology, 56*(11 Suppl. 4), S16–S20.

Dixon, R. M., Bradley, K. M., Budge, M. M., Styles, P., & Smith, A. D. (2002). Longitudinal quantitative proton magnetic resonance spectroscopy of the hippocampus in Alzheimer's disease. *Brain: A Journal of Neurology, 125*(Pt 10), 2332–2341.

Duchesne, S., Valdivia, F., Robitaille, N., Mouiha, A., Valdivia, F. A., Bocchetta, M., et al. (2015). Segmentation E-AWGoTHPfMH, for the Alzheimer's Disease Neuroimaging I. Manual segmentation qualification platform for the EADC-ADNI harmonized protocol for hippocampal segmentation project. *Alzheimer's & Dementia: The Journal of the Alzheimer's Association, 11*(2), 161–174.

Dysken, M. W., Nelson, M. J., Hoover, K. M., Kuskowski, M., & McGeachie, R. (1990). Rapid dynamic CT scanning in primary degenerative dementia and age-matched controls. *Biological Psychiatry, 28*(5), 425–434.

Edison, P., Archer, H. A., Gerhard, A., Hinz, R., Pavese, N., Turkheimer, F. E., et al. (2008). Microglia, amyloid, and cognition in Alzheimer's disease: an [11C](R)PK11195-PET and [11C]PIB-PET study. *Neurobiology of Disease, 32*(3), 412–419.

Farrall, A. J., & Wardlaw, J. M. (2009). Blood–brain barrier: ageing and microvascular disease–systematic review and meta-analysis. *Neurobiology of Aging, 30*(3), 337–352.

Fellgiebel, A., & Yakushev, I. (2011). Diffusion tensor imaging of the hippocampus in MCI and early Alzheimer's disease. *Journal of Alzheimer's Disease, 26*(Suppl. 3), 257–262.

Fox, N. C., & Freeborough, P. A. (1997). Brain atrophy progression measured from registered serial MRI: validation and application to Alzheimer's disease. *Journal of Magnetic Resonance Imaging: JMRI, 7*(6), 1069–1075.

Fox, N. C., Freeborough, P. A., & Rossor, M. N. (1996). Visualisation and quantification of rates of atrophy in Alzheimer's disease. *Lancet, 348*(9020), 94–97.

Fox, N. C., & Schott, J. M. (2004). Imaging cerebral atrophy: normal ageing to Alzheimer's disease. *Lancet, 363*(9406), 392–394.

Frederick, B. D., Lyoo, I. K., Satlin, A., Ahn, K. H., Kim, M. J., Yurgelun-Todd, D. A., et al. (2004). In vivo proton magnetic resonance spectroscopy of the temporal lobe in Alzheimer's disease. *Progress in Neuro-psychopharmacology & Biological Psychiatry, 28*(8), 1313–1322.

Frederick, B., Satlin, A., Wald, L. L., Hennen, J., Bodick, N., & Renshaw, P. F. (2002). Brain proton magnetic resonance spectroscopy in Alzheimer disease: changes after treatment with xanomeline. *The American Journal of Geriatric Psychiatry: Official Journal of the American Association for Geriatric Psychiatry, 10*(1), 81–88.

Freeborough, P. A., & Fox, N. C. (1997). The boundary shift integral: an accurate and robust measure of cerebral volume changes from registered repeat MRI. *IEEE Transactions on Medical Imaging, 16*(5), 623–629.

Frisoni, G. B., Jack, C. R., Jr., Bocchetta, M., Bauer, C., Frederiksen, K. S., Liu, Y., et al. (2015). The EADC-ADNI Harmonized Protocol for manual hippocampal segmentation on magnetic resonance: evidence of validity. *Alzheimer's & Dementia: The Journal of the Alzheimer's Association, 11*(2), 111–125.

Glodzik, L., King, K. G., Gonen, O., Liu, S., De Santi, S., & de Leon, M. J. (2008). Memantine decreases hippocampal glutamate levels: a magnetic resonance spectroscopy study. *Progress in Neuro-psychopharmacology & Biological Psychiatry, 32*(4), 1005–1012.

Gosche, K. M., Mortimer, J. A., Smith, C. D., Markesbery, W. R., & Snowdon, D. A. (2002). Hippocampal volume as an index of Alzheimer neuropathology: findings from the nun study. *Neurology, 58*(10), 1476–1482.

Griffith, H. R., den Hollander, J. A., Okonkwo, O. C., O'Brien, T., Watts, R. L., & Marson, D. C. (2008). Brain N-acetylaspartate is reduced in Parkinson disease with dementia. *Alzheimer Disease and Associated Disorders, 22*(1), 54–60.

Griffith, H. R., Stewart, C. C., & den Hollander, J. A. (2009). Proton magnetic resonance spectroscopy in dementias and mild cognitive impairment. *International Review of Neurobiology, 84*, 105–131.

Gusnard, D. A., Raichle, M. E., & Raichle, M. E. (2001). Searching for a baseline: functional imaging and the resting human brain. *Nature Reviews, 2*(10), 685–694.

Haass, C., & Selkoe, D. J. (2007). Soluble protein oligomers in neurodegeneration: lessons from the Alzheimer's amyloid beta-peptide. *Nature Reviews Molecular Cell Biology, 8*(2), 101–112.

Harms, L., Meierkord, H., Timm, G., Pfeiffer, L., & Ludolph, A. C. (1997). Decreased N-acetylaspartate/choline ratio and increased lactate in the frontal lobe of patients with Huntington's disease: a proton magnetic resonance spectroscopy study. *Journal of Neurology, Neurosurgery & Psychiatry, 62*(1), 27–30.

Hattori, N., Abe, K., Sakoda, S., & Sawada, T. (2002). Proton MR spectroscopic study at 3 Tesla on glutamate/glutamine in Alzheimer's disease. *Neuroreport, 13*(1), 183–186.

Hoang, T. Q., Bluml, S., Dubowitz, D. J., Moats, R., Kopyov, O., Jacques, D., et al. (1998). Quantitative proton-decoupled ^{31}P MRS and ^{1}H MRS in the evaluation of Huntington's and Parkinson's diseases. *Neurology, 50*(4), 1033–1040.

Hsu, Y. Y., Du, A. T., Schuff, N., & Weiner, M. W. (2001). Magnetic resonance imaging and magnetic resonance spectroscopy in dementias. *Journal of Geriatric Psychiatry and Neurology, 14*(3), 145–166.

Hugg, J. W., Kuzniecky, R. I., Gilliam, F. G., Morawetz, R. B., Fraught, R. E., & Hetherington, H. P. (1996). Normalization of contralateral metabolic function following temporal lobectomy demonstrated by ^{1}H magnetic resonance spectroscopic imaging. *Annals of Neurology, 40*(2), 236–239.

Iqbal, K., Liu, F., Gong, C. X., & Grundke-Iqbal, I. (2010). Tau in Alzheimer disease and related tauopathies. *Current Alzheimer Research, 7*(8), 656–664.

Jack, C. R., Jr., Albert, M. S., Knopman, D. S., McKhann, G. M., Sperling, R. A., Carrillo, M. C., et al. (2011). Introduction to the recommendations from the National Institute on Aging-Alzheimer's Association workgroups on diagnostic guidelines for Alzheimer's disease. *Alzheimer's & Dementia: The Journal of the Alzheimer's Association, 7*(3), 257–262.

Jack, C. R., Jr., Petersen, R. C., Xu, Y. C., Waring, S. C., O'Brien, P. C., Tangalos, E. G., et al. (1997). Medial temporal atrophy on MRI in normal aging and very mild Alzheimer's disease. *Neurology, 49*(3), 786–794.

Jack, C. R., Jr., Shiung, M. M., Gunter, J. L., O'Brien, P. C., Weigand, S. D., Knopman, D. S., et al. (2004). Comparison of different MRI brain atrophy rate measures with clinical disease progression in AD. *Neurology, 62*(4), 591–600.

James, O. G., Doraiswamy, P. M., & Borges-Neto, S. (2015). PET Imaging of Tau Pathology in Alzheimer's Disease and Tauopathies. *Frontiers in Neurology, 6*, 38. http://dx.doi.org/10.3389/fneur.2015.00038.

Jenkins, B. G., Koroshetz, W. J., Beal, M. F., & Rosen, B. R. (1993). Evidence for impairment of energy metabolism in vivo in Huntington's disease using localized ^{1}H NMR spectroscopy. *Neurology, 43*(12), 2689–2695.

Jenkins, B. G., Rosas, H. D., Chen, Y. C., Makabe, T., Myers, R., MacDonald, M., et al. (1998). ^{1}H NMR spectroscopy studies of Huntington's disease: correlations with CAG repeat numbers. *Neurology, 50*(5), 1357–1365.

Jessen, F., Block, W., Traber, F., Keller, E., Flacke, S., Lamerichs, R., et al. (2001). Decrease of *N*-acetylaspartate in the MTL correlates with cognitive decline of AD patients. *Neurology, 57*(5), 930–932.

Jung, R. E., Yeo, R. A., Chiulli, S. J., Sibbitt, W. L., Jr., Weers, D. C., Hart, B. L., et al. (1999). Biochemical markers of cognition: a proton MR spectroscopy study of normal human brain. *Neuroreport, 10*(16), 3327–3331.

Kantarci, K. (2007). [1]H magnetic resonance spectroscopy in dementia. *The British Journal of Radiology, 80*(Spec No. 2), S146–S152.

Kantarci, K., Petersen, R. C., Boeve, B. F., Knopman, D. S., Tang-Wai, D. F., O'Brien, P. C., et al. (2004). [1]H MR spectroscopy in common dementias. *Neurology, 63*(8), 1393–1398.

Kantarci, K., Reynolds, G., Petersen, R. C., Boeve, B. F., Knopman, D. S., Edland, S. D., et al. (2003). Proton MR spectroscopy in mild cognitive impairment and Alzheimer disease: comparison of 1.5 and 3 T. *AJNR. American Journal of Neuroradiology, 24*(5), 843–849.

Katzman, R., Terry, R., DeTeresa, R., Brown, T., Davies, P., Fuld, P., et al. (1988). Clinical, pathological, and neurochemical changes in dementia: a subgroup with preserved mental status and numerous neocortical plaques. *Annals of Neurology, 23*(2), 138–144.

Khan, O., Shen, Y., Caon, C., Bao, F., Ching, W., Reznar, M., et al. (2005). Axonal metabolic recovery and potential neuroprotective effect of glatiramer acetate in relapsing-remitting multiple sclerosis. *Multiple Sclerosis: Clinical and Laboratory Research, 11*(6), 646–651.

Koennecke, H. C. (2006). Cerebral microbleeds on MRI: prevalence, associations, and potential clinical implications. *Neurology, 66*(2), 165–171.

Krishnan, K. R., Charles, H. C., Doraiswamy, P. M., Mintzer, J., Weisler, R., Yu, X., et al. (2003). Randomized, placebo-controlled trial of the effects of donepezil on neuronal markers and hippocampal volumes in Alzheimer's disease. *The American Journal of Psychiatry, 160*(11), 2003–2011.

Le Bihan, D., Mangin, J. F., Poupon, C., Clark, C. A., Pappata, S., Molko, N., et al. (2001). Diffusion tensor imaging: concepts and applications. *Journal of Magnetic Resonance Imaging: JMRI, 13*(4), 534–546.

Leinsinger, G., Teipel, S., Wismuller, A., Born, C., Meindl, T., Flatz, W., et al. (2003). Volumetric MRI for evaluation of regional pattern and progression of neocortical degeneration in Alzheimer's disease. *Der Radiologe, 43*(7), 537–542.

Leung, K. K., Ridgway, G. R., Ourselin, S., & Fox, N. C. (2012). Alzheimer's disease neuroimaging. I. Consistent multi-time-point brain atrophy estimation from the boundary shift integral. *Neuroimage, 59*(4), 3995–4005.

Lind, J., Persson, J., Ingvar, M., Larsson, A., Cruts, M., Van Broeckhoven, C., et al. (2006). Reduced functional brain activity response in cognitively intact apolipoprotein E epsilon 4 carriers. *Brain: A Journal of Neurology, 129*(Pt 5), 1240–1248.

Logothetis, N. K. (2003). The underpinnings of the BOLD functional magnetic resonance imaging signal. *The Journal of Neuroscience: The Official Journal of the Society for Neuroscience, 23*(10), 3963–3971.

Maier, F. C., Wehrl, H. F., Schmid, A. M., Mannheim, J. G., Wiehr, S., Lerdkrai, C., et al. (2014). Longitudinal PET-MRI reveals beta-amyloid deposition and rCBF dynamics and connects vascular amyloidosis to quantitative loss of perfusion. *Nature Medicine, 20*(12), 1485–1492.

Mandrekar-Colucci, S., & Landreth, G. E. (2010). Microglia and inflammation in Alzheimer's disease. *CNS Neurological Disorders Drug Targets, 9*(2), 156–167.

Maniega, S. M., Valdes Hernandez, M. C., Clayden, J. D., Royle, N. A., Murray, C., Morris, Z., et al. (2015). White matter hyperintensities and normal-appearing white matter integrity in the aging brain. *Neurobiology of Aging, 36*(2), 909–918.

Mankoff, D. A., Dunnwald, L. K., Gralow, J. R., Ellis, G. K., Charlop, A., Lawton, T. J., et al. (2002). Blood flow and metabolism in locally advanced breast cancer: relationship to response to therapy. *Journal of Nuclear Medicine: Official Publication, Society of Nuclear Medicine, 43*(4), 500–509.

Marizzoni, M., Antelmi, L., Bosch, B., Bartres-Faz, D., Muller, B. W., Wiltfang, J., et al. (2015). Longitudinal reproducibility of automatically segmented hippocampal subfields: a multisite European 3T study on healthy elderly. *Human Brain Mapping, 36*(9), 3516–3527.

Marquie, M., Normandin, M. D., Vanderburg, C. R., Costantino, I. M., Bien, E. A., Rycyna, L. G., et al. (2015). Validating novel tau positron emission tomography tracer [F-18]-AV-1451 (T807) on postmortem brain tissue. *Annals of Neurology, 78*(5), 787–800.

Maruyama, M., Shimada, H., Suhara, T., Shinotoh, H., Ji, B., Maeda, J., et al. (2013). Imaging of tau pathology in a tauopathy mouse model and in Alzheimer patients compared to normal controls. *Neuron, 79*(6), 1094–1108.

Matsuda, H. (2001). Cerebral blood flow and metabolic abnormalities in Alzheimer's disease. *Annals of Nuclear Medicine, 15*(2), 85–92.

Mattsson, N., Tosun, D., Insel, P. S., Simonson, A., Jack, C. R., Jr., Beckett, L. A., et al. (2014). Alzheimer's disease neuroimaging. I. Association of brain amyloid-beta with cerebral perfusion and structure in Alzheimer's disease and mild cognitive impairment. *Brain: A Journal of Neurology, 137*(Pt 5), 1550–1561.

McKhann, G. M., Knopman, D. S., Chertkow, H., Hyman, B. T., Jack, C. R., Jr., Kawas, C. H., et al. (2011). The diagnosis of dementia due to Alzheimer's disease: recommendations from the National Institute on Aging-Alzheimer's Association workgroups on diagnostic guidelines for Alzheimer's disease. *Alzheimer's & Dementia: The Journal of the Alzheimer's Association, 7*(3), 263–269.

Metastasio, A., Rinaldi, P., Tarducci, R., Mariani, E., Feliziani, F. T., Cherubini, A., et al. (2006). Conversion of MCI to dementia: role of proton magnetic resonance spectroscopy. *Neurobiology of Aging, 27*(7), 926–932.

Miles, K. A., & Williams, R. E. (2008). Warburg revisited: imaging tumour blood flow and metabolism. *Cancer Imaging: The Official Publication of the International Cancer Imaging Society [Electronic Resource], 8*, 81–86.

Miller, B. L., Moats, R. A., Shonk, T., Ernst, T., Woolley, S., & Ross, B. D. (1993). Alzheimer disease: depiction of increased cerebral myo-inositol with proton MR spectroscopy. *Radiology, 187*(2), 433–437.

Mizrahi, R., Rusjan, P. M., Kennedy, J., Pollock, B., Mulsant, B., Suridjan, I., et al. (2012). Translocator protein (18 kDa) polymorphism (rs6971) explains in-vivo brain binding affinity of the PET radioligand [(18)F]-FEPPA. *Journal of Cerebral Blood Flow & Metabolism, 32*(6), 968–972.

Modrego, P. J., Fayed, N., & Pina, M. A. (2005). Conversion from mild cognitive impairment to probable Alzheimer's disease predicted by brain magnetic resonance spectroscopy. *The American Journal of Psychiatry, 162*(4), 667–675.

Mosconi, L. (2005). Brain glucose metabolism in the early and specific diagnosis of Alzheimer's disease: FDG-PET studies in MCI and AD. *European Journal of Nuclear Medicine and Molecular Imaging, 32*(4), 486–510.

Nestor, S. M., Gibson, E., Gao, F. Q., Kiss, A., & Black, S. E. (2013). Alzheimer's disease neuroimaging. I. A direct morphometric comparison of five labeling protocols for multi-atlas driven automatic segmentation of the hippocampus in Alzheimer's disease. *Neuroimage, 66*, 50–70.

Nestor, S. M., Rupsingh, R., Borrie, M., Smith, M., Accomazzi, V., Wells, J. L., et al. (2008). Ventricular enlargement as a possible measure of Alzheimer's disease progression validated using the Alzheimer's disease neuroimaging initiative database. *Brain: A Journal of Neurology, 131*(Pt 9), 2443–2454.

Okamura, N., Furumoto, S., Fodero-Tavoletti, M. T., Mulligan, R. S., Harada, R., Yates, P., et al. (2014). Non-invasive assessment of Alzheimer's disease neurofibrillary pathology using 18F-THK5105 PET. *Brain: A Journal of Neurology, 137*(Pt 6), 1762–1771.

Okamura, N., Furumoto, S., Harada, R., Tago, T., Yoshikawa, T., Fodero-Tavoletti, M., et al. (2013). Novel 18F-labeled arylquinoline derivatives for noninvasive imaging of tau pathology in Alzheimer disease. *Journal of Nuclear Medicine: Official Publication, Society of Nuclear Medicine, 54*(8), 1420–1427.

Okazawa, H., Ikawa, M., Tsujikawa, T., Kiyono, Y., & Yoneda, M. (2014). Brain imaging for oxidative stress and mitochondrial dysfunction in neurodegenerative diseases. *The Quarterly Journal of Nuclear Medicine and Molecular Imaging: Official Publication of the Italian Association of Nuclear Medicine (AIMN) [and] the International Association of Radiopharmacology (IAR), [and] Section of the Society of Radiopharmaceutical Chemistry and Biology, 58*(4), 387–397.

Owen, D. R., Gunn, R. N., Rabiner, E. A., Bennacef, I., Fujita, M., Kreisl, W. C., et al. (2011). Mixed-affinity binding in humans with 18-kDa translocator protein ligands. *Journal of Nuclear Medicine: Official Publication, Society of Nuclear Medicine, 52*(1), 24–32.

Oz, G., Alger, J. R., Barker, P. B., Bartha, R., Bizzi, A., Boesch, C., et al. (2014). Clinical proton MR spectroscopy in central nervous system disorders. *Radiology, 270*(3), 658–679.

Pan, L., Alagapan, S., Franca, E., Brewer, G. J., & Wheeler, B. C. (2011). Propagation of action potential activity in a predefined microtunnel neural network. *Journal of Neural Engineering, 8*(4), 046031.

Panza, F., Frisardi, V., Imbimbo, B. P., Seripa, D., Solfrizzi, V., & Pilotto, A. (2011). Monoclonal antibodies against beta-amyloid (Abeta) for the treatment of Alzheimer's disease: the Abeta target at a crossroads. *Expert Opinion on Biological Therapy, 11*(6), 679–686.

Panza, F., Solfrizzi, V., Frisardi, V., Capurso, C., D'Introno, A., Colacicco, A. M., et al. (2009). Disease-modifying approach to the treatment of Alzheimer's disease: from alpha-secretase activators to gamma-secretase inhibitors and modulators. *Drugs & Aging, 26*(7), 537–555.

Parnetti, L., Tarducci, R., Presciutti, O., Lowenthal, D. T., Pippi, M., Palumbo, B., et al. (1997). Proton magnetic resonance spectroscopy can differentiate Alzheimer's disease from normal aging. *Mechanisms of Ageing and Development, 97*(1), 9–14.

Penner, J., Rupsingh, R., Smith, M., Wells, J. L., Borrie, M. J., & Bartha, R. (2010). Increased glutamate in the hippocampus after galantamine treatment for Alzheimer disease. *Progress in Neuro-Psychopharmacology & Biological Psychiatry, 34*(1), 104–110.

Peterson, E. C., Wang, Z., & Britz, G. (2011). Regulation of cerebral blood flow. *International Journal of Vascular Medicine, 2011*:823525.

Phelps, M. E., Huang, S. C., Hoffman, E. J., Selin, C., Sokoloff, L., & Kuhl, D. E. (1979). Tomographic measurement of local cerebral glucose metabolic rate in humans with (F-18)2-fluoro-2-deoxy-D-glucose: validation of method. *Annals of Neurology, 6*(5), 371–388.

Poloni, G., Minagar, A., Haacke, E. M., & Zivadinov, R. (2011). Recent developments in imaging of multiple sclerosis. *The Neurologist, 17*(4), 185–204.

Pouwels, P. J., & Frahm, J. (1998). Regional metabolite concentrations in human brain as determined by quantitative localized proton MRS. *Magnetic Resonance in Medicine, 39*(1), 53–60.

Ramirez, J., Scott, C. J., McNeely, A. A., Berezuk, C., Gao, F., Szilagyi, G. M., et al. (2014). Lesion Explorer: a video-guided, standardized protocol for accurate and reliable MRI-derived volumetrics in Alzheimer's disease and normal elderly. *Journal of Visualized Experiments, 86.*

Rapoport, S. I. (2002). Hydrogen magnetic resonance spectroscopy in Alzheimer's disease. *Lancet Neurology, 1*(2), 82.

Reese, T. S., & Karnovsky, M. J. (1967). Fine structural localization of a blood–brain barrier to exogenous peroxidase. *The J cell biol, 34*(1), 207–217.

Reynolds, G. P., & Pearson, S. J. (1994). Glutamate in Huntington's disease. *Lancet, 344*(8916), 189–190.

Rogers, J., Luber-Narod, J., Styren, S. D., & Civin, W. H. (1988). Expression of immune system-associated antigens by cells of the human central nervous system: relationship to the pathology of Alzheimer's disease. *Neurobiology of Aging, 9*(4), 339–349.

Rose, S. E., Chen, F., Chalk, J. B., Zelaya, F. O., Strugnell, W. E., Benson, M., et al. (2000). Loss of connectivity in Alzheimer's disease: an evaluation of white matter tract integrity with colour coded MR diffusion tensor imaging. *Journal of Neurology, Neurosurgery & Psychiatry, 69*(4), 528–530.

Rose, S. E., Janke, A. L., & Chalk, J. B. (2008). Gray and white matter changes in Alzheimer's disease: a diffusion tensor imaging study. *Journal of Magnetic Resonance Imaging: JMRI, 27*(1), 20–26.

Rupsingh, R., Borrie, M., Smith, M., Wells, J. L., & Bartha, R. (2011). Reduced hippocampal glutamate in Alzheimer disease. *Neurobiology of Aging, 32*(5), 802–810.

Sanchez-Pernaute, R., Garcia-Segura, J. M., del Barrio Alba, A., Viano, J., & de Yebenes, J. G. (1999). Clinical correlation of striatal ^{1}H MRS changes in Huntington's disease. *Neurology, 53*(4), 806–812.

Scheff, S. W., Price, D. A., Schmitt, F. A., DeKosky, S. T., & Mufson, E. J. (2007). Synaptic alterations in CA1 in mild Alzheimer disease and mild cognitive impairment. *Neurology, 68*(18), 1501–1508.

Scheff, S. W., Price, D. A., Schmitt, F. A., & Mufson, E. J. (2006). Hippocampal synaptic loss in early Alzheimer's disease and mild cognitive impairment. *Neurobiology of Aging, 27*(10), 1372–1384.

Schlageter, N. L., Carson, R. E., & Rapoport, S. I. (1987). Examination of blood–brain barrier permeability in dementia of the Alzheimer type with [68Ga]EDTA and positron emission tomography. *Journal of Cerebral Blood Flow & Metabolism, 7*(1), 1–8.

Schott, J. M., Price, S. L., Frost, C., Whitwell, J. L., Rossor, M. N., & Fox, N. C. (2005). Measuring atrophy in Alzheimer disease: a serial MRI study over 6 and 12 months. *Neurology, 65*(1), 119–124.

Schuff, N., Capizzano, A. A., Du, A. T., Amend, D. L., O'Neill, J., Norman, D., et al. (2003). Different patterns of N-acetylaspartate loss in subcortical ischemic vascular dementia and AD. *Neurology, 61*(3), 358–364.

Shonk, T. K., Moats, R. A., Gifford, P., Michaelis, T., Mandigo, J. C., Izumi, J., et al. (1995). Probable Alzheimer disease: diagnosis with proton MR spectroscopy. *Radiology, 195*(1), 65–72.

Siger, M., Schuff, N., Zhu, X., Miller, B. L., & Weiner, M. W. (2009). Regional myo-inositol concentration in mild cognitive impairment using ^{1}H magnetic resonance spectroscopic imaging. *Alzheimer Disease and Associated Disorders, 23*(1), 57–62.

Smith, S. M., Fox, P. T., Miller, K. L., Glahn, D. C., Fox, P. M., Mackay, C. E., et al. (2009). Correspondence of the brain's functional architecture during activation and rest. *Proceedings of the National Academy of Sciences of the United States of America, 106*(31), 13040–13045.

Sperling, R. A., Aisen, P. S., Beckett, L. A., Bennett, D. A., Craft, S., Fagan, A. M., et al. (2011). Toward defining the preclinical stages of Alzheimer's disease: recommendations from the National Institute on Aging-Alzheimer's association workgroups on diagnostic guidelines for Alzheimer's disease. *Alzheimer's & Dementia: The Journal of the Alzheimer's Association, 7*(3), 280–292.

Stoppe, G., Bruhn, H., Pouwels, P. J., Hanicke, W., & Frahm, J. (2000). Alzheimer disease: absolute quantification of cerebral metabolites in vivo using localized proton magnetic resonance spectroscopy. *Alzheimer Disease and Associated Disorders*, *14*(2), 112–119.

Summerfield, C., Gomez-Anson, B., Tolosa, E., Mercader, J. M., Marti, M. J., Pastor, P., et al. (2002). Dementia in Parkinson disease: a proton magnetic resonance spectroscopy study. *Archives of Neurology*, *59*(9), 1415–1420.

Taylor-Robinson, S. D., Weeks, R. A., Bryant, D. J., Sargentoni, J., Marcus, C. D., Harding, A. E., et al. (1996). Proton magnetic resonance spectroscopy in Huntington's disease: evidence in favour of the glutamate excitotoxic theory. *Movement Disorders: Official Journal of the Movement Disorder Society*, *11*(2), 167–173.

Taylor-Robinson, S. D., Weeks, R. A., Sargentoni, J., Marcus, C. D., Bryant, D. J., Harding, A. E., et al. (1994). Evidence for glutamate excitotoxicity in Huntington's disease with proton magnetic resonance spectroscopy. *Lancet*, *343*(8906), 1170.

Thompson, P. M., Hayashi, K. M., De Zubicaray, G. I., Janke, A. L., Rose, S. E., Semple, J., et al. (2004). Mapping hippocampal and ventricular change in Alzheimer disease. *Neuroimage*, *22*(4), 1754–1766.

de la Torre, J. C., Butler, K., Kozlowski, P., Fortin, T., & Saunders, J. K. (1995). Correlates between nuclear magnetic resonance spectroscopy, diffusion weighted imaging, and CA1 morphometry following chronic brain ischemia. *Journal of Neuroscience Research*, *41*(2), 238–245.

Travers, B. G., Adluru, N., Ennis, C., Tromp do, P. M., Destiche, D., Doran, S., et al. (2012). Diffusion tensor imaging in autism spectrum disorder: a review. *Autism Research: Official Journal of the International Society for Autism Research*, *5*(5), 289–313.

Valenzuela, M. J., & Sachdev, P. (2001). Magnetic resonance spectroscopy in AD. *Neurology*, *56*(5), 592–598.

van Berckel, B. N., Ossenkoppele, R., Tolboom, N., Yaqub, M., Foster-Dingley, J. C., Windhorst, A. D., et al. (2013). Longitudinal amyloid imaging using ^{11}C-PiB: methodologic considerations. *Journal of Nuclear Medicine: Official Publication, Society of Nuclear Medicine*, *54*(9), 1570–1576.

Villemagne, V. L., Pike, K. E., Chetelat, G., Ellis, K. A., Mulligan, R. S., Bourgeat, P., et al. (2011). Longitudinal assessment of Abeta and cognition in aging and Alzheimer disease. *Annals of Neurology*, *69*(1), 181–192.

Villemagne, V. L., Pike, K. E., Darby, D., Maruff, P., Savage, G., Ng, S., et al. (2008). Abeta deposits in older non-demented individuals with cognitive decline are indicative of preclinical Alzheimer's disease. *Neuropsychologia*, *46*(6), 1688–1697.

Villemagne, V. L., & Rowe, C. C. (2013). Long night's journey into the day: amyloid-beta imaging in Alzheimer's disease. *Journal of Alzheimer's Disease*, *33*(Suppl. 1), S349–S359.

Wang, H., Golob, E. J., & Su, M. Y. (2006). Vascular volume and blood–brain barrier permeability measured by dynamic contrast enhanced MRI in hippocampus and cerebellum of patients with MCI and normal controls. *Journal of Magnetic Resonance Imaging: JMRI*, *24*(3), 695–700.

Wang, K., Liang, M., Wang, L., Tian, L., Zhang, X., Li, K., et al. (2007). Altered functional connectivity in early Alzheimer's disease: a resting-state fMRI study. *Human Brain Mapping*, *28*(10), 967–978.

Wermke, M., Sorg, C., Wohlschlager, A. M., & Drzezga, A. (2008). A new integrative model of cerebral activation, deactivation and default mode function in Alzheimer's disease. *European Journal of Nuclear Medicine and Molecular Imaging*, *35*(Suppl. 1), S12–S24.

Wiley, C. A., Lopresti, B. J., Venneti, S., Price, J., Klunk, W. E., DeKosky, S. T., et al. (2009). Carbon 11-labeled Pittsburgh Compound B and carbon 11-labeled (R)-PK11195 positron emission tomographic imaging in Alzheimer disease. *Archives of Neurology*, *66*(1), 60–67.

Willette, A. A., Bendlin, B. B., Starks, E. J., Birdsill, A. C., Johnson, S. C., Christian, B. T., et al. (2015). Association of insulin resistance with cerebral glucose uptake in late middle-aged adults at risk for Alzheimer disease. *JAMA Neurology*, *72*(9), 1013–1020.

Wong, D. F., Rosenberg, P. B., Zhou, Y., Kumar, A., Raymont, V., Ravert, H. T., et al. (2010). In vivo imaging of amyloid deposition in Alzheimer disease using the radioligand 18F-AV-45 (florbetapir [corrected] F 18). *Journal of Nuclear Medicine*, *51*(6), 913–920.

Xia, C. F., Arteaga, J., Chen, G., Gangadharmath, U., Gomez, L. F., Kasi, D., et al. (2013). [(18) F]T807, a novel tau positron emission tomography imaging agent for Alzheimer's disease. *Alzheimer's & Dementia: The Journal of the Alzheimer's Association*, *9*(6), 666–676.

Yates, P. A., Desmond, P. M., Phal, P. M., Steward, C., Szoeke, C., Salvado, O., et al. (2014). Incidence of cerebral microbleeds in preclinical Alzheimer disease. *Neurology*, *82*(14), 1266–1273.

Yates, P. A., Villemagne, V. L., Ellis, K. A., Desmond, P. M., Masters, C. L., & Rowe, C. C. (2014). Cerebral microbleeds: a review of clinical, genetic, and neuroimaging associations. *Frontiers in Neurology*, *4*, 205.

Yoshii, Y., Yoneda, M., Ikawa, M., Furukawa, T., Kiyono, Y., Mori, T., et al. (2012). Radiolabeled Cu-ATSM as a novel indicator of overreduced intracellular state due to mitochondrial dysfunction: studies with mitochondrial DNA-less rho0 cells and cybrids carrying MELAS mitochondrial DNA mutation. *Nuclear Medicine and Biology*, *39*(2), 177–185.

Zhang, H. Y., Wang, S. J., Xing, J., Liu, B., Ma, Z. L., Yang, M., et al. (2009). Detection of PCC functional connectivity characteristics in resting-state fMRI in mild Alzheimer's disease. *Behavioural Brain Research*, *197*(1), 103–108.

Zlokovic, B. V. (2011). Neurovascular pathways to neurodegeneration in Alzheimer's disease and other disorders. *Nature Reviews*, *12*(12), 723–738.

Part II

The Cerebral Cortex in Neurodegenerative Disorders

Chapter 4

Alzheimer's Disease

J.H.K. Tam, S.H. Pasternak
Western University, London, ON, Canada

CLINICAL MANIFESTATIONS

Alzheimer's disease (AD) is the most common form of dementia and presents clinically as a progressive decline in memory and cognition. The latest data from the Alzheimer's Association estimated that over 5 million Americans have AD. This number is expected to rise to 14 million by 2050 unless therapeutics are designed to slow or stop the disease (Alzheimer's Association, 2014). The current total cost of caring for Americans with AD is over $200 billion, and that number is expected to rise to over $1 trillion by 2050 (Alzheimer's Association, 2015). The main risk factor for AD is age, with the incidence of AD increasing exponentially with age (Bachman et al., 1993; Hebert et al., 1995; Higdon et al., 2002; Jorm & Jolley, 1998; Kawas, Gray, Brookmeyer, Fozard, & Zonderman, 2000).

In most patients, the earliest signs of AD are typically loss of short-term episodic memory, with preserved long-term memory. As AD progresses, patients experience deficits in all spheres of cognition, including language, visuospatial function, frontal executive function, and praxis. Language impairment commonly begins with deficits in word finding but eventually evolves into a fluent aphasia with progressive deficits in word finding, agrammatism, and loss of nouns. In addition, there is progressive impairment in visuospatial function, resulting in progressive difficulties in recognizing and understanding what they see. Frontal executive function (the ability to reason and plan) and praxis (the ability to make controlled motor movements) are also affected. With disease progression, language is reduced to simple utterances (short phrases, single words) and patients lose the ability to make simple motor movements. The end stage of the disease is marked by complete failure of all of these systems, resulting in akinetic mutism. Eventually, the patient succumbs to AD or an immobility-related comorbidity. The prognosis from diagnosis till death is approximately 5–8 years (Förstl & Kurz, 1999).

The progression of outward clinical signs in AD mirrors the brain areas affected. Typically the earliest sign of incipient AD is found in the entorhinal cortex (EC) and adjacent hippocampus; the seat of short-term episodic

The Cerebral Cortex in Neurodegenerative and Neuropsychiatric Disorders.
http://dx.doi.org/10.1016/B978-0-12-801942-9.00004-5

83

memory (Fig. 4.3A) (Tomlinson, Blessed, & Roth, 1970). The EC and hippo-campus are among the first to accumulate neurofibrillary tangles (NFTs) and amyloid plaques, which are hallmarks of AD. From the hippocampus, NFT pathosis appears to spread to physically and functionally connected brain areas, such as the frontal, parietal, and temporal cortices (Braak & Braak, 1991; Hof, Bouras, Constantinidis, & Morrison, 1989; Hyman, Kromer, & Van Hoesen, 1988; Hyman, Van Hoesen, Kromer, & Damasio, 1986). Early studies of amy-loid plaques did not show the same pattern as found with NFTs. Conversely, deposition of insoluble amyloid first appeared in the frontal, temporal, and occipital lobes (Braak & Braak, 1991). However, recent work has shown that insoluble aggregates of amyloid may not be the most pathologically relevant form. Rather, soluble-oligomeric forms of amyloid are likely the pathologically relevant aggregate. When soluble forms of β-amyloid (Aβ) are considered, a pattern similar to that found with NFTs emerges. The soluble forms of amyloid rise first in the hippocampus and the EC before increasing in other brain areas (Naslund et al., 2000). The purpose of this chapter is to summarize the current knowledge of tau, the precursor to NFTs, and Aβ, the major constituent of amy-loid plaques, and attempt to explain how these pathological findings, which start in the hippocampus, can give rise to cortical signs of AD.

Tau and Neurofibrillary Tangles

One of the major histopathological findings during the postmortem examination of an AD brain are NFTs and senile plaques that accompany the pronounced loss of neurons (Ball, 1977) (see examples of plaques and tangles in Fig. 4.1). Electron microscopy studies in the 1960s revealed that NFTs were composed of a number of smaller paired helical filaments (PHFs) (Kidd, 1963). It was not until the 1980s that the biochemical identity of Alzheimer filaments was unveiled. The first hints to the identity of the protein core of PHFs came from immunological studies that found the microtubule-associated protein tau might share epitopes with PHFs. By breaking down the insoluble PHFs with the aid of proteases and formic acid extraction, a 12-kDa band was isolated (Wischik et al., 1988). The discovery of this 12-kDa band helped reveal that PHFs were composed of the protein tau (Goedert, Wischik, Crowther, Walker, & Klug, 1988).

Tau was discovered as a protein factor that promoted the polymeriza-tion of tubulin isolated from porcine brain (Weingarten, Lockwood, Hwo, & Kirschner, 1975). The role of tau in microtubule polymerization and stability was confirmed by later studies (Cleveland, Hwo, & Kirschner, 1977a, 1977b). Six different isoforms of tau, ranging from 352 residues to 441 residues were isolated from a normal human complementary DNA library (Goedert, Spillan-tini, Jakes, Rutherford, & Crowther, 1989). Recombinant versions of the six isoforms of tau segregate into six distinct bands ranging from 48 to 67 kDa when undergoing sodium dodecyl sulfate polyacrylamide gel electrophoresis

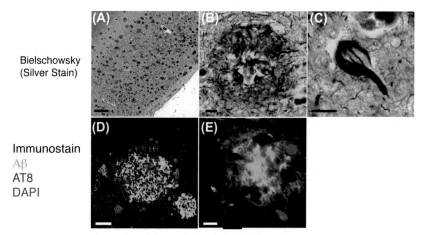

FIGURE 4.1 Extracellular Alzheimer's disease (AD) pathology. (A–C) Modified Bielschowsky silver stain of a human brain with AD. (A) Lower power view of the temporal cortex. (B) Higher magnification from the same case showing an amyloid plaque, with amyloid appearing *brown* and dystrophic neuritis in *black* (scale bar = 10 μm). (C) A high-power view of the same case showing an neurofibrillary tangle (NFT) (scale bar = 10 μm). (D, E) Immunohistochemistry after formic acid antigen retrieval. (D) An amyloid plaque stained for Aβ42 *(green)*. AT8 stains *(red)* for abnormally phosphorylated tau. Nuclei are in *blue* (scale bar = 30 μm). (E) An amyloid plaque stained for Aβ42 *(green)* in the brain of an *APP*$_{Swe}$*/PSEN1*Δ exon 9 mouse. Nuclei are in *blue (DAPI stain)* (scale bar = 10 μm). *Modified from Tam, J.H., & Pasternak, S.H. (2012). Amyloid and Alzheimer's disease: inside and out.* The Canadian Journal of Neurological Sciences. Le Journal Canadien Des Sciences Neurologiques, 39(3), 286–298.

(Goedert, Spillantini, Cairns, & Crowther, 1992b). Despite being antigenically related to tau, solubilized PHFs isolated from the brains of AD patients migrate in three distinct bands, ranging from 57 to 68 kDa (Greenberg & Davies, 1990). Phosphatase treatment of the PHF-derived bands recapitulated the six bands with the same size as recombinant tau (Goedert et al., 1992b), suggesting that tau is abnormally phosphorylated and may contribute to AD pathology. Indeed, tau from the brains of patients with AD contains 2–3 times the number of phosphates/mol as that found in age-matched controls (Köpke, Tung, Shaikh, Iqbal, & Grundke-Iqbal, 1993). Phosphorylated tau cannot promote microtubule assembly and formation (Biernat, Gustke, Drewes, Mandelkow, & Mandelkow, 1993; Lindwall & Cole, 1984; Mandelkow et al., 1992; Utton et al., 1997; Zaidi, Grundke-Iqbal, & Iqbal, 1994). In addition, tau phosphorylated in vitro by protein kinases assembles into PHFs reminiscent of species found in the brains of patients who have AD (Alonso, Zaidi, Novak, Grundke-Iqbal, & Iqbal, 2001; Wang, Grundke-Iqbal, & Iqbal, 2007).

The phosphorylation state of tau is the result of a balance of the activities of kinases and phosphatases that act upon tau. Therefore there is an imbalance of phosphorylation and dephosphorylation in AD. Tau can be phosphorylated by a large number of serine/threonine kinases, including PKA (protein kinase A),

AMPK (5′adenosine monophosphate-activated protein kinase), GSK3β (glycogen synthase kinase 3β), CDK5 (cyclin dependent kinase 5), MARK (microtubule affinity regulating kinase), ERK2 (extracellular signal regulated kinase), and CaMKII (Ca^{2+}/calmodulin-dependent protein kinase II) (Drewes, Ebneth, Preuss, Mandelkow, & Mandelkow, 1997; Goedert, Cohen, Jakes, & Cohen, 1992; Goedert, Jakes, Qi, Wang, & Cohen, 1995; Mandelkow et al., 1992; Pei et al., 1998; Vingtdeux, Davies, Dickson, & Marambaud, 2010; Xiao, Perry, Troncoso, & Monteiro, 1996). Tau kinases may work cooperatively to regulate the function of tau. For example, tau phosphorylation by PKA potentiates the tau phosphorylation by GSK3β and has the greatest inhibition of tau binding and polymerization of microtubules (Wang, Wu, Smith, Grundke-Iqbal, & Iqbal, 1998).

Dephosphorylation can also influence phosphorylated tau levels. In the brain, the main enzyme responsible for tau dephosphorylation is protein phosphatase 2A (PP-2A) (Bennecib, Gong, Grundke-Iqbal, & Iqbal, 2000; Goedert et al., 1995; Goedert et al., 1992; Gong et al., 2000). Inhibition of PP-2A activity results in tau hyperphosphorylation. PP-2A activity is significantly decreased in the brains of AD patients (Gong et al., 1995; Gong, Singh, Grundke-Iqbal, & Iqbal, 1993), suggesting that decreased PP-2A activity contributes to the accumulation of hyperphosphorylated tau in AD.

Amyloid and Plaques

Another hallmark of AD is the accumulation of the 4-kDa fragment known as *Aβ*. The amyloid hypothesis states that Aβ accumulation is central to the etiology of AD, and leads to NFTs, cell loss, vascular damage, and dementia (Hardy & Higgins, 1992). Despite its role in the pathology of AD, Aβ is normally and constitutively produced in human and rat cortical cultures (Haass et al., 1992; Moghekar et al., 2011; Seubert et al., 1993), suggesting physiological roles for Aβ (reviewed in Ref. Pearson & Peers, 2006).

Aβ was first sequenced from amyloid plaques in the brains of patients with AD and from patients with Down syndrome (Glenner & Wong, 1984; Masters et al., 1985). Those with Down syndrome invariably accumulate Aβ with age and usually show symptoms of AD (Mann, Yates, & Marcyniuk, 1984; Wisniewski, Wisniewski, & Wen, 1985). Down syndrome is caused by trisomy 21 (the chromosome containing the *APP* gene), which suggests a gene–dosage effect. Subsequent studies have identified families with familial AD (FAD) that have gene duplication only of the *APP* gene. In addition, overexpression of *APP* causes cognitive deficits, Aβ deposition, and early death in mouse models overexpressing *APP* (Moechars et al., 1999).

APP can undergo nonamyloidogenic or amyloidogenic processing. Nonamyloidogenic processing results in cleavage by α-secretase in the Aβ region, which precludes the formation of Aβ (Lammich et al., 1999). In contrast, amyloidogenic cleavage of *APP* begins with β-secretase cleavage, which releases an amino-terminal ectodomain (Lin et al., 2000; Vassar et al., 1999). The 99-residue carboxyl-terminal fragment is cleaved by γ-secretase

(A)

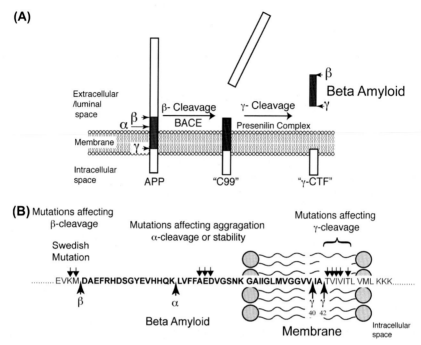

(B)

FIGURE 4.2   (A) Schematic depicting amyloidogenic processing of *APP*. The α-secretase cleavage site is also indicated. BACE1 is the beta secretase. C99 is the 99 amino acid C-terminal of APP produced by BACE cleavage. γ-CTF is the C-terminal 57 amino acids fragment of APP that results from beta and gamma cleavage of APP. (B) The sequence of the transmembrane span region of APP including the β- and γ-cleavage sites. Examples of Alzheimer's disease (AD)–causing familial AD (FAD) mutations are also indicated. *Modified from Tam, J.H., & Pasternak, S.H. (2012). Amyloid and Alzheimer's disease: inside and out.* The Canadian Journal of Neurological Sciences. Le Journal Canadien Des Sciences Neurologiques, 39(3), *286–298.*

to produce Aβ species ranging from 38 to 43 residues (Fig. 4.2A) (Sisodia & St George-Hyslop, 2002). Mutations in *APP* are associated with 10–15% of early-onset familial AD cases (Pagon et al., 1993) and further implicate a role for *APP* in AD. One such mutation, the Swedish mutation *(APP_Swe)*, is located at the β-secretase cleavage site (see Fig. 4.2B). This mutation increases β-cleavage, resulting in increased production of all Aβ species (Citron et al., 1994; Perez, Squazzo, & Koo, 1996; Thinakaran, Teplow, Siman, Greenberg, & Sisodia, 1996). A number of other mutations are near the γ-cleavage site, such as the London mutation *(APP_Lon)*, and preferentially increase the production of Aβ42 as compared to other Aβ species (Maruyama et al., 1996; Suzuki et al., 1994) (see Fig. 4.2B). Transgenic mice overexpressing human *APP_Swe* or *APP_Lon* demonstrate Aβ deposits in the brain parenchyma, synaptic loss, and memory deficits reminiscent of AD (Games et al., 1995; Kawarabayashi et al., 2001; Lamb et al., 1997; Rustay et al., 2010; Sturchler-Pierrat et al., 1997).

In addition to FAD mutations in *APP*, mutations were also mapped to a locus on chromosome 14, which codes for presenilin 1 *(PSEN1)* (Sherrington et al., 1995). A homolog of *PSEN1,* called *presenilin 2 (PSEN2),* was found on chromosome 1. Presenilins are a member of the γ-secretase enzyme complex (De Strooper, 2003), which cleaves *APP* at a γ-cleavage site to release Aβ. Presenilin 1 contains aspartic acid residues that comprise the catalytic site of the enzyme. Mutations in presenilins increase the relative amounts of Aβ42 in the brain. Plasma and fibroblasts from patients with clinical FAD mutations in *PSEN1* and *PSEN2* also show increased Aβ42 levels relative to Aβ40 (Scheuner et al., 1996). The increased Aβ42/Aβ40 ratio is recapitulated in a number of cell lines and mouse models bearing clinical mutations in *Psen1* and *Psen2* (Bentahir et al., 2006; Borchelt et al., 1996; Scheuner et al., 1996). The effect of *PSEN1* mutations could be either a gain or loss of function. Loss-of-function mutations in presenilin might function by decreasing Aβ40 production, and gain-of-function mutations increase the production of Aβ42 (Bentahir et al., 2006). Mutations to *PSEN1* and *PSEN2* are not associated with specific regions of the protein, which suggests multiple possible mechanisms for regulating Aβ levels. However, it is evident that mutations in either *APP* or *PSEN1* shift the promiscuous γ -cleavage site on *APP* in preference of Aβ42 production.

Whereas the evidence from early-onset FAD implicates Aβ42 in the etiology of AD, FAD only accounts for 1% of AD cases. The vast majority of AD cases are late-onset AD (LOAD). Although a number of genome-wide association studies have been performed, the locus for apolipoprotein E (ApoE) has the best correlation with AD (Kamboh et al., 2012). There are three alleles for *APOE* (ε2, ε3, and ε4). The ε2 allele is known to have a protective affect in AD and the ε4 allele exacerbates AD. Individuals homozygous for ε4 have a 12-fold increased risk for developing AD (Kim et al., 2009).

The mechanism by which ApoE increases brain deposition of Aβ is unclear. Some studies suggest that ApoE is critical for Aβ fibrillogenesis. The presence of ApoE accelerates Aβ fibrillization, and is significantly increased by the presence of the ε4 isoform (Ma, Yee, Brewer, Das, & Potter, 1994; Wisniewski, Castaño, Golabek, Vogel, & Frangione, 1994). Transgenic *ApoE* knockout (KO) mice expressing APP_{Lon} have fewer amyloid deposits, and reintroduction of human *APOE* recapitulates amyloid deposition (Holtzman et al., 2000). The ε4 allele causes increased Aβ deposition in human AD patients and mouse models of AD (Castellano et al., 2011; Holtzman et al., 2000; Schmechel et al., 1993). Other research has implicated ApoE in the clearance of Aβ from the brain parenchyma. In transgenic mice expressing a FAD mutation of *APP* and the different isoforms of *ApoE*, the ε4 allele increases the half-life of Aβ in brain interstitial fluid (Castellano et al., 2011). Aβ clearance by microglia is dependent on ApoE (Jiang et al., 2008). Regardless of the mechanism of action, the evidence from ApoE studies suggests that Aβ deposition is also an important part of LOAD pathology.

Originally, the amyloid hypothesis focused on Aβ fibrils. In early experiments, Yankner, Duffy, and Kirschner (1990) showed that Aβ40 fibrils were neurotoxic to hippocampal cultures and other neuronal cell types (Li, Bushnell, Lee, Perlmutter, & Wong, 1996). Inhibition of Aβ fibrillization rescued cell viability (Lorenzo & Yankner, 1994; Monji et al., 2000; Soto et al., 1998) and prevented Aβ accumulation in a transgenic mouse model (Chacón, Barría, Soto, & Inestrosa, 2004). The idea that fibrillogenic Aβ was the neurotoxic species dominated the field for some time. However, the pattern of Aβ deposition in AD corresponded poorly with cognitive deficits (Dickson & Yen, 1989; Katzman et al., 1988; Terry et al., 1991; Thal, Rüb, Orantes, & Braak, 2002). Furthermore, acute passive immunization of mice against Aβ reversed memory deficits but did not decrease the Aβ plaque burden (Dodart et al., 2002). More recent work suggests that soluble oligomers of Aβ are the important neurotoxic species in AD (discussed in Soluble β-Amyloid and Alzheimer's Disease Pathology and reviewed in Ref. Klein, 2002).

CEREBRAL CORTEX PATTERN OF ALZHEIMER'S DISEASE PROGRESSION

Tauopathy in Clinical Alzheimer's Disease

Tauopathy in AD patients follows a selective and predictable course, beginning in the allocortex before spreading to neocortical multimodal association regions and finally primary cortical areas (Bouras, Hof, & Morrison, 1993; Braak & Braak, 1991; Tomlinson et al., 1970; Tomlinson, Blessed, & Roth, 1968). Although some NFT pathosis can be found in brains from patients without dementia, it appears in the brains of AD patients at much higher levels (Braak & Del Tredici, 2010; Tomlinson et al., 1968, 1970). NFT pathological changes are evaluated globally by areas of the brain affected, and can be organized into six stages, (referred to as *Braak staging*) (Fig. 4.3) (Braak & Braak, 1991). The first two stages are also referred to as the *transentorhinal stages* of AD. The main finding in patients with AD is the development of NFTs in the transentorhinal cortex and layers two and four of the EC (see Fig. 4.3E) (Braak & Braak, 1991). The transentorhinal stage is characterized by the absence of clinical signs and is regarded as the preclinical stage of AD (Braak & Braak, 1991; Sperling et al., 2011). During the limbic stages (stages III and IV), the NFT pathology in the transentorhinal cortex and EC becomes more severe (see Fig. 4.3F) (Braak & Braak, 1991). NFT pathosis also spreads to the subiculum and the *cornu Ammonis* (CA) 1 region. Patients in the limbic stages have mild cognitive decline in a range of cognitive domains including memory and executive function, but do not meet the criteria for AD diagnosis. Rather, it is thought to represent the symptomatic predementia phase referred to as mild cognitive impairment (MCI) (Albert et al., 2011; Khachaturian, 1985; McKhann et al., 2011; Mirra et al., 1991; Tierney et al., 1988).

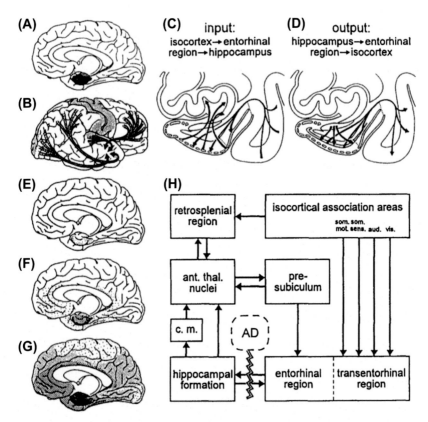

FIGURE 4.3 Braak staging and entorhinal cortex (EC) connectivity. (A) The human neocortex and allocortex (neocortex, *white*; hippocampus, *hatched*; presubiculum and EC, *black*). (B) Sensory input from various sensory modalities converges on the EC. (C) Neurons in layer 2 of the EC receive neocortical information and relay the information to the hippocampus (ie, via the perforant pathway). (D) In turn, the hippocampus projects feedback input via the subiculum into the Pri alpha region of the EC. The Pri alpha region sends feedback projections to the neocortex. (E, G) The six Braak stages of NFT pathology in AD. Neurofibrillary changes are shown by increased shading. (E) The transentorhinal stages (stages I and II). (F) The limbic stages (stages III and IV). (G) The neocortical stages (stages V and VI). (H) Schematic of limbic and neocortical input to the EC. Note that damage to the EC, during Alzheimer's disease *(AD)* or otherwise, can interfere with information transfer between the EC and hippocampus. *ant. thal. nuclei*, Anterior thalamic nuclei; *aud.*, auditory; *c.m.*, mammillary body; *som. mot.*, somatomotor; *som. sens.*, somatosensory; *vis.*, visual. *From Braak, H., & Braak, E. (1995). Staging of Alzheimer's disease-related neurofibrillary changes. Neurobiology of Aging, 16(3), 271–278– discussion 278–84.* http://dx.doi.org/10.1016/0197-4580(95)00021-6.

The progression of NFT pathosis from the EC to the hippocampus appears to be dependent on neuronal connections between these brain areas, which are important for memory formation (see Fig. 4.3C–H) (Damasio, Eslinger, Damasio, Van Hoesen, & Cornell, 1985; Scoville & Milner, 1957). Memory formation depends upon reciprocal connections between the EC to the hippocampus and multimodal association cortices (see Fig. 4.3B) (Van Hoesen & Pandya, 1975b, 1975a; Van Hoesen, Pandya, & Butters, 1975; Witter et al., 2000). Axons from layers 2 and 3 of the EC form the major projection to the hippocampus. From the EC, these axons transverse the angular bundle and "perforate" the subiculum to reach termination zones in the dentate gyrus (DG), CA1, and CA3. The laminar appearance of plaques in the brains of AD patients is based on the interconnectedness between the EC and the hippocampus, and is a common theme that dictates eventual progression into neocortical areas.

Clinical Evidence for Interneuronal Spreading of Tauopathy in Alzheimer's Disease

The neurons that are preferentially afflicted in AD patients are layer-3 pyramidal neurons, which project to other brain areas (Mountjoy, Roth, Evans, & Evans, 1983; Terry et al., 1991). The pattern of neuronal susceptibility in AD gives rise to the characteristic laminar NFT pathological disorder and neuron loss found in AD, and is evident in the neurons connecting the EC and the hippocampus. Pyramidal neurons in layer 2 and the superficial areas of layer 3 of the EC are preferentially lost in AD, with their efferent axons along the perforant pathway demonstrating prominent degeneration. The cellular degeneration is reflected in NFT staining and mirrors the findings of Braak & Braak (1991) (Hyman et al., 1986, 1988). Furthermore, a histopathological study of termination zones in the perforant pathway of AD patients are inundated with neuritic plaques (Hyman et al., 1986). These findings suggest that localized AD pathosis in the EC can spread along axonal pathways from one brain area to the next (see Fig. 4.3).

Axonal spread of AD-related pathological changes between interconnected neurons is not restricted to just the EC and hippocampal formation, but there is also evidence that AD pathological changes spread transneuronally in neocortical regions. During the neocortical stages of AD (Braak stages V and VI), NFTs severely affect the neocortical association areas, but the primary sensory areas appear resistant to pathological changes (see Fig. 4.3G) (Braak & Braak, 1991). The neocortical stage is associated with a diagnosis of dementia and the associated cortical signs (Khachaturian, 1985; McKhann et al., 2011, 1984). In particular, cortical layers 3 and 5 have the highest number of tangles, with layer 4 virtually unaffected (Lewis, Campbell, Terry, & Morrison, 1987; Wilcock, 1985). In the cerebral cortex, neurons responsible for long corticocortical connections reside in layers 3 and 5 (Desimone, Fleming, & Gross, 1980; Pandya, Hallett, & Kmukherjee, 1969; Rockland & Pandya, 1979). Furthermore, these neurons have the same size and laminar location as the large neurons that are preferentially lost over the course of AD (Mountjoy et al., 1983; Terry et al., 1991).

Our understanding of brain connections has been revealed by studies in Rhesus monkeys. The large pyramidal neurons in layers 3 and 5 provide the biological substrate for hierarchical connections between interconnected brain areas. Sensory information is first processed in primary sensory areas (visual, auditory, and sensory cortices). Sensory information spreads from primary sensory areas to multimodal association areas (see Fig. 4.3B). Interestingly, the EC serves as a multimodal association area that receives input from several other association areas, serving as a central hub (see Fig. 4.3B–D) (Jones & Powell, 1970a, 1970b). In the neocortex, feed-forward projections from primary sensory areas originate from layer 3. These efferent axons project to the input layer (layer 4) of downstream multimodal association areas. Neurons in association areas can reciprocate these connections from pyramidal neurons originating from layer 5 (reviewed in Ref. De Lacoste & White, 1993).

NFT pathology also follows the laminar pattern based on brain interconnectivity. In brain areas closer to primary sensory areas, layer-3 pyramidal neurons are more heavily affected than neurons arising from layer 5. However, in downstream association areas, layer 5 becomes more heavily afflicted with NFTs. The principle of transneuronal spread of NFT pathology also appears in noncanonical presentations of AD, such as AD with Balint syndrome (ADB). In ADB, the occipital–parietal pathway is preferentially affected, which results in concurrent presentation of visuospatial deficits and the neurological deficits traditionally seen in AD. Corresponding with these visuospatial deficits, visual areas such as Brodmann areas 17, 18, and 19 have higher levels of NFTs in ADB as compared with AD. Prefrontal areas are relatively spared in ADB, unlike traditional AD (Hof et al., 1989; Hof, Bouras, Constantinidis, & Morrison, 1990).

Transsynaptic Spreading? In Vitro and Animal Models

These findings suggest that NFT pathosis can spread transsynaptically from the EC anterogradely (to the hippocampus) and retrogradely (to neocortical association areas) (see Fig. 4.3D). In vitro experiments show that tau oligomers can be transferred from cell to cell and promote the formation of intracellular aggregates (Frost, Jacks, & Diamond, 2009; Kfoury, Holmes, Jiang, Holtzman, & Diamond, 2012). These results were later confirmed in elegant studies with primary neuronal cultures. Primary mouse neurons were cultured in microfluidic chambers that separated the somatodendritic and axonal compartments. Low–molecular-weight aggregates of tau were shown to be transported anterogradely or retrogradely by lysosomes (Wu et al., 2013).

Whereas these studies provided a plausible mechanism for transmission of tau aggregates, they did not demonstrate that tau transfer occurs in vivo. Injection of insoluble tau aggregates into transgenic mice bearing human tau suggested that tau could spread transsynaptically from the injection site to distant brain areas (Clavaguera et al., 2009). In an attempt to recapitulate the course of NFT spread in AD, two independent groups overexpressed human tau in the EC of mice (de Calignon et al., 2012; Liu et al., 2012). In one set of experiments, transgenic mice were designed to express human tau in pyramidal neurons in layer 2 of the transentorhinal cortex. In these aged mice, neurons in the connected regions of the DG, CA1, and parietal cortex stained for tangles and hyperphosphorylated tau (Liu et al., 2012). De Calignon and co-workers found similar findings when they expressed human tau, bearing the P301L mutation, found in familial frontal temporal dementia (de Calignon et al., 2012). Importantly, these findings recapitulated NFT conditions found in AD patients (Braak & Braak, 1991).

Soluble β-Amyloid and Alzheimer's Disease Pathology

Although tau pathology appears to be highly correlated with AD pathology, the tau hypothesis cannot fully explain all the pathological changes found in AD. Although tau overexpression recapitulates the NFTs seen in AD, transgenic mice take 22 months to recapitulate the pathosis found in stages II–III of AD (Liu et al., 2012). Furthermore, despite the correlation of tangles and neurological deficits, tangle formation on its own does not appear to disrupt neuronal networks in mice (Kuchibhotla et al., 2014; Rudinskiy et al., 2014). This idea is also supported by the discovery of tau mutations in humans, which cause NFT pathological changes without amyloid deposition. These mutations do not cause AD, but instead diseases with differing phenotypes including frontotemporal dementia and amyotrophic lateral sclerosis. Therefore tau deposition alone does not sufficiently account for all the pathological findings in AD.

There is a body of evidence that suggests tau pathological changes are downstream of amyloid pathosis. When transgenic mouse models of AD were crossed with a tau KO mouse, they were protected from cognitive decline (Roberson, Scearce-Levie, Palop, & Yan, 2007). Cells treated with fibrillar Aβ generate phosphorylated tau (Busciglio, Lorenzo, Yeh, & Yankner, 1995; Götz, Chen, van Dorpe, & Nitsch, 2001). However, amyloid plaques in AD patients, unlike tangles, did not correlate with the progression of cognitive deficits. Whereas appearance of tangles in the EC and the hippocampus was associated with memory loss, amyloid plaques are initially deposited in the frontal, temporal, and occipital cortices (Braak & Braak, 1991). In addition to the spatial separation of neurological deficits and Aβ deposition, this was further confounded by deposition of Aβ in clinically normal individuals (Blessed, Tomlinson, & Roth, 1968; Dickson & Yen, 1989; Katzman et al., 1988; Terry et al., 1991; Tomlinson et al., 1968, 1970). Despite the ability of Aβ solutions to cause neurotoxicity (Glabe & Cotman, 1993; Harrigan, Kunkel, Nguyen, & Malouf, 1995; Lorenzo & Yankner, 1994; Takadera, Sakura, Mohri, & Hashimoto, 1993), an apparent paradox arose. If Aβ is critical to neurotoxicity and appears to be the key to AD pathogenesis, why is there such a poor correlation with cognition in dementia?

Are Soluble Aggregates of β-Amyloid the Answer?

The first hints came from studies of apolipoprotein J (ApoJ), which prevented Aβ fibrillization yet resulted in increased toxicity (Oda et al., 1995). Structural analysis of ApoJ-treated Aβ solutions revealed the absence of fibrillar rodlike structures, but instead revealed small globular aggregates of Aβ oligomers (AβOs) (Stine et al., 1996). Water-soluble Aβ species are detectable in the brains of AD and Down syndrome patients, but not in cognitively normal controls (Kayed et al., 2003; Kuo et al., 1996; Teller et al., 1996). These soluble species range in size from 10 to 100 kDa (Teller et al., 1996) and were shown to be neurotoxic to hippocampal slices and cultured cells (Kayed et al., 2003; Kim et al., 2003; Lambert et al., 1998). In addition to their neurotoxic properties, AβOs disrupt synaptic spines and synaptic vesicle release in cultured hippocampal cells (Lacor et al., 2004, 2007; Park, Jang, & Chang, 2013; Zempel et al., 2013). Furthermore, AβOs disrupt long-term potentiation (LTP) in hippocampal slices (Jo et al., 2011; Lambert et al., 1998; Ostapchenko et al., 2013; Walsh et al., 2002; Wang et al., 2002). Furthermore, when soluble AβOs species are injected into the ventricles of mice, they profoundly disrupt synaptic plasticity and memory (Shankar et al., 2008).

Evidence From Patients With Alzheimer's Disease

In addition to their neurotoxic and synaptotoxic effects, AβOs also correlate with the onset of cognitive decline. When total levels of Aβ40 and Aβ 42 (aggregates and soluble AβOs) are accounted for, Aβ levels correlate well with progression of AD. As patients transition from a clinical dementia rating 0 (cognitively normal) to 0.5 (MCI), there is a sixfold to sevenfold increase in the levels of Aβ in the EC (Naslund et al., 2000). With disease progression, total Aβ levels increase in association areas before afflicting the primary visual cortex. Like NFT pathology, this provides evidence that Aβ levels also correlate with neurologically affected areas in AD (Braak & Braak, 1991).

Although soluble levels of Aβ are correlated with cognitive decline, the specific oligomeric species involved responsible for AD pathosis remains unclear. Dimers and dodecamers of Aβ have been suggested as the neurotoxic species (Lesné et al., 2013; Murphy et al., 2007; Reed et al., 2011; Renner et al., 2010; Shankar et al., 2008). Transgenic mice expressing *APP* bearing the Swedish mutation showed that an increase in dodecameric AβOs was correlated with the appearance of cognitive deficits in these mice (Murphy et al., 2007). These findings were recapitulated in similar studies of human brains. Lesné and colleagues demonstrated that dodecamers increased gradually during the first 6 decades of life, but increased rapidly thereafter. The increase in the dodecameric species was correlated with the appearance of hyperphosphorylated tau (Lesné et al., 2013). Other studies have suggested that dimeric Aβ species may also be neurotoxic (Larson et al., 2012; Reed et al., 2011; Um et al., 2012). Therefore the pathologically relevant species remains to be determined, and the differences between different investigations may be the result of different methods of preparing AβOs or that there are multiple subtypes of pathological AβO.

In Vitro Models and Animal Models of Soluble β-Amyloid Toxicity

One proposed receptor for AβO-mediated LTP impairment is the cellular prion protein (PrPᶜ) (Laurén, Gimbel, Nygaard, Gilbert, & Strittmatter, 2009;

Ostapchenko et al., 2013). Aβ binding to PrP^c promotes clustering of PrP^c and mGluR5 at the cell surface and pathologically increases intracellular calcium (Renner et al., 2010; Um et al., 2013). This dysregulated calcium influx may result in the appearance of extrasynaptic N-methyl-D-aspartate receptors (NMDARs), which can then generate spurious (nonsynaptic) signaling. Tonic overactivation of NMDARs may create "synaptic noise" (Parsons, Stöffler, & Danysz, 2007). Furthermore, activation of NR2b subunit containing NMDARs may also result in cell death (Amadoro et al., 2006; Hardingham, Fukunaga, & Bading, 2002). AβO binding to the PrP^c/mGluR5 receptor has been shown to activate Fyn (a Src family tyrosine-kinase), which can phosphorylate the NR2b subunit of the NMDAR, and increase these receptors at the synapse (Larson et al., 2012; Um et al., 2013). Translocation of Fyn to NMDARs is dependent on tau translocation into the dendritic spine. With tau KO or loss of Fyn/tau interaction, Fyn is uncoupled from NMDARs and prevents excitotoxicity and improves transgenic *APP* mouse survival (Ittner et al., 2010).

As discussed earlier, tau can be phosphorylated by a number of serine/threonine kinases. AβOs can lead to GSK3β activation (Chong et al., 2006; Jo et al., 2011; Tokutake et al., 2012). GSK3β activation also impairs LTP (Jo et al., 2011) and can lead to tau hyperphosphorylation (discussed earlier and in Ref. Tokutake et al., 2012). Indeed, neuronal cultures from a tau KO animal are nearly completely protected from Aβ-induced toxicity (Rapoport, Dawson, Binder, Vitek, & Ferreira, 2002). Furthermore, when tau KO mice were crossed with Aβ-producing transgenic mice, the crossed animals were protected from premature mortality and memory impairment (Ittner et al., 2010). Although the exact mechanism linking AβOs to tau is not yet fully elucidated, these findings demonstrate a potential therapeutically accessible connection between amyloid and tau pathology in AD.

Are Lysosomes the Source of Soluble β-Amyloid?

Just as lysosomes may play a role in transneuronal spread of NFTs (Wu et al., 2013), emerging evidence suggests that the endosomal/lysosomal system may also be central to amyloid pathology. Synaptic activity increases the release of Aβ into the cerebrospinal fluid in an endocytosis-dependent manner (Cirrito et al., 2008, 2005). APP and PSEN1 (the catalytic component of γ-secretase) are resident proteins of the lysosome and function optimally at an acidic pH (Pasternak et al., 2003). Alkalinization of endosomal/lysosomal pH by chloroquine or ammonium chloride can decrease Aβ production (Schrader-Fischer & Paganetti, 1996). Indeed, unprocessed APP can be visualized in the lysosomal compartment after loss of γ-secretase function (Chen, 2000; Tam, Seah, & Pasternak, 2014). Furthermore, multiple investigators have found that diverting APP away from the endosomal/lysosomal system can decrease amyloid production (Cirrito et al., 2008; Tam et al., 2014). Endosomes and lysosomes also provide the optimal subcellular milieu for Aβ aggregation (Su & Chang, 2001).

Intracellular Aβ
Tam and Pasternak

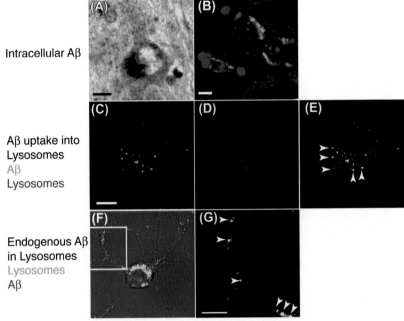

Intracellular Aβ

Aβ uptake into
Lysosomes
Aβ
Lysosomes

Endogenous Aβ
in Lysosomes
Lysosomes
Aβ

FIGURE 4.4 Lysosomal Aβ42 in Alzheimer's disease (AD). (A) and (B) Intracellular amyloid is detected using heat treatment (Retriever 2100) to immunostain intracellular accumulations of Aβ42 in humans (A, *brown*; scale bar = 10 μm) and in mice (B, *green*; Nuclei are *blue*). (C–E) SN56 cells were exposed to 250 nM HiLyte Fluor 488 labeled for 24 h to allow uptake of Aβ42 into lysosomes. (C) Aβ42 is shown in *green*. (D) Lysosomes labeled with transfected Lysosomal associated membrane protein 1 tagged with monomeric red fluorescent protein (LAMP1-mRFP) *(red)*. (E) A merge of *C* and *D*. Colocalized pixels are *yellow* and denoted by an *arrowhead* (scale bar = 10 μm). (F) A neuron from a mouse expressing human *APP_Swe/PSEN1Δ* exon 9 and immunostained for β-amyloid *(Aβ, red)* and LAMP1-labeled lysosomes *(green)*. Colocalized pixels are *yellow* (scale bar = 10 μm). The box in *F* is magnified in (G). Colocalized pixels are yellow and denoted by *arrowheads* (scale bar = 5 μm). *Modified from Tam, J.H., & Pasternak, S.H. (2012). Amyloid and Alzheimer's disease: inside and out.* The Canadian Journal of Neurological Sciences. Le Journal Canadien Des Sciences Neurologiques, 39(3), 286–298.

Intracellular accumulations of Aβ have been detected in animal models and human patients (Iulita et al., 2014). Examples of intracellular amyloid, predominately localized to lysosomes, are shown in Fig. 4.4. These lysosomal aggregates of Aβ can destabilize the lysosomal membrane, leading to the release of lysosomal proteases into the cytosol (Liu et al., 2010). In addition to disrupting the lysosomal membrane, Aβ may be secreted from intraluminal vesicles known as exosomes, which are found in endosomes and lysosomes (Rajendran et al., 2006). Soluble Aβ aggregates derived from lysosomes can "seed" fibrillization of extracellular Aβ (Hu et al., 2009). The finding that endosome-/

lysosome-derived vesicles are capable of secreting aggregated amyloid leads us to the tempting solution that lysosomes produce and secrete Aβ.

IMAGING ALZHEIMER'S DISEASE PATHOLOGY

Work from the imaging field studying the morphology, connectivity, functionality, and localization of Aβ and tau has been illuminating. These studies have furthered our understanding of AD disease progression and provided methods to diagnose AD earlier. Magnetic resonance imaging (MRI) of brain structure has confirmed atrophy in areas previously seen histologically. During early AD, the brain areas experiencing the highest rates of atrophy are located in the hippocampus and EC (Frisoni, Prestia, Rasser, Bonetti, & Thompson, 2009; Rowe et al., 2010; Vemuri et al., 2011). From the medial temporal lobe, pathosis spreads to multimodal association areas such as the frontal cortex and parietal cortex (Frisoni et al., 2009; Thompson et al., 2003). Using the Mini Mental State Exam (MMSE) as a measure of cognition, Shi, Liu, Zhou, Yu, and Jiang (2009) found that decreased hippocampal volumes were associated with lower scores on the MMSE. These changes precede a clinical diagnosis of AD (Bateman et al., 2012; Ridha et al., 2006).

Newer imaging modalities have taken advantage of the presence of amyloid and tau in the brains of AD patients. One of the biggest advancements was the development of a specific positron emission tomography (PET) imaging agent that stained specifically for fibrillar Aβ. Modification of thioflavine-T created 2-(4-methylaminophenyl)benzothiazole (BTA-1) (Klunk et al., 2001, 2003). BTA-1 crossed the blood–brain barrier and bound specifically to fibrillar amyloid in postmortem AD brains (Klunk et al., 2003). BTA-1 was developed into the PET imaging dye, Pittsburgh-B compound (PiB), and was shown to accumulate in areas where amyloid has been found histologically (Klunk et al., 2004).

Pike et al. (2007) demonstrated the potential of PiB as a biomarker for AD. Patients with MCI and AD were imaged using PiB-PET, and PiB-positive patients with MCI were shown to perform significantly worse on episodic memory tasks (Pike et al., 2007). These findings were echoed by Chételat et al. (2011), who found that Aβ deposition in the temporal cortex, detected by PiB, had a direct relationship to episodic memory deficits. PiB also accumulates in other pathologically relevant brain areas (hippocampus, temporal lobe, frontal lobe, parietal lobe) (Klunk et al., 2003, 2004; Niedowicz et al., 2012). Indeed, PiB binding associates well with cortical atrophy, as detected by MRI (Jack et al., 2008; Rowe et al., 2010).

Changes in neuronal activity can be measured by ^{18}F-fluorodeoxyglucose (FDG) PET. Hypometabolism, as detected by FDG, occurs in defined brain regions over the course of AD. In a similar pattern to the results seen with structural MRI, hypometabolism begins in the hippocampus before proceeding to temporal and parietal cortices and finally affecting other brain areas (Mosconi et al., 2009, 2005). Hypometabolism in AD correlates with maps of altered cortical connectivity (Buckner et al., 2009; Zhou, Gennatas, Kramer, Miller, & Seeley, 2012). Functional MRI (fMRI) can measure brain activity by measuring levels of deoxygenated blood [blood oxygenation level–dependent (BOLD) fMRI]. By correlating the brain areas that are active at the same time, maps of cortical connectivity can be created. BOLD fMRI has found that the default-mode network (DMN) has lower connectivity in the brains of AD patients (Hedden et al., 2009; Sheline et al., 2010), although one study has found an increase in activity in association with PiB (Lim et al., 2014). The DMN is typically engaged when the subject is not actively engaged in a task, such as during episodic memory (reviewed in Ref. Buckner, Buckner, Hanna, Andrews Hanna, & Schacter, 2008). The presence of Aβ may lead to cortical network correlation remodeling (Oh & Jagust, 2013). Human *APP* overexpression in a transgenic mouse model resulted in structural changes that increased the activity of dentate granule cells in the hippocampus. These structural changes can be recapitulated by treatment with kainate, to mimic excitotoxicity in the hippocampus (Wang et al., 2007). This suggests that an excitotoxic assault may be sufficient to initiate the cortical changes seen in AD. This is in agreement with the possibility that AβOs can cause aberrant excitation in neurons (discussed earlier). The deposition of Aβ also seems to follow functionally connected networks (Iturria-Medina, Sotero, Toussaint, & Evans, 2014; Sheline et al., 2010). For example, important areas of the DMN such as the cingulate cortex, hippocampus, EC, and parahippocampal gyrus appear to be affected early in AD (Iturria-Medina et al., 2014; Sheline et al., 2010). These appear to be focal points from which Aβ pathological change and, possibly, AD pathosis spread to afflict other interconnected brain areas (Iturria-Medina et al., 2014). Therefore it seems that Aβ causes an aberrant increase in brain activity and eventually results in network remodeling and network dysfunction.

Imaging agents that bind specifically to PHFs have also been designed, with success in both animal and human tauopathies. Currently, a definite diagnosis of AD can only be made postmortem by detecting senile plaques and NFTs in the brain. Two of the most promising molecules for imaging tau were found after screening a novel class of compounds known as *benzo[4,5]imidazo[1,2a] pyrimidines*, which were chosen for their potential for binding to PHF tau (Zhang et al., 2012). [^{18}F]T807and [^{18}F]T808 were found in the screen and showed high colocalization with PHF tau and phosphorylated tau, but not amyloid plaques. Exploratory studies in a small sample of human subjects also shows higher retention of both [^{18}F]T807 and [^{18}F]T808 in the brains of AD patients. Interestingly, the retention of both [^{18}F]T807 and [^{18}F]T808 was highest in the hippocampus, temporal cortex, and parietal cortex in patients with MCI or mild AD. In agreement with Braak staging, the retention of the agent increased in the frontal and occipital lobe in more severe cases of AD (Chien et al., 2013, 2014). Another class of compounds, phenyl/pyridinylbutadienyl-benzothiazoles/

benzothiazoliums (PBBs), was also screened based on the ability of PBBs to bind to β-sheets of aggregated tau. [^{11}C]PBB3 arose from this screen, and could stain phosphorylated tau and PHF tau. It also showed higher retention in mouse models of AD and human AD patients. Strikingly the tau binding pattern is reminiscent of Braak staging (Maruyama et al., 2013). The further development of tau staining will improve our ability to determine the severity of disease and will further development of antitau therapies in AD and other neurological disorders.

ALZHEIMER'S DISEASE THERAPEUTICS

There is currently no cure for AD—only pharmacological treatments to stall the progression of AD—but the inevitable progression of AD continues nonetheless. The most common treatments are acetylcholinesterase (AChE) inhibitors, such as donepezil, rivastigmine, and galantamine, which block the breakdown of the neurotransmitter acetylcholine (ACh), thereby raising the levels of ACh in the brain. The role of ACh in normal cognition and memory has been well documented (reviewed in Ref. Kása, Rakonczay, & Gulya, 1997). The nucleus basalis represents a major cholinergic input to the cortex (Mesulam & Geula, 1988). Controlled ablation of a limited number neurons in the nucleus basalis of rats resulted in a significant impairment in aged rats (31 months of age) (Burk, Herzog, Porter, & Sarter, 2002). Many of the current pharmacological treatments are based on the cholinergic hypothesis. The cholinergic hypothesis was developed because of the loss of cholinergic neurons commonly observed in AD (Kása et al., 1997). In AD patients, AChE inhibitors typically cause modest increases in cognitive ability and stall the progression of AD by raising the cortical levels of ACh (Farlow, 2004; Hsiung & Feldman, 2004; Möbius, 2004).

AD can also be treated by memantine, which blocks spurious activation of the NMDARs (Xia, Chen, Zhang, & Lipton, 2010). As discussed, excessive NMDAR activity can lead to excitotoxicity. The goal of N-methyl-D-aspartate (NMDA)-based therapeutics is to avoid pathological signaling at the synapse while being permissive to physiological stimulus (Lipton, 2006; Parsons et al., 2007; Xia et al., 2010). Memantine acts by blocking extrasynaptic NMDAR activity but preserving the activity of synaptic NMDARs for neuronal transmission (Xia et al., 2010). 3xTg-AD mice treated with memantine had improved cognition, and also had lower levels of phosphorylated tau and AβOs. Strikingly the effects were strongest for the 3xTg-AD mice with the most advanced impairments (Martinez-Coria et al., 2010). The beneficial effects of memantine were seen in clinical trials of human patients and memantine was the first clinical treatment that showed benefit for severe AD (Möbius, 2004).

Although the current treatment modalities can stall disease progression, a cure remains elusive. Several experimental treatment modalities focus on findings based on the amyloid cascade hypothesis and tau hypothesis. There are several treatments at different stages of development, which have furthered our understanding of AD pathology. Over the past 2 decades, the amyloid cascade hypothesis has been the dominant theory driving AD research and therapeutic innovation. Based on this hypothesis, effective treatments would decrease the production of Aβ or increase the clearance of Aβ. The main therapeutics designed have focused on β- or γ-secretase inhibition to lower Aβ production, and on reducing Aβ aggregation using small molecule drugs or immunotherapy.

γ-Secretase, which produces that final cleavage of *APP* to produce Aβ, is an attractive target for AD therapeutics. Indeed, inhibition of γ-secretase in AD transgenic mice reduces cortical Aβ and improved memory in a fear-conditioning test (Comery et al., 2005; Dovey et al., 2001), suggesting γ-secretase inhibition as a viable therapeutic target. However, in addition to *APP*, γ-secretase can cleave a large number of additional substrates, including the developmental regulatory receptor, Notch. Indeed, *Psen1* KO is embryonically lethal. The broad substrate specificity of γ-secretase increases the complexity in targeting this complex. These complexities were illustrated in the recent failures of avagacestat, semagacestat, and tarenflurbil in clinical trials (Coric et al., 2012; Doody et al., 2013; Green et al., 2009). Avagacestat did not continue to phase 3 trials, and tarenflurbil showed no benefit. Semagacestat caused a worsening in cognition and in the ability to perform activities of daily living in the treatment groups compared with placebo. Semagacestat trials were ended prematurely because of an increased risk for skin cancer and gastrointestinal effects (Doody et al., 2014).

The amyloid cascade hypothesis has also been tested clinically through the use of amyloid immunotherapies. Following the narrative of the failed γ-secretase inhibitors, amyloid immunotherapies had dramatically promising starts in animal models of AD, but so far have shown no benefit in humans in phase 3 trials. Active immunization of mice with Aβ peptides reduced cortical amyloid plaque burden and also improved cognition in animal models (Janus et al., 2000; Morgan et al., 2000; Schenk et al., 1999). However, immunization of AD patients did not improve cognition and increased the incidence of infection, headache, encephalitis, and diarrhea (Gilman et al., 2005). Despite these failures, a faint glimmer of hope is on the horizon. A small subset of patients that responded to Aβ immunization seemed to have a slower decline in cognition, suggesting a possible role in long-term treatment of Aβ (Vellas et al., 2009).

Passive immunization of mice also drastically reduced cortical amyloid burden and improved cognition (DeMattos et al., 2001; Dodart et al., 2002). One antibody was humanized and developed as solanezumab by Eli Lily (Indianapolis, IN, United States). Unfortunately, patients who received solanezumab did not have improved cognition or functional ability, although there may have been some benefit in patients with mild disease. Similarly, another passive antibody, bapineuzimab (Janssen Immunotherapy, New York, NY, United States and Pfizer, San Francisco, CA, United States), also failed a large randomized phase 3 trial, although there were some patients who showed improvements based on biomarker levels (Salloway et al., 2014). Both of these treatments also had a risk for hemorrhage and focal cerebral edema (Doody et al., 2014). Recently, Biogen Inc. (Cambridge, MA, United States) announced phase I data for aducanumab, demonstrating that this passive immunotherapy resulted in dramatic clearance of amyloid and improved cognition ("Biogen Antibody Buoyed by Phase1 Data and Hungry Investors", 2015). Needless to say, the results of phase 3 trials are anxiously awaited.

Another potential therapeutic is aimed at inhibiting the aggregation of tau (Wischik, Harrington, & Storey, 2014). Several families of compounds have been shown to solubilize aggregated tau and prevent the formation of PHFs (Pickhardt et al., 2007; Wischik, Edwards, Lai, Roth, & Harrington, 1996). Methylene blue (methylthionium chloride) was developed to a novel, stable, reduced form (LMTX). In phase II clinical trials, LMTX showed benefit for mild and moderate cases of AD (Wischik et al., 2015). The drug has entered phase 3 clinical trials and results are eagerly expected in 2016.

FUTURE DIRECTIONS

These clinical experiences with antiamyloid therapies emphasize the difficulties in translating potential therapeutics discovered in mice to treatments for AD, suggesting that our mouse models of AD may not be completely representative of the human condition. Wild-type mice do not develop AD, and only transgenic mice expressing human *APP*, which also incorporate FAD-causing mutations, develop plaques. Even then, robust development of amyloid plaques typically requires the addition of a human *PSEN* gene, also bearing FAD mutation(s). These mice are still limited, because for the most part they do not develop cell death or NFTs. The development of NFTs requires the addition of yet another transgene for the human protein tau, also bearing a disease-causing mutation. Therefore it can be argued that these animal models are quite artificial. In addition, FAD only represents a small percentage of all AD cases; these models may not be representative of the vast majority of the human condition. Furthermore, more recent discoveries suggest that AβOs are pathologically the most relevant form of Aβ. Thus, treatments that successfully reduce amyloid plaque load in mice may not be targeting the most important form of Aβ.

If there is one thing to be learned from the recent failure of Aβ-modifying treatments, it is the complexity of human biology. A single treatment modality will likely not be able to alter, cure, or modify the disease on its own. The complexity is evident in the cellular response to AβOs, which requires multiple proteins working in concert to produce a downstream response. *APP* may serve as a scaffold for some of the proteins involved (Hoe et al., 2008), adding further complexity to this system. It is interesting that tau appears to be involved in synaptic changes in response to AβOs (Ittner et al., 2010). This discovery provides a chance to reconcile the tau and amyloid aspects of the disease (Mudher & Lovestone, 2002). Despite these promising advances, the pathologically relevant AβOs species is/are still unclear. Furthermore, the identity of the AβO receptor is still undergoing fierce debate, with some investigators suggesting PrP^c and others suggesting a synaptic surface protein (Wilcox et al., 2015; Laurén et al., 2009). The next generation of disease-modifying drugs may depend on the precise modification of the AβOs' signaling network.

The recent advances in imaging techniques for AD have been truly exciting. The development of imaging agents specific to amyloid plaques and PHF tau has deepened our understanding of the disease process. For the first time, we are capable of observing the disease progression in living patients and animal models, allowing us to perform longitudinal studies on the accumulation of amyloid and tau over the course of AD. Importantly, this will allow an earlier diagnosis of AD. Endosomal and lysosomal dysfunction has been suggested to precede the appearance of plaques and tangles in AD (Cataldo et al., 2000; Nixon & Yang, 2011). Designing imaging agents to detect lysosomal pathology may be a promising research avenue (Ta et al., 2013). The efficacy of AD treatments may depend upon the early detection of AD.

Additionally, new experimental techniques have furthered our understanding of disease progression and the underlying molecular biology. For example, the recent MRI- and PET-based studies have confirmed the pattern of amyloid deposition and neuronal loss reported from histological studies over 20 years ago. Furthermore, these studies have also provided functional evidence that interconnected areas appear to spread amyloid pathosis along axonal connections between brain regions. The interneuronal transmission of AD pathosis may explain the eventual development of cortical symptoms in AD. Clinically, AD begins with mild memory loss, and this is likely because of initial disease beginning in the limbic system (hippocampus, entorhinal cortex, cingulate cortex, and parahippocampal cortex). As a result of this region's interconnectedness to many other regions, this may lead to the appearance of AD pathological changes in cortical regions of the brain.

Despite the disappointment in our clinical experience with Aβ modification, we do appear to be entering a period where several clinical trials that are likely to yield positive results. The discovery of imaging agents specific to amyloid plaques and PHF tau may allow for an earlier diagnosis of AD and earlier intervention. Furthermore, our understanding of the cellular basis of AD has never been greater, which may yield more precise methods of modifying AD. Hopefully, the first disease-modifying treatments for AD are only a few years away.

REFERENCES

Albert, M. S., DeKosky, S. T., Dickson, D., Dubois, B., Feldman, H. H., Gamst, A., et al. (2011). The diagnosis of mild cognitive impairment due to Alzheimer's disease: recommendations from the National Institute on Aging-Alzheimer's Association workgroups on diagnostic guidelines for Alzheimer's disease. *Alzheimer's & Dementia, 7*(3), 270–279.

Alonso, A., Zaidi, T., Novak, M., Grundke-Iqbal, I., & Iqbal, K. (2001). Hyperphosphorylation induces self-assembly of tau into tangles of paired helical filaments/straight filaments. *Proceedings of the National Academy of Sciences of the United States of America, 98*(12), 6923–6928. http://dx.doi.org/10.1073/pnas.121119298.

Alzheimer's Association. (2014). 2014 Alzheimer's disease facts and figures. *Alzheimer's & Dementia, 10*(2), e47–92.

Alzheimer's Association. (2015). Changing the trajectory of Alzheimer's disease: how a treatment by 2025 saves lives and dollars. *Alzheimer's & Dementia, 10*(2), e47–92.

Amadoro, G., Ciotti, M. T., Costanzi, M., Cestari, V., Calissano, P., & Canu, N. (2006). NMDA receptor mediates tau-induced neurotoxicity by calpain and *ERK/MAPK* activation. *Proceedings of the National Academy of Sciences of the United States of America, 103*(8), 2892–2897. http://dx.doi.org/10.1073/pnas.0511065103.

Bachman, D. L., Wolf, P. A., Linn, R. T., Knoefel, J. E., Cobb, J. L., Belanger, A. J., et al. (1993). Incidence of dementia and probable Alzheimer's disease in a general population the Framingham Study. *Neurology, 43*(3 Part 1), 515. http://dx.doi.org/10.1212/WNL.43.3_Part_1.515.

Ball, M. J. (1977). Neuronal loss, neurofibrillary tangles and granulovacuolar degeneration in the hippocampus with ageing and dementia: a quantitative study. *Acta Neuropathologica, 37*(2), 111–118. http://dx.doi.org/10.1007/BF00692056.

Bateman, R. J., Xiong, C., Benzinger, T. L. S., Fagan, A. M., Goate, A., Fox, N. C., et al. (2012). Clinical and biomarker changes in dominantly inherited Alzheimer's disease. *New England Journal of Medicine, 367*(9), 795–804. http://dx.doi.org/10.1056/NEJMoa1202753.

Bennecib, M., Gong, C. X., Grundke-Iqbal, I., & Iqbal, K. (2000). Role of protein phosphatase-2A and -1 in the regulation of GSK-3, CDK5 and CDC2 and the phosphorylation of tau in rat forebrain. *FEBS Letters, 485*(1), 87–93.

Bentahir, M., Nyabi, O., Verhamme, J., Tolia, A., Horre, K., Wiltfang, J., et al. (2006). Presenilin clinical mutations can affect gamma-secretase activity by different mechanisms. *Journal of Neurochemistry, 96*(3), 732–742. http://dx.doi.org/10.1111/j.1471-4159.2005.03578.x.

Biernat, J., Gustke, N., Drewes, G., Mandelkow, E. M., & Mandelkow, E. (1993). Phosphorylation of Ser262 strongly reduces binding of tau to microtubules: distinction between PHF-like immunoreactivity and microtubule binding. *Neuron, 11*(1), 153–163.

Biogen antibody buoyed by phase1 data and hungry investors. (March 25, 2015). *Biogen antibody buoyed by Phase 1 data and hungry investors*. From http://www.alzforum.org/news/conference-coverage/biogen-antibody-buoyed-phase-1-data-and-hungry-investors. Retrieved May 11, 2015.

Blessed, G., Tomlinson, B. E., & Roth, M. (1968). The association between quantitative measures of dementia and of senile change in the cerebral grey matter of elderly subjects. *The British Journal of Psychiatry, 114*(512), 797–811.

Borchelt, D. R., Thinakaran, G., Eckman, C. B., Lee, M. K., Davenport, F., Ratovitsky, T., et al. (1996). Familial Alzheimer's disease–linked presenilin 1 variants elevate Aβ1–42/1–40 ratio in vitro and in vivo. *Neuron, 17*(5), 1005–1013. http://dx.doi.org/10.1016/S0896-6273(00)80230-5.

Bouras, C., Hof, P. R., & Morrison, J. H. (1993). Neurofibrillary tangle densities in the hippocampal formation in a non-demented population define subgroups of patients with differential early pathologic changes. *Neuroscience Letters, 153*(2), 131–135. http://dx.doi.org/10.1016/0304-3940(93)90305-5.

Braak, H., & Braak, E. (1991). Neuropathological staging of Alzheimer-related changes. *Acta Neuropathologica, 82*(4), 239–259.

Braak, H., & Braak, E. (1995). Staging of Alzheimer's disease-related neurofibrillary changes. *Neurobiology of Aging, 16*(3), 271–278. http://dx.doi.org/10.1016/0197-4580(95)00021-6 discussion 278–84.

Braak, H., & Del Tredici, K. (2010). The pathological process underlying Alzheimer's disease in individuals under thirty. *Acta Neuropathologica, 121*(2), 171–181. http://dx.doi.org/10.1007/s00401-010-0789-4.

Buckner, R. L., Buckner, R. L., Hanna, J. A., Andrews Hanna, J. R., & Schacter, D. L. (2008). The brain's default network. *Annals of the New York Academy of Sciences, 1124*(1), 1–38. http://dx.doi.org/10.1196/annals.1440.011.

Buckner, R. L., Sepulcre, J., Talukdar, T., Krienen, F. M., Liu, H., Hedden, T., et al. (2009). Cortical hubs revealed by intrinsic functional connectivity: mapping, assessment of stability, and relation to Alzheimer's disease. *Journal of Neuroscience, 29*(6), 1860–1873. http://dx.doi.org/10.1523/JNEUROSCI.5062-08.2009.

Burk, J. A., Herzog, C. D., Porter, M. C., & Sarter, M. (2002). Interactions between aging and cortical cholinergic deafferentation on attention. *Neurobiology of Aging, 23*(3), 467–477.

Busciglio, J., Lorenzo, A., Yeh, J., & Yankner, B. A. (1995). Beta-amyloid fibrils induce tau phosphorylation and loss of microtubule binding. *Neuron, 14*(4), 879–888.

de Calignon, A., Polydoro, M., Suárez-Calvet, M., William, C., Adamowicz, D. H., Kopeikina, K. J., et al. (2012). Propagation of tau pathology in a model of early Alzheimer's disease. *Neuron, 73*(4), 685–697. http://dx.doi.org/10.1016/j.neuron.2011.11.033.

Castellano, J. M., Kim, J., Stewart, F. R., Jiang, H., DeMattos, R. B., Patterson, B. W., et al. (2011). Human ApoE isoforms differentially regulate brain amyloid-β peptide clearance. *Science Translational Medicine, 3*(89), 89ra57. http://dx.doi.org/10.1126/scitranslmed.3002156.

Cataldo, A. M., Peterhoff, C. M., Troncoso, J. C., Gomez-Isla, T., Hyman, B. T., & Nixon, R. A. (2000). Endocytic pathway abnormalities precede amyloid beta deposition in sporadic Alzheimer's disease and Down syndrome: differential effects of APOE genotype and presenilin mutations. *The American Journal of Pathology, 157*(1), 277–286.

Chacón, M. A., Barría, M. I., Soto, C., & Inestrosa, N. C. (2004). Beta-sheet breaker peptide prevents Aβ-induced spatial memory impairments with partial reduction of amyloid deposits. *Molecular Psychiatry, 9*(10), 953–961. http://dx.doi.org/10.1038/sj.mp.4001516.

Chen, F. (2000). Carboxyl-terminal fragments of Alzheimer beta-amyloid precursor protein accumulate in restricted and unpredicted intracellular compartments in presenilin 1-deficient cells. *Journal of Biological Chemistry, 275*(47), 36794–36802. http://dx.doi.org/10.1074/jbc.M006986200.

Chételat, G., Villemagne, V. L., Pike, K. E., Ellis, K. A., Bourgeat, P., Jones, G., et al. (2011). Independent contribution of temporal beta-amyloid deposition to memory decline in the pre-dementia phase of Alzheimer's disease. *Brain: a Journal of Neurology, 134*(Pt 3), 798–807. http://dx.doi.org/10.1093/brain/awq383.

Chien, D. T., Bahri, S., Szardenings, A. K., Walsh, J. C., Mu, F., Su, M.-Y., et al. (2013). Early clinical PET imaging results with the novel PHF-tau radioligand [F-18]-T807. *Journal of Alzheimer's Disease, 34*(2), 457–468. http://dx.doi.org/10.3233/JAD-122059.

Chien, D. T., Szardenings, A. K., Bahri, S., Walsh, J. C., Mu, F., Xia, C., et al. (2014). Early clinical PET imaging results with the novel PHF-tau radioligand [F18]-T808. *Journal of Alzheimer's Disease, 38*(1), 171–184. http://dx.doi.org/10.3233/JAD-130098.

Chong, Y. H., Shin, Y. J., Lee, E. O., Kayed, R., Glabe, C. G., & Tenner, A. J. (2006). ERK1/2 activation mediates Aβ oligomer-induced neurotoxicity via caspase-3 activation and tau cleavage in rat organotypic hippocampal slice cultures. *Journal of Biological Chemistry, 281*(29), 20315–20325. http://dx.doi.org/10.1074/jbc.M601016200.

Cirrito, J. R., Kang, J.-E., Lee, J., Stewart, F. R., Verges, D. K., Silverio, L. M., et al. (2008). Endocytosis is required for synaptic activity-dependent release of amyloid-β in vivo. *Neuron, 58*(1), 42–51. http://dx.doi.org/10.1016/j.neuron.2008.02.003.

Cirrito, J. R., Yamada, K. A., Finn, M. B., Sloviter, R. S., Bales, K. R., May, P. C., et al. (2005). Synaptic activity regulates interstitial fluid amyloid-β levels in vivo. *Neuron, 48*(6), 913–922. http://dx.doi.org/10.1016/j.neuron.2005.10.028.

Citron, M., Vigo-Pelfrey, C., Teplow, D. B., Miller, C., Schenk, D., Johnston, J., et al. (1994). Excessive production of amyloid beta-protein by peripheral cells of symptomatic and presymptomatic patients carrying the Swedish familial Alzheimer disease mutation. *Proceedings of the National Academy of Sciences of the United States of America, 91*(25), 11993–11997.

Clavaguera, F., Bolmont, T., Crowther, R. A., Abramowski, D., Frank, S., Probst, A., et al. (2009). Transmission and spreading of tauopathy in transgenic mouse brain. *Nature Cell Biology, 11*(7), 909–913. http://dx.doi.org/10.1038/ncb1901.

Cleveland, D. W., Hwo, S. Y., & Kirschner, M. W. (1977a). Physical and chemical properties of purified tau factor and the role of tau in microtubule assembly. *Journal of Molecular Biology, 116*(2), 227–247.

Cleveland, D. W., Hwo, S. Y., & Kirschner, M. W. (1977b). Purification of tau, a microtubule-associated protein that induces assembly of microtubules from purified tubulin. *Journal of Molecular Biology, 116*(2), 207–225.

Comery, T. A., Martone, R. L., Aschmies, S., Atchison, K. P., Diamantidis, G., Gong, X., et al. (2005). Acute gamma-secretase inhibition improves contextual fear conditioning in the Tg2576 mouse model of Alzheimer's disease. *Journal of Neuroscience, 25*(39), 8898–8902. http://dx.doi.org/10.1523/JNEUROSCI.2693-05.2005.

Coric, V., van Dyck, C. H., Salloway, S., Andreasen, N., Brody, M., Richter, R. W., et al. (2012). Safety and tolerability of the γ-secretase inhibitor avagacestat in a phase 2 study of mild to moderate Alzheimer disease. *Archives of Neurology, 69*(11), 1430–1440. http://dx.doi.org/10.1001/archneurol.2012.2194.

Damasio, A. R., Eslinger, P. J., Damasio, H., Van Hoesen, G. W., & Cornell, S. (1985). Multimodal amnesic syndrome following bilateral temporal and basal forebrain damage. *Archives of Neurology, 42*(3), 252–259.

De Lacoste, M. C., & White, C. L. (1993). The role of cortical connectivity in Alzheimer's disease pathogenesis: a review and model system. *Neurobiology of Aging, 14*(1), 1–16.

DeMattos, R. B., Bales, K. R., Cummins, D. J., Dodart, J. C., Paul, S. M., & Holtzman, D. M. (2001). Peripheral anti-A beta antibody alters CNS and plasma A beta clearance and decreases brain A beta burden in a mouse model of Alzheimer's disease. *Proceedings of the National Academy of Sciences of the United States of America, 98*(15), 8850–8855. http://dx.doi.org/10.1073/pnas.151261398.

De Strooper, B. (2003). Aph-1, Pen-2, and nicastrin with presenilin generate an active gamma-secretase complex. *Neuron, 38*(1), 9–12.

Desimone, R., Fleming, J., & Gross, C. G. (1980). Prestriate afferents to inferior temporal cortex: an HRP study. *Brain Research, 184*(1), 41–55.

Dickson, D. W., & Yen, S. H. (1989). Beta-amyloid deposition and paired helical filament formation: which histopathological feature is more significant in Alzheimer's disease? *Neurobiology of Aging, 10*(5), 402–404 discussion 412–4.

Dodart, J.-C., Bales, K. R., Gannon, K. S., Greene, S. J., DeMattos, R. B., Mathis, C., et al. (2002). Immunization reverses memory deficits without reducing brain Aβ burden in Alzheimer's disease model. *Nature Neuroscience* 5. http://dx.doi.org/10.1038/nn842.

Doody, R. S., Raman, R., Farlow, M., Iwatsubo, T., Vellas, B., Joffe, S., et al. (2013). A phase 3 trial of semagacestat for treatment of Alzheimer's disease. *New England Journal of Medicine, 369*(4), 341–350. http://dx.doi.org/10.1056/NEJMoa1210951.

Doody, R. S., Thomas, R. G., Farlow, M., Iwatsubo, T., Vellas, B., Joffe, S., et al. (2014). Phase 3 trials of solanezumab for mild-to-moderate Alzheimer's disease. *New England Journal of Medicine, 370*(4), 311–321. http://dx.doi.org/10.1056/NEJMoa1312889.

Dovey, H. F., John, V., Anderson, J. P., Chen, L. Z., De Saint Andrieu, P., Fang, L. Y., et al. (2001). Functional gamma-secretase inhibitors reduce beta-amyloid peptide levels in brain. *Journal of Neurochemistry, 76*(1), 173–181. http://dx.doi.org/10.1046/j.1471-4159.2001.00012.x.

Drewes, G., Ebneth, A., Preuss, U., Mandelkow, E. M., & Mandelkow, E. (1997). MARK, a novel family of protein kinases that phosphorylate microtubule-associated proteins and trigger microtubule disruption. *Cell, 89*(2), 297–308.

Farlow, M. R. (2004). Rivastigmine for treatment of AD. In R. W. Richter, & B. Z. Richter (Eds.), *Alzheimer's disease* (pp. 187–192). Totowa, New Jersey: Humana Press.

Förstl, H., & Kurz, A. (1999). Clinical features of Alzheimer's disease. *European Archives of Psychiatry and Clinical Neuroscience, 249*(6), 288–290. http://dx.doi.org/10.1038/nn.2785.

Frisoni, G. B., Prestia, A., Rasser, P. E., Bonetti, M., & Thompson, P. M. (2009). In vivo mapping of incremental cortical atrophy from incipient to overt Alzheimer's disease. *Journal of Neurology, 256*(6), 916–924. http://dx.doi.org/10.1007/s00415-009-5040-7.

Frost, B., Jacks, R. L., & Diamond, M. I. (2009). Propagation of tau misfolding from the outside to the inside of a cell. *Journal of Biological Chemistry, 284*(19), 12845–12852. http://dx.doi.org/10.1074/jbc.M808759200.

Games, D., Adams, D., Alessandrini, R., Barbour, R., Berthelette, P., Blackwell, C., et al. (1995). Alzheimer-type neuropathology in transgenic mice overexpressing V717F beta-amyloid precursor protein. *Nature, 373*(6514), 523–527. http://dx.doi.org/10.1038/373523a0.

Gilman, S., Koller, M., Black, R. S., Jenkins, L., Griffith, S. G., Fox, N. C., et al. (2005). Clinical effects of Aβ immunization (AN1792) in patients with AD in an interrupted trial. *Neurology, 64*(9), 1553–1562. http://dx.doi.org/10.1212/01.WNL.0000159740.16984.3C.

Glabe, C. G., & Cotman, C. W. (1993). Neurodegeneration induced by beta-amyloid peptides in vitro: the role of peptide assembly state. *The Journal of Neuroscience, 13*(4), 1676–1687.

Glenner, G. G., & Wong, C. W. (1984). Alzheimer's disease: initial report of the purification and characterization of a novel cerebrovascular amyloid protein. *Biochemical and Biophysical Research Communications, 120*(3), 885–890.

Goedert, M., Cohen, E. S., Jakes, R., & Cohen, P. (1992). p42 MAP kinase phosphorylation sites in microtubule-associated protein tau are dephosphorylated by protein phosphatase 2A1: implications for Alzheimer's disease [corrected]. *FEBS Letters, 312*(1), 95–99.

Goedert, M., Jakes, R., Qi, Z., Wang, J. H., & Cohen, P. (1995). Protein phosphatase 2A is the major enzyme in brain that dephosphorylates tau protein phosphorylated by proline-directed protein kinases or cyclic AMP-dependent protein kinase. *Journal of Neurochemistry, 65*(6), 2804–2807.

Goedert, M., Spillantini, M. G., Cairns, N. J., & Crowther, R. A. (1992). Tau proteins of Alzheimer paired helical filaments: abnormal phosphorylation of all six brain isoforms. *Neuron, 8*(1), 159–168. http://dx.doi.org/10.1007/978-1-59745-324-0_9.

Goedert, M., Spillantini, M. G., Jakes, R., Rutherford, D., & Crowther, R. A. (1989). Multiple isoforms of human microtubule-associated protein tau: sequences and localization in neurofibrillary tangles of Alzheimer's disease. *Neuron, 3*(4), 519–526.

Goedert, M., Wischik, C. M., Crowther, R. A., Walker, J. E., & Klug, A. (1988). Cloning and sequencing of the cDNA encoding a core protein of the paired helical filament of Alzheimer disease: identification as the microtubule-associated protein tau. *Proceedings of the National Academy of Sciences of the United States of America, 85*(11), 4051–4055.

Gong, C. X., Lidsky, T., Wegiel, J., Zuck, L., Grundke-Iqbal, I., & Iqbal, K. (2000). Phosphorylation of microtubule-associated protein tau is regulated by protein phosphatase 2A in mammalian brain: implications for neurofibrillary degeneration in Alzheimer's disease. *Journal of Biological Chemistry, 275*(8), 5535–5544.

Gong, C. X., Shaikh, S., Wang, J. Z., Zaidi, T., Grundke-Iqbal, I., & Iqbal, K. (1995). Phosphatase activity toward abnormally phosphorylated tau: decrease in Alzheimer disease brain. *Journal of Neurochemistry, 65*(2), 732–738.

Gong, C. X., Singh, T. J., Grundke-Iqbal, I., & Iqbal, K. (1993). Phosphoprotein phosphatase activities in Alzheimer disease brain. *Journal of Neurochemistry, 61*(3), 921–927.

Götz, J., Chen, F., van Dorpe, J., & Nitsch, R. M. (2001). Formation of neurofibrillary tangles in P301l tau transgenic mice induced by Aβ 42 fibrils. *Science, 293*(5534), 1491–1495. http://dx.doi.org/10.1126/science.1062097.

Green, R. C., Schneider, L. S., Amato, D. A., Beelen, A. P., Wilcock, G., Swabb, E. A., et al. (2009). Effect of tarenflurbil on cognitive decline and activities of daily living in patients with mild Alzheimer disease: a randomized controlled trial. *JAMA, 302*(23), 2557–2564. http://dx.doi.org/10.1001/jama.2009.1866.

Greenberg, S. G., & Davies, P. (1990). A preparation of Alzheimer paired helical filaments that displays distinct tau proteins by polyacrylamide gel electrophoresis. *Proceedings of the National Academy of Sciences of the United States of America, 87*(15), 5827–5831.

Haass, C., Schlossmacher, M. G., Hung, A. Y., Vigo-Pelfrey, C., Mellon, A., Ostaszewski, B. L., et al. (1992). Amyloid beta-peptide is produced by cultured cells during normal metabolism. *Nature, 359*(6393), 322–325. http://dx.doi.org/10.1038/359322a0.

Hardingham, G. E., Fukunaga, Y., & Bading, H. (2002). Extrasynaptic NMDARs oppose synaptic NMDARs by triggering CREB shut-off and cell death pathways. *Nature Neuroscience, 5*(5), 405–414. http://dx.doi.org/10.1038/nn835.

Hardy, J. A., & Higgins, G. A. (1992). Alzheimer's disease: the amyloid cascade hypothesis. *Science, 256*(5054), 184–185.

Harrigan, M. R., Kunkel, D. D., Nguyen, L. B., & Malouf, A. T. (1995). Beta amyloid is neurotoxic in hippocampal slice cultures. *Neurobiology of Aging, 16*(5), 779–789.

Hebert, L. E., Scherr, P. A., Beckett, L. A., Albert, M. S., Pilgrim, D. M., Chown, M. J., et al. (1995). Age-specific incidence of Alzheimer's disease in a community population. *JAMA, 273*(17), 1354–1359.

Hedden, T., Van Dijk, K. R. A., Becker, J. A., Mehta, A., Sperling, R. A., Johnson, K. A., et al. (2009). Disruption of functional connectivity in clinically normal older adults harboring amyloid burden. *Journal of Neuroscience, 29*(40), 12686–12694. http://dx.doi.org/10.1523/JNEUROSCI.3189-09.2009.

Higdon, R., Bowen, J. D., McCormick, W. C., Teri, L., Schellenberg, G. D., van Belle, G., et al. (2002). Dementia and Alzheimer disease incidence: a prospective cohort study. *Archives of Neurology, 59*(11), 1737–1746.

Hoe, H.-S., Minami, S. S., Makarova, A., Lee, J., Hyman, B. T., Matsuoka, Y., et al. (2008). Fyn modulation of Dab1 effects on amyloid precursor protein and ApoE receptor 2 processing. *Journal of Biological Chemistry, 283*(10), 6288–6299. http://dx.doi.org/10.1074/jbc.M704140200.

Hof, P. R., Bouras, C., Constantinidis, J., & Morrison, J. H. (1989). Balint's syndrome in Alzheimer's disease: specific disruption of the occipito-parietal visual pathway. *Brain Research, 493*(2), 368–375.

Hof, P. R., Bouras, C., Constantinidis, J., & Morrison, J. H. (1990). Selective disconnection of specific visual association pathways in cases of Alzheimer's disease presenting with Balint's syndrome. *Journal of Neuropathology and Experimental Neurology, 49*(2), 168–184.

Holtzman, D. M., Bales, K. R., Tenkova, T., Fagan, A. M., Parsadanian, M., Sartorius, L. J., et al. (2000). Apolipoprotein E isoform-dependent amyloid deposition and neuritic degeneration in a mouse model of Alzheimer's disease. *Proceedings of the National Academy of Sciences of the United States of America*, *97*(6), 2892–2897. http://dx.doi.org/10.1073/pnas.050004797.

Hsiung, G.-Y. R., & Feldman, H. (2004). Donepezil in treatment of AD. In R. W. Richter, & B. Z. Richter (Eds.), *Alzheimer's disease* (pp. 179–185). Totowa, New Jersey: Humana Press.

Hu, X., Crick, S. L., Bu, G., Frieden, C., Pappu, R. V., & Lee, J.-M. (2009). Amyloid seeds formed by cellular uptake, concentration, and aggregation of the amyloid-beta peptide. *Proceedings of the National Academy of Sciences*, *106*(48), 20324–20329. http://dx.doi.org/10.1073/pnas.0911281106.

Hyman, B. T., Kromer, L. J., & Van Hoesen, G. W. (1988). A direct demonstration of the perforant pathway terminal zone in Alzheimer's disease using the monoclonal antibody Alz-50. *Brain Research*, *450*(1–2), 392–397.

Hyman, B. T., Van Hoesen, G. W., Kromer, L. J., & Damasio, A. R. (1986). Perforant pathway changes and the memory impairment of Alzheimer's disease. *Annals of Neurology*, *20*(4), 472–481. http://dx.doi.org/10.1002/ana.410200406.

Ittner, L. M., Ke, Y. D., Delerue, F., Bi, M., Gladbach, A., van Eersel, J., et al. (2010). Dendritic function of tau mediates amyloid-beta toxicity in Alzheimer's disease mouse models. *Cell*, *142*(3), 387–397. http://dx.doi.org/10.1016/j.cell.2010.06.036.

Iturria-Medina, Y., Sotero, R. C., Toussaint, P. J., & Evans, A. C. (2014). Epidemic spreading model to characterize misfolded proteins propagation in aging and associated neurodegenerative disorders. *PLoS Computational Biology*, *10*(11), e1003956. http://dx.doi.org/10.1371/journal.pcbi.1003956.

Iulita, M. F., Allard, S., Richter, L., Munter, L.-M., Ducatenzeiler, A., Weise, C., et al. (2014). Intracellular Aβ pathology and early cognitive impairments in a transgenic rat overexpressing human amyloid precursor protein: a multidimensional study. *Acta Neuropathologica Communications*, *2*(1), 61. http://dx.doi.org/10.1186/2051-5960-2-61.

Jack, C. R., Lowe, V. J., Senjem, M. L., Weigand, S. D., Kemp, B. J., Shiung, M. M., et al. (2008). 11C PiB and structural MRI provide complementary information in imaging of Alzheimer's disease and amnestic mild cognitive impairment. *Brain: a Journal of Neurology*, *131*(Pt 3), 665–680. http://dx.doi.org/10.1093/brain/awm336.

Janus, C., Pearson, J., McLaurin, J., Mathews, P. M., Jiang, Y., Schmidt, S. D., et al. (2000). A beta peptide immunization reduces behavioural impairment and plaques in a model of Alzheimer's disease. *Nature*, *408*(6815), 979–982. http://dx.doi.org/10.1038/35050110.

Jiang, Q., Lee, C. Y. D., Mandrekar, S., Wilkinson, B., Cramer, P., Zelcer, N., et al. (2008). ApoE promotes the proteolytic degradation of Aβ. *Neuron*, *58*(5), 681–693. http://dx.doi.org/10.1016/j.neuron.2008.04.010.

Jo, J., Whitcomb, D. J., Olsen, K. M., Kerrigan, T. L., Lo, S.-C., Bru-Mercier, G., et al. (2011). Aβ(1-42) inhibition of LTP is mediated by a signaling pathway involving caspase-3, Akt1 and GSK-3β. *Nature Neuroscience*, *14*(5), 545–547. http://dx.doi.org/10.1038/nn.2785.

Jones, E. G., & Powell, T. P. (1970a). An anatomical study of converging sensory pathways within the cerebral cortex of the monkey. *Brain: a Journal of Neurology*, *93*(4), 793–820.

Jones, E. G., & Powell, T. P. (1970b). Connections of the somatic sensory cortex of the rhesus monkey. 3. Thalamic connections. *Brain: a Journal of Neurology*, *93*(1), 37–56.

Jorm, A. F., & Jolley, D. (1998). The incidence of dementia: a meta-analysis. *Neurology*, *51*(3), 728–733.

Kamboh, M. I., Demirci, F. Y., Wang, X., Minster, R. L., Carrasquillo, M. M., Pankratz, V. S., et al. (2012). Genome-wide association study of Alzheimer's disease. *Translational Psychiatry*, *2*, e117. http://dx.doi.org/10.1038/tp.2012.45.

Kása, P., Rakonczay, Z., & Gulya, K. (1997). The cholinergic system in Alzheimer's disease. *Progress in Neurobiology*, *52*(6), 511–535. http://dx.doi.org/10.1016/S0301-0082(97)00028-2.

Katzman, R., Terry, R., DeTeresa, R., Brown, T., Davies, P., Fuld, P., et al. (1988). Clinical, pathological, and neurochemical changes in dementia: a subgroup with preserved mental status and numerous neocortical plaques. *Annals of Neurology*, *23*(2), 138–144. http://dx.doi.org/10.1002/ana.410230206.

Kawarabayashi, T., Younkin, L. H., Saido, T. C., Shoji, M., Ashe, K. H., & Younkin, S. G. (2001). Age-dependent changes in brain, CSF, and plasma amyloid (beta) protein in the Tg2576 transgenic mouse model of Alzheimer's disease. *Journal of Neuroscience*, *21*(2), 372–381.

Kawas, C., Gray, S., Brookmeyer, R., Fozard, J., & Zonderman, A. (2000). Age-specific incidence rates of Alzheimer's disease: the Baltimore longitudinal study of aging. *Neurology*, *54*(11), 2072–2077.

Kayed, R., Head, E., Thompson, J. L., McIntire, T. M., Milton, S. C., Cotman, C. W., et al. (2003). Common structure of soluble amyloid oligomers implies common mechanism of pathogenesis. *Science*, *300*(5618), 486–489. http://dx.doi.org/10.1126/science.1079469.

Kfoury, N., Holmes, B. B., Jiang, H., Holtzman, D. M., & Diamond, M. I. (2012). Trans-cellular propagation of tau aggregation by fibrillar species. *The Journal of Biological Chemistry*, *287*(23), 19440–19451. http://dx.doi.org/10.1074/jbc.M112.346072.

Khachaturian, Z. S. (1985). Diagnosis of Alzheimer's disease. *Archives of Neurology*, *42*(11), 1097–1105.

Kidd, M. (1963). Paired helical filaments in electron microscopy of Alzheimer's disease. *Nature*, *197*, 192–193. http://dx.doi.org/10.1038/197192b0.

Kim, J., Castellano, J. M., Jiang, H., Basak, J. M., Parsadanian, M., Pham, V., et al. (2009). Overexpression of low-density lipoprotein receptor in the brain markedly inhibits amyloid deposition and increases extracellular aβ clearance. *Neuron*, *64*(5), 632–644. http://dx.doi.org/10.1016/j.neuron.2009.11.013.

Kim, H.-J., Chae, S.-C., Lee, D.-K., Chromy, B., Lee, S. C., Park, Y.-C., et al. (2003). Selective neuronal degeneration induced by soluble oligomeric amyloid beta protein. *The FASEB Journal*, *17*(1), 118–120. http://dx.doi.org/10.1096/fj.01-0987fje.

Klein, W. L. (2002). Aβ toxicity in Alzheimer's disease: globular oligomers (ADDLs) as new vaccine and drug targets. *Neurochemistry International*, *41*(5), 345–352.

Klunk, W. E., Engler, H., Nordberg, A., Wang, Y., Blomqvist, G., Holt, D. P., et al. (2004). Imaging brain amyloid in Alzheimer's disease with Pittsburgh compound-B. *Annals of Neurology*, *55*(3), 306–319. http://dx.doi.org/10.1002/ana.20009.

Klunk, W. E., Wang, Y., Huang, G. F., Debnath, M. L., Holt, D. P., & Mathis, C. A. (2001). Uncharged thioflavine-T derivatives bind to amyloid-beta protein with high affinity and readily enter the brain. *Life Sciences*, *69*(13), 1471–1484.

Klunk, W. E., Wang, Y., Huang, G.-F., Debnath, M. L., Holt, D. P., Shao, L., et al. (2003). The binding of 2-(4'-methylaminophenyl)benzothiazole to postmortem brain homogenates is dominated by the amyloid component. *Journal of Neuroscience*, *23*(6), 2086–2092.

Köpke, E., Tung, Y. C., Shaikh, S., Iqbal, K., & Grundke-Iqbal, I. (1993). Microtubule-associated protein tau: abnormal phosphorylation of a non-paired helical filament pool in Alzheimer disease. *Journal of Biological Chemistry*, *268*(32), 24374–24384.

Kuchibhotla, K. V., Wegmann, S., Kopeikina, K. J., Hawkes, J., Rudinskiy, N., Andermann, M. L., et al. (2014). Neurofibrillary tangle-bearing neurons are functionally integrated in cortical circuits in vivo. *Proceedings of the National Academy of Sciences of the United States of America, 111*(1), 510–514. http://dx.doi.org/10.1073/pnas.1318807111.

Kuo, Y.-M., Emmerling, M. R., Vigo-Pelfrey, C., Kasunic, T. C., Kirkpatrick, J. B., Murdoch, G. H., et al. (1996). Water-soluble A (N-40, N-42) oligomers in normal and Alzheimer disease brains. *The Journal of Biological Chemistry, 271*(8), 4077–4081.

Lacor, P. N., Buniel, M. C., Chang, L., Fernandez, S. J., Gong, Y., Viola, K. L., et al. (2004). Synaptic targeting by Alzheimer's-related amyloid beta oligomers. *Journal of Neuroscience, 24*(45), 10191–10200. http://dx.doi.org/10.1523/JNEUROSCI.3432-04.2004.

Lacor, P. N., Buniel, M. C., Furlow, P. W., Clemente, A. S., Velasco, P. T., Wood, M., et al. (2007). Aβ oligomer-induced aberrations in synapse composition, shape, and density provide a molecular basis for loss of connectivity in Alzheimer's disease. *Journal of Neuroscience, 27*(4), 796–807. http://dx.doi.org/10.1523/JNEUROSCI.3501-06.2007.

Lamb, B. T., Call, L. M., Slunt, H. H., Bardel, K. A., Lawler, A. M., Eckman, C. B., et al. (1997). Altered metabolism of familial Alzheimer's disease-linked amyloid precursor protein variants in yeast artificial chromosome transgenic mice. *Human Molecular Genetics, 6*(9), 1535–1541. http://dx.doi.org/10.1093/hmg/6.9.1535.

Lambert, M. P., Barlow, A. K., Chromy, B. A., Edwards, C., Freed, R., Liosatos, M., et al. (1998). Diffusible, nonfibrillar ligands derived from Aβ1-42 are potent central nervous system neurotoxins. *Proceedings of the National Academy of Sciences of the United States of America, 95*(11), 6448–6453.

Lammich, S., Kojro, E., Postina, R., Gilbert, S., Pfeiffer, R., Jasionowski, M., et al. (1999). Constitutive and regulated alpha-secretase cleavage of Alzheimer's amyloid precursor protein by a disintegrin metalloprotease. *Proceedings of the National Academy of Sciences of the United States of America, 96*(7), 3922–3927.

Larson, M., Sherman, M. A., Amar, F., Nuvolone, M., Schneider, J. A., Bennett, D. A., et al. (2012). The complex PrP^c-Fyn couples human oligomeric a with pathological tau changes in Alzheimer's disease. *Journal of Neuroscience, 32*(47), 16857–16871. http://dx.doi.org/10.1523/JNEUROSCI.1858-12.2012.

Laurén, J., Gimbel, D. A., Nygaard, H. B., Gilbert, J. W., & Strittmatter, S. M. (2009). Cellular prion protein mediates impairment of synaptic plasticity by amyloid-β oligomers. *Nature, 457*(7233), 1128–1132. http://dx.doi.org/10.1038/nature07761.

Lesné, S. E., Sherman, M. A., Grant, M., Kuskowski, M., Bennett, D. A., & Ashe, K. H. (2013). Brain amyloid-β oligomers in ageing and Alzheimer's disease. *Brain: a Journal of Neurology, 136*(5), awt062–1398. http://dx.doi.org/10.1093/brain/awt062.

Lewis, D. A., Campbell, M. J., Terry, R. D., & Morrison, J. H. (1987). Laminar and regional distributions of neurofibrillary tangles and neuritic plaques in Alzheimer's disease: a quantitative study of visual and auditory cortices. *The Journal of Neuroscience, 7*(6), 1799–1808.

Li, Y. P., Bushnell, A. F., Lee, C. M., Perlmutter, L. S., & Wong, S. K. (1996). Beta-amyloid induces apoptosis in human-derived neurotypic SH-SY5Y cells. *Brain Research, 738*(2), 196–204.

Lim, H. K., Nebes, R., Snitz, B., Cohen, A., Mathis, C., Price, J., et al. (2014). Regional amyloid burden and intrinsic connectivity networks in cognitively normal elderly subjects. *Brain: a Journal of Neurology, 137*(12), awu271–3338. http://dx.doi.org/10.1093/brain/awu271.

Lin, X., Koelsch, G., Wu, S., Downs, D., Dashti, A., & Tang, J. (2000). Human aspartic protease memapsin 2 cleaves the beta-secretase site of beta-amyloid precursor protein. *Proceedings of the National Academy of Sciences of the United States of America, 97*(4), 1456–1460.

Lindwall, G., & Cole, R. D. (1984). Phosphorylation affects the ability of tau protein to promote microtubule assembly. *Journal of Biological Chemistry, 259*(8), 5301–5305.

Lipton, S. A. (2006). Paradigm shift in neuroprotection by NMDA receptor blockade: memantine and beyond. *Nature Reviews Drug Discovery, 5*(2), 160–170. http://dx.doi.org/10.1038/nrd1958.

Liu, L., Drouet, V., Wu, J. W., Witter, M. P., Small, S. A., & Clelland, C. (2012). Trans-synaptic spread of tau pathology in vivo. *PLoS One, 7*(2), e31302. http://dx.doi.org/10.1371/journal. pone.0031302.

Liu, R.-Q., Zhou, Q.-H., Ji, S.-R., Zhou, Q., Feng, D., Wu, Y., et al. (2010). Membrane localization of beta-amyloid 1-42 in lysosomes: a possible mechanism for lysosome labilization. *The Journal of Biological Chemistry, 285*(26), 19986–19996. http://dx.doi.org/10.1074/jbc.M109.036798.

Lorenzo, A., & Yankner, B. A. (1994). Beta-amyloid neurotoxicity requires fibril formation and is inhibited by congo red. *Proceedings of the National Academy of Sciences of the United States of America, 91*(25), 12243–12247.

Ma, J., Yee, A., Brewer, H. B., Das, S., & Potter, H. (1994). Amyloid-associated proteins alpha 1-antichymotrypsin and apolipoprotein E promote assembly of Alzheimer beta-protein into filaments. *Nature, 372*(6501), 92–94. http://dx.doi.org/10.1038/372092a0.

Mandelkow, E. M., Drewes, G., Biernat, J., Gustke, N., Van Lint, J., Vandenheede, J. R., et al. (1992). Glycogen synthase kinase-3 and the Alzheimer-like state of microtubule-associated protein tau. *FEBS Letters, 314*(3), 315–321.

Mann, D. M., Yates, P. O., & Marcyniuk, B. (1984). Alzheimer's presenile dementia, senile dementia of Alzheimer type and Down's syndrome in middle age form an age related continuum of pathological changes. *Neuropathology and Applied Neurobiology, 10*(3), 185–207. http://dx.doi.org/10.1111/j.1365-2990.1984.tb00351.x.

Martinez-Coria, H., Green, K. N., Billings, L. M., Kitazawa, M., Albrecht, M., Rammes, G., et al. (2010). Memantine improves cognition and reduces Alzheimer's-like neuropathology in transgenic mice. *The American Journal of Pathology, 176*(2), 870–880. http://dx.doi.org/10.2353/ajpath.2010.090452.

Maruyama, K., Tomita, T., Shinozaki, K., Kume, H., Asada, H., Saido, T. C., et al. (1996). Familial Alzheimer's disease-linked mutations at val 717 of amyloid precursor protein are specific for the increased secretion of Aβ42(43). *Biochemical and Biophysical Research Communications, 227*(3), 730–735.

Maruyama, M., Shimada, H., Suhara, T., Shinotoh, H., Ji, B., Maeda, J., et al. (2013). Imaging of tau pathology in a tauopathy mouse model and in Alzheimer patients compared to normal controls. *Neuron, 79*(6), 1094–1108. http://dx.doi.org/10.1016/j.neuron.2013.07.037.

Masters, C. L., Simms, G., Weinman, N. A., Multhaup, G., McDonald, B. L., & Beyreuther, K. (1985). Amyloid plaque core protein in Alzheimer disease and Down syndrome. *Proceedings of the National Academy of Sciences of the United States of America, 82*(12), 4245–4249.

McKhann, G., Drachman, D., Folstein, M., Katzman, R., Price, D., & Stadlan, E. M. (July 1984). Clinical diagnosis of Alzheimer's disease: report of the NINCDS-ADRDA work group under the auspices of Department of Health and human Services task force on Alzheimer's disease. *Neurology, 34*(7), 939–944.

McKhann, G. M., Chertkow, H., Hyman, B. T., Jack, C. R., Kawas, C. H., Klunk, W. E., et al. (2011). The diagnosis of dementia due to Alzheimer's disease: recommendations from the National Institute on Aging-Alzheimer's Association workgroups on diagnostic guidelines for Alzheimer's disease. *Alzheimer's & Dementia, 7*, 263–269. http://dx.doi.org/10.1016/j.jalz.2011.03.005.

Mesulam, M. M., & Geula, C. (1988). Nucleus basalis (Ch4) and cortical cholinergic innervation in the human brain: observations based on the distribution of acetylcholinesterase and choline acetyltransferase. *The Journal of Comparative Neurology*, *275*(2), 216–240. http://dx.doi.org/10.1002/cne.902750205.

Mirra, S. S., Heyman, A., McKeel, D., Sumi, S. M., Crain, B. J., Brownlee, L. M., et al. (1991). The Consortium to Establish a Registry for Alzheimer's Disease (CERAD). Part II. Standardization of the neuropathologic assessment of Alzheimer's disease. *Neurology*, *41*(4), 479–486.

Möbius, H. J. (2004). Memantine in treatment of AD. In R. W. Richter, & B. Z. Richter (Eds.), *Alzheimer's disease* (pp. 203–209). Totowa, New Jersey: Humana Press.

Moechars, D., Dewachter, I., Lorent, K., Reversé, D., Baekelandt, V., Naidu, A., et al. (1999). Early phenotypic changes in transgenic mice that overexpress different mutants of amyloid precursor protein in brain. *The Journal of Biological Chemistry*, *274*(10), 6483–6492.

Moghekar, A., Rao, S., Li, M., Ruben, D., Mammen, A., Tang, X., et al. (2011). Large quantities of Aβ peptide are constitutively released during amyloid precursor protein metabolism in vivo and in vitro. *Journal of Biological Chemistry*, *286*(18), 15989–15997. http://dx.doi.org/10.1074/jbc.M110.191262.

Monji, A., Yoshida, I., Tashiro, K., Hayashi, Y., Matsuda, K., & Tashiro, N. (2000). Inhibition of A beta fibril formation and A beta-induced cytotoxicity by senile plaque-associated proteins. *Neuroscience Letters*, *278*(1–2), 81–84. http://dx.doi.org/10.1016/S0304-3940(99)00899-X.

Morgan, D., Diamond, D. M., Gottschall, P. E., Ugen, K. E., Dickey, C., Hardy, J., et al. (2000). A beta peptide vaccination prevents memory loss in an animal model of Alzheimer's disease. *Nature*, *408*(6815), 982–985. http://dx.doi.org/10.1038/35050116.

Mosconi, L., Mistur, R., Switalski, R., Tsui, W. H., Glodzik, L., Li, Y., et al. (2009). FDG-PET changes in brain glucose metabolism from normal cognition to pathologically verified Alzheimer's disease. *European Journal of Nuclear Medicine and Molecular Imaging*, *36*(5), 811–822. http://dx.doi.org/10.1007/s00259-008-1039-z.

Mosconi, L., Tsui, W.-H., De Santi, S., Li, J., Rusinek, H., Convit, A., et al. (2005). Reduced hippocampal metabolism in MCI and AD: automated FDG-PET image analysis. *Neurology*, *64*(11), 1860–1867. http://dx.doi.org/10.1212/01.WNL.0000163856.13524.08.

Mountjoy, C. Q., Roth, M., Evans, N. J., & Evans, H. M. (1983). Cortical neuronal counts in normal elderly controls and demented patients. *Neurobiology of Aging*, *4*(1), 1–11.

Mudher, A., & Lovestone, S. (2002). Alzheimer's disease: do tauists and baptists finally shake hands? *Trends in Neurosciences*, *25*(1), 22–26.

Murphy, M. P., Beckett, T. L., Ding, Q., Patel, E., Markesbery, W. R., St Clair, D. K., et al. (2007). Aβ solubility and deposition during AD progression and in APPxPS-1 knock-in mice. *Neurobiology of Disease*, *27*(3), 301–311. http://dx.doi.org/10.1016/j.nbd.2007.06.002.

Naslund, J., Haroutunian, V., Mohs, R., Davis, K. L., Davies, P., Greengard, P., et al. (2000). Correlation between elevated levels of amyloid beta-peptide in the brain and cognitive decline. *JAMA*, *283*(12), 1571–1577.

Niedowicz, D. M., Beckett, T. L., Matveev, S., Weidner, A. M., Baig, I., Kryscio, R. J., et al. (2012). Pittsburgh compound B and the postmortem diagnosis of Alzheimer disease. *Annals of Neurology*, *72*(4), 564–570. http://dx.doi.org/10.1002/ana.23633.

Nixon, R. A., & Yang, D.-S. (2011). Autophagy failure in Alzheimer's disease: locating the primary defect. *Neurobiology of Disease*, *43*(1), 38–45. http://dx.doi.org/10.1016/j.nbd.2011.01.021.

Oda, T., Wals, P., Osterburg, H. H., Johnson, S. A., Pasinetti, G. M., Morgan, T. E., et al. (1995). Clusterin (apoJ) alters the aggregation of amyloid beta-peptide (A beta 1-42) and forms slowly sedimenting A beta complexes that cause oxidative stress. *Experimental Neurology*, *136*(1), 22–31.

Oh, H., & Jagust, W. J. (2013). Frontotemporal network connectivity during memory encoding is increased with aging and disrupted by beta-amyloid. *Journal of Neuroscience*, *33*(47), 18425–18437. http://dx.doi.org/10.1523/JNEUROSCI.2775-13.2013.

Ostapchenko, V. G., Beraldo, F. H., Mohammad, A. H., Xie, Y.-F., Hirata, P. H. F., Magalhaes, A. C., et al. (2013). The prion protein ligand, stress-inducible phosphoprotein 1, regulates amyloid-β oligomer toxicity. *Journal of Neuroscience, 33*(42), 16552–16564. http://dx.doi.org/10.1523/JNEUROSCI.3214-13.2013.

Pagon, R. A., Adam, M. P., Bird, T. D., Dolan, C. R., Fong, C.-T., Smith, R. J., et al. (1993). *Early-onset familial Alzheimer disease.* Seattle, WA: University of Washington (Seattle).

Pandya, D. N., Hallett, M., & Kmukherjee, S. K. (1969). Intra- and interhemispheric connections of the neocortical auditory system in the rhesus monkey. *Brain Research, 14*(1), 49–65.

Park, J., Jang, M., & Chang, S. (2013). Deleterious effects of soluble amyloid-β oligomers on multiple steps of synaptic vesicle trafficking. *Neurobiology of Disease, 55*, 129–139. http://dx.doi.org/10.1016/j.nbd.2013.03.004.

Parsons, C. G., Stöffler, A., & Danysz, W. (2007). Memantine: a NMDA receptor antagonist that improves memory by restoration of homeostasis in the glutamatergic system–too little activation is bad, too much is even worse. *Neuropharmacology, 53*(6), 699–723. http://dx.doi.org/10.1016/j.neuropharm.2007.07.013.

Pasternak, S. H., Bagshaw, R. D., Guiral, M., Zhang, S., Ackerley, C. A., Pak, B. J., et al. (2003). Presenilin-1, nicastrin, amyloid precursor protein, and gamma-secretase activity are co-localized in the lysosomal membrane. *The Journal of Biological Chemistry, 278*(29), 26687–26694. http://dx.doi.org/10.1074/jbc.M212192200.

Pearson, H. A., & Peers, C. (2006). Physiological roles for amyloid beta peptides. *The Journal of Physiology, 575*(Pt 1), 5–10. http://dx.doi.org/10.1113/jphysiol.2006.111203.

Pei, J. J., Grundke-Iqbal, I., Iqbal, K., Bogdanovic, N., Winblad, B., & Cowburn, R. F. (1998). Accumulation of cyclin-dependent kinase 5 (CDK5) in neurons with early stages of Alzheimer's disease neurofibrillary degeneration. *Brain Research, 797*(2), 267–277.

Perez, R. G., Squazzo, S. L., & Koo, E. H. (1996). Enhanced release of amyloid beta-protein from codon 670/671 "Swedish" mutant beta-amyloid precursor protein occurs in both secretory and endocytic pathways. *The Journal of Biological Chemistry, 271*(15), 9100–9107.

Pickhardt, M., Larbig, G., Khlistunova, I., Coksezen, A., Meyer, B., Mandelkow, E.-M., et al. (2007). Phenylthiazolyl-hydrazide and its derivatives are potent inhibitors of τ aggregation and toxicity in vitro and in cells. *Biochemistry, 46*(35), 10016–10023. http://dx.doi.org/10.1021/bi700878g.

Pike, K. E., Savage, G., Villemagne, V. L., Ng, S., Moss, S. A., Maruff, P., et al. (2007). β-amyloid imaging and memory in non-demented individuals: evidence for preclinical Alzheimer's disease. *Brain: a Journal of Neurology, 130*(11), 2837–2844. http://dx.doi.org/10.1093/brain/awm238.

Rajendran, L., Honsho, M., Zahn, T. R., Keller, P., Geiger, K. D., Verkade, P., et al. (2006). Alzheimer's disease beta-amyloid peptides are released in association with exosomes. *Proceedings of the National Academy of Sciences of the United States of America, 103*(30), 11172–11177. http://dx.doi.org/10.1073/pnas.0603838103.

Rapoport, M., Dawson, H. N., Binder, L. I., Vitek, M. P., & Ferreira, A. (2002). Tau is essential to beta -amyloid-induced neurotoxicity. *Proceedings of the National Academy of Sciences of the United States of America, 99*(9), 6364–6369. http://dx.doi.org/10.1073/pnas.092136199.

Reed, M. N., Hofmeister, J. J., Jungbauer, L., Welzel, A. T., Yu, C., Sherman, M. A., et al. (2011). Cognitive effects of cell-derived and synthetically derived Aβ oligomers. *Neurobiology of Aging, 32*(10), 1784–1794. http://dx.doi.org/10.1016/j.neurobiolaging.2009.11.007.

Renner, M., Lacor, P. N., Velasco, P. T., Xu, J., Contractor, A., Klein, W. L., et al. (2010). Deleterious effects of amyloid beta oligomers acting as an extracellular scaffold for mGluR5. *Neuron, 66*(5), 739–754. http://dx.doi.org/10.1016/j.neuron.2010.04.029.

Ridha, B.H., Barnes, J., Bartlett, J.W., Godbolt, A., Pepple, T., & Rossor, M.N.. (2006). Tracking atrophy progression in familial Alzheimer's disease: a serial MRI study.,The Lancet. Neurology 5(10), 828–834. http://doi.org/10.1016/S1474-4422(06)70550-6.

Roberson, E. D., Scearce-Levie, K., Palop, J. J., & Yan, F. (2007). Reducing endogenous tau ameliorates amyloid ß-induced deficits in an Alzheimer's disease mouse model. *Science, 316*(5825), 750–754. http://dx.doi.org/10.1126/science.1141736.

Rockland, K. S., & Pandya, D. N. (1979). Laminar origins and terminations of cortical connections of the occipital lobe in the rhesus monkey. *Brain Research, 179*(1), 3–20.

Rowe, C. C., Ellis, K. A., Rimajova, M., Bourgeat, P., Pike, K. E., Jones, G., et al. (2010). Amyloid imaging results from the Australian imaging, biomarkers and lifestyle (AIBL) study of aging. *Neurobiology of Aging, 31*(8), 1275–1283. http://dx.doi.org/10.1016/j.neurobiolaging.2010.04.007.

Rudinskiy, N., Hawkes, J. M., Wegmann, S., Kuchibhotla, K. V., Muzikansky, A., Betensky, R. A., et al. (2014). Tau pathology does not affect experience-driven single-neuron and network-wide Arc/Arg3.1 responses. *Acta Neuropathologica Communications, 2*(1), 63. http://dx.doi.org/10.1186/2051-5960-2-63.

Rustay, N. R., Cronin, E. A., Curzon, P., Markosyan, S., Bitner, R. S., Ellis, T. A., et al. (2010). Mice expressing the Swedish APP mutation on a 129 genetic background demonstrate consistent behavioral deficits and pathological markers of Alzheimer's disease. *Brain Research, 1311*, 136–147. http://dx.doi.org/10.1016/j.brainres.2009.11.040.

Salloway, S., Sperling, R., Fox, N. C., Blennow, K., Klunk, W., Raskind, M., et al. (2014). Two phase 3 trials of bapineuzumab in mild-to-moderate Alzheimer's disease. *New England Journal of Medicine, 370*(4), 322–333. http://dx.doi.org/10.1056/NEJMoa1304839.

Schenk, D., Barbour, R., Dunn, W., Gordon, G., Grajeda, H., Guido, T., et al. (1999). Immunization with amyloid-beta attenuates Alzheimer-disease-like pathology in the PDAPP mouse. *Nature, 400*(6740), 173–177. http://dx.doi.org/10.1038/22124.

Scheuner, D., Eckman, C., Jensen, M., Song, X., Citron, M., Suzuki, N., et al. (1996). Secreted amyloid beta-protein similar to that in the senile plaques of Alzheimer's disease is increased in vivo by the presenilin 1 and 2 and APP mutations linked to familial Alzheimer's disease. *Nature Medicine, 2*(8), 864–870.

Schmechel, D. E., Saunders, A. M., Strittmatter, W. J., Crain, B. J., Hulette, C. M., Joo, S. H., et al. (1993). Increased amyloid beta-peptide deposition in cerebral cortex as a consequence of apolipoprotein E genotype in late-onset Alzheimer disease. *Proceedings of the National Academy of Sciences of the United States of America, 90*(20), 9649–9653.

Schrader-Fischer, G., & Paganetti, P. A. (1996). Effect of alkalizing agents on the processing of the beta-amyloid precursor protein. *Brain Research, 716*(1–2), 91–100. http://dx.doi.org/10.1016/0006-8993(96)00002-9.

Scoville, W. B., & Milner, B. (1957). Loss of recent memory after bilateral hippocampal lesions. *Journal of Neurology, Neurosurgery, and Psychiatry, 20*(1), 11–21.

Seubert, P., Oltersdorf, T., Lee, M. G., Barbour, R., Blomquist, C., Davis, D. L., et al. (1993). Secretion of beta-amyloid precursor protein cleaved at the amino terminus of the beta-amyloid peptide. *Nature, 361*(6409), 260–263. http://dx.doi.org/10.1038/361260a0.

Shankar, G. M., Li, S., Mehta, T. H., Garcia-Munoz, A., Shepardson, N. E., Smith, I., et al. (2008). Amyloid-beta protein dimers isolated directly from Alzheimer's brains impair synaptic plasticity and memory. *Nature Medicine, 14*(8), 837–842. http://dx.doi.org/10.1038/nm1782.

Sheline, Y. I., Raichle, M. E., Snyder, A. Z., Morris, J. C., Head, D., Wang, S., et al. (2010). Amyloid plaques disrupt resting state default mode network connectivity in cognitively normal elderly. *Biological Psychiatry, 67*(6), 584–587. http://dx.doi.org/10.1016/j.biopsych.2009.08.024.

Sherrington, R., Rogaev, E. I., Liang, Y., Rogaeva, E. A., Levesque, G., Ikeda, M., et al. (1995). Cloning of a gene bearing missense mutations in early-onset familial Alzheimer's disease. *Nature*, *375*(6534), 754–760. http://dx.doi.org/10.1038/375754a0.

Shi, F., Liu, B., Zhou, Y., Yu, C., & Jiang, T. (2009). Hippocampal volume and asymmetry in mild cognitive impairment and Alzheimer's disease: meta-analyses of MRI studies. *Hippocampus*, *19*(11), 1055–1064. http://dx.doi.org/10.1002/hipo.20573.

Sisodia, S. S., & St George-Hyslop, P. H. (2002). γ-Secretase, notch, aβ and Alzheimer's disease: where do the presenilins fit in? *Nature Reviews Neuroscience*, *3*(4), 281–290. http://dx.doi. org/10.1038/nrn785.

Soto, C., Sigurdsson, E. M., Morelli, L., Kumar, R. A., Castaño, E. M., & Frangione, B. (1998). Beta-sheet breaker peptides inhibit fibrillogenesis in a rat brain model of amyloidosis: implications for Alzheimer's therapy. *Nature Medicine*, *4*(7), 822–826. http://dx.doi.org/10.1038/ nm0798-822.

Sperling, R. A., Beckett, L. A., Bennett, D. A., Craft, S., Fagan, A. M., Iwatsubo, T., et al. (2011). Toward defining the preclinical stages of Alzheimer's disease: recommendations from the National Institute on Aging-Alzheimer's Association workgroups on diagnostic guidelines for Alzheimer's disease. *Alzheimer's & Dementia*, *7*, 280–292. http://dx.doi.org/10.1016/j. jalz.2011.03.003.

Stine, W. B., Snyder, S. W., Ladror, U. S., Wade, W. S., Miller, M. F., Perun, T. J., et al. (1996). The nanometer-scale structure of amyloid-beta visualized by atomic force microscopy. *Journal of Protein Chemistry*, *15*(2), 193–203. Retrieved from http://www.metapress.com.proxy2.lib. uwo.ca:2048/content/p71h74j46028123h/fulltext.pdf.

Sturchler-Pierrat, C., Abramowski, D., Duke, M., Wiederhold, K. H., Mistl, C., Rothacher, S., et al. (1997). Two amyloid precursor protein transgenic mouse models with Alzheimer disease-like pathology. *Proceedings of the National Academy of Sciences of the United States of America*, *94*(24), 13287–13292.

Su, Y., & Chang, P. T. (2001). Acidic pH promotes the formation of toxic fibrils from beta-amyloid peptide. *Brain Research*, *893*(1–2), 287–291.

Suzuki, N., Cheung, T. T., Cai, X. D., Odaka, A., Otvos, L., Eckman, C., et al. (1994). An increased percentage of long amyloid beta protein secreted by familial amyloid beta protein precursor (beta APP717) mutants. *Science*, *264*(5163), 1336–1340.

Ta, R., Suchy, M., Tam, J. H., Li, A. X., Martinez-Santiesteban, F. S., Scholl, T. J., et al. (2013). A dual magnetic resonance imaging/fluorescent contrast agent for Cathepsin-D detection. *Contrast Media & Molecular Imaging*, *8*(2), 127–139. http://dx.doi.org/10.1002/ cmmi.1502.

Takadera, T., Sakura, N., Mohri, T., & Hashimoto, T. (1993). Toxic effect of a beta-amyloid peptide (beta 22-35) on the hippocampal neuron and its prevention. *Neuroscience Letters*, *161*(1), 41–44.

Tam, J. H., & Pasternak, S. H. (2012). Amyloid and Alzheimer's disease: inside and out. *The Canadian Journal of Neurological Sciences. Le Journal Canadien Des Sciences Neurologiques*, *39*(3), 286–298.

Tam, J. H., Seah, C., & Pasternak, S. H. (2014). The amyloid precursor protein is rapidly transported from the Golgi apparatus to the lysosome and where it is processed into beta-amyloid. *Molecular Brain*, *7*(1), 54. http://dx.doi.org/10.1186/s13041-014-0054-1.

Teller, J. K., Russo, C., Debusk, L. M., Angelini, G., Zaccheo, D., Dagna-Bricarelli, F., et al. (1996). Presence of soluble amyloid beta-peptide precedes amyloid plaque formation in Down's syndrome. *Nature Medicine*, *2*(1), 93–95. http://dx.doi.org/10.1038/nm0196-93.

Terry, R. D., Masliah, E., Salmon, D. P., Butters, N., DeTeresa, R., Hill, R., et al. (1991). Physical basis of cognitive alterations in Alzheimer's disease: synapse loss is the major correlate of cognitive impairment. *Annals of Neurology, 30*(4), 572–580. http://dx.doi.org/10.1002/ana.410300410.

Thal, D. R., Rüb, U., Orantes, M., & Braak, H. (2002). Phases of A beta-deposition in the human brain and its relevance for the development of AD. *Neurology, 58*(12), 1791–1800.

Thinakaran, G., Teplow, D. B., Siman, R., Greenberg, B., & Sisodia, S. S. (1996). Metabolism of the "Swedish" amyloid precursor protein variant in neuro2a (N2a) cells: evidence that cleavage at the "beta-secretase" site occurs in the Golgi apparatus. *The Journal of Biological Chemistry, 271*(16), 9390–9397.

Thompson, P. M., Hayashi, K. M., de Zubicaray, G., Janke, A. L., Rose, S. E., Semple, J., et al. (2003). Dynamics of gray matter loss in Alzheimer's disease. *Journal of Neuroscience, 23*(3), 994–1005.

Tierney, M. C., Fisher, R. H., Lewis, A. J., Zorzitto, M. L., Snow, W. G., Reid, D. W., et al. (1988). The NINCDS-ADRDA Work Group criteria for the clinical diagnosis of probable Alzheimer's disease: a clinicopathologic study of 57 cases. *Neurology, 38*(3), 359. http://dx.doi.org/10.1212/wnl.38.3.359.

Tokutake, T., Kasuga, K., Yajima, R., Sekine, Y., Tezuka, T., Nishizawa, M., et al. (2012). Hyperphosphorylation of tau induced by naturally secreted amyloid-β at nanomolar concentrations is modulated by insulin-dependent Akt-GSK3β signaling pathway. *The Journal of Biological Chemistry, 287*(42), 35222–35233. http://dx.doi.org/10.1074/jbc.M112.348300.

Tomlinson, B. E., Blessed, G., & Roth, M. (1968). Observations on the brains of non-demented old people. *Journal of the Neurological Sciences, 7*(2), 331–356. http://dx.doi.org/10.1016/0022-510X(68)90154-8.

Tomlinson, B. E., Blessed, G., & Roth, M. (1970). Observations on the brains of demented old people. *Journal of the Neurological Sciences, 11*(3), 205–242. http://dx.doi.org/10.1016/0022-510X(70)90063-8.

Um, J. W., Kaufman, A. C., Kostylev, M., Heiss, J. K., Stagi, M., Takahashi, H., et al. (2013). Metabotropic glutamate receptor 5 is a coreceptor for Alzheimer aβ oligomer bound to cellular prion protein. *Neuron, 79*(5), 887–902. http://dx.doi.org/10.1016/j.neuron.2013.06.036.

Um, J. W., Nygaard, H. B., Heiss, J. K., Kostylev, M. A., Stagi, M., Vortmeyer, A., et al. (2012). Alzheimer amyloid-β oligomer bound to postsynaptic prion protein activates Fyn to impair neurons. *Nature Neuroscience, 15*(9), 1227–1235. http://dx.doi.org/10.1038/nn.3178.

Utton, M. A., Vandecandelaere, A., Wagner, U., Reynolds, C. H., Gibb, G. M., Miller, C. C., et al. (1997). Phosphorylation of tau by glycogen synthase kinase 3beta affects the ability of tau to promote microtubule self-assembly. *Biochemical Journal, 323*(Pt 3), 741–747.

Van Hoesen, G. W., & Pandya, D. N. (1975a). Some connections of the entorhinal (area 28) and perirhinal (area 35) cortices of the rhesus monkey. I. Temporal lobe afferents. *Brain Research, 95*(1), 1–24. http://dx.doi.org/10.1016/0006-8993(75)90204-8.

Van Hoesen, G. W., & Pandya, D. N. (1975b). Some connections of the entorhinal (area 28) and perirhinal (area 35) cortices of the Rhesus monkey. III. Efferent connections. *Brain Research, 95*(1), 39–59. http://dx.doi.org/10.1016/0006-8993(75)90206-1.

Van Hoesen, G. W., Pandya, D. N., & Butters, N. (1975). Some connections of the entorhinal (area 28) and perirhinal (area 35) cortices of the Rhesus monkey. II. Frontal lobe afferents. *Brain Research, 95*(1), 25–38. http://dx.doi.org/10.1016/0006-8993(75)90205-X.

Vassar, R., Bennett, B. D., Babu-Khan, S., Kahn, S., Mendiaz, E. A., Denis, P., et al. (1999). Beta-secretase cleavage of Alzheimer's amyloid precursor protein by the transmembrane aspartic protease BACE. *Science, 286*(5440), 735–741.

Vellas, B., Black, R., Thal, L. J., Daniels, M., McLennan, G., Tompkins, C., et al. (2009). Long-term follow-up of patients immunized with AN1792: reduced functional decline in antibody responders. *Current Alzheimer Research, 6*(2), 144–151. http://dx.doi.org/10.1001/jama.2009.1866.

Vemuri, P., Weigand, S. D., Przybelski, S. A., Smith, G. E., Shaw, L. M., Decarli, C. S., et al. (2011). Cognitive reserve and Alzheimer's disease biomarkers are independent determinants of cognition. *Brain: a Journal of Neurology, 134*(Pt 5), 1479–1492. http://dx.doi.org/10.1093/brain/awr049.

Vingtdeux, V., Davies, P., Dickson, D. W., & Marambaud, P. (2010). *AMPK is abnormally activated in tangle- and pre-tangle-bearing neurons in Alzheimer's disease and other tauopathies. Acta Neuropathologica, 121*(3), 337–349. http://dx.doi.org/10.1007/s00401-010-0759-x.

Walsh, D. M., Klyubin, I., Fadeeva, J. V., Cullen, W. K., Anwyl, R., Wolfe, M. S., et al. (2002). Naturally secreted oligomers of amyloid beta protein potently inhibit hippocampal long-term potentiation in vivo. *Nature, 416*(6880), 535–539. http://dx.doi.org/10.1038/416535a.

Wang, H.-W., Pasternak, J. F., Kuo, H., Ristic, H., Lambert, M. P., Chromy, B., et al. (2002). Soluble oligomers of beta amyloid (1-42) inhibit long-term potentiation but not long-term depression in rat dentate gyrus. *Brain Research, 924*(2), 133–140. http://dx.doi.org/10.1016/S0006-8993(01)03058-X.

Wang, J., Thwin, M. T., Bien-Ly, N., Yoo, J., Ho, K. O., Kreitzer, A., et al. (2007). Aberrant excitatory neuronal activity and compensatory remodeling of inhibitory hippocampal circuits in mouse models of Alzheimer's disease. *Neuron, 55*(5), 697–711. http://dx.doi.org/10.1016/j.neuron.2007.07.025.

Wang, J.-Z., Grundke-Iqbal, I., & Iqbal, K. (2007). Kinases and phosphatases and tau sites involved in Alzheimer neurofibrillary degeneration. *European Journal of Neuroscience, 25*(1), 59–68. http://dx.doi.org/10.1111/j.1460-9568.2006.05226.x.

Wang, J. Z., Wu, Q., Smith, A., Grundke-Iqbal, I., & Iqbal, K. (1998). Tau is phosphorylated by GSK-3 at several sites found in Alzheimer disease and its biological activity markedly inhibited only after it is prephosphorylated by A-kinase. *FEBS Letters, 436*(1), 28–34.

Weingarten, M. D., Lockwood, A. H., Hwo, S. Y., & Kirschner, M. W. (1975). A protein factor essential for microtubule assembly. *Proceedings of the National Academy of Sciences of the United States of America, 72*(5), 1858–1862.

Wilcox, K. C., Marunde, M. R., Das, A., Velasco, P. T., Kuhns, B. D., Marty, M. T., et al. (2015). Nanoscale synaptic membrane mimetic allows unbiased high throughput screen that targets binding sites for Alzheimer's-associated aβ oligomers. *PLoS One, 10*(4), e0125263. http://dx.doi.org/10.1371/journal.pone.0125263.

Wilcock, G. K. (1985). Anatomical correlates of the distribution of the pathological changes in the neocortex in Alzheimer disease. *Proceedings of the National Academy of Sciences of the United States of America, 82*(13), 4531–4534.

Wischik, C. M., Edwards, P. C., Lai, R. Y., Roth, M., & Harrington, C. R. (1996). Selective inhibition of Alzheimer disease-like tau aggregation by phenothiazines. *Proceedings of the National Academy of Sciences of the United States of America, 93*(20), 11213–11218.

Wischik, C. M., Harrington, C. R., & Storey, J. M. D. (2014). Tau-aggregation inhibitor therapy for Alzheimer's disease. *Biochemical Pharmacology, 88*(4), 529–539. http://dx.doi.org/10.1016/j.bcp.2013.12.008.

Wischik, C. M., Novak, M., Thøgersen, H. C., Edwards, P. C., Runswick, M. J., Jakes, R., et al. (1988). Isolation of a fragment of tau derived from the core of the paired helical filament of

Alzheimer disease. *Proceedings of the National Academy of Sciences of the United States of America*, *85*(12), 4506–4510.

Wischik, C. M., Staff, R. T., Wischik, D. J., Bentham, P., Murray, A. D., Storey, J. M. D., et al. (2015). Tau aggregation inhibitor therapy: an exploratory phase 2 study in mild or moderate Alzheimer's disease. *Journal of Alzheimer's Disease*, *44*(2), 705–720. http://dx.doi.org/10.3233/JAD-142874.

Wisniewski, K. E., Wisniewski, H. M., & Wen, G. Y. (1985). Occurrence of neuropathological changes and dementia of Alzheimer's disease in Down's syndrome. *Annals of Neurology*, *17*(3), 278–282. http://dx.doi.org/10.1002/ana.410170310.

Wisniewski, T., Castaño, E. M., Golabek, A., Vogel, T., & Frangione, B. (1994). Acceleration of Alzheimer's fibril formation by apolipoprotein E in vitro. *The American Journal of Pathology*, *145*(5), 1030–1035.

Witter, M. P., Naber, P. A., van Haeften, T., Machielsen, W. C., Rombouts, S. A., Barkhof, F., et al. (2000). Cortico-hippocampal communication by way of parallel parahippocampal-subicular pathways. *Hippocampus*, *10*(4), 398–410. http://dx.doi.org/10.1002/1098-1063(2000)10:4<398::AID-HIPO6>3.0.CO;2-K.

Wu, J. W., Herman, M., Liu, L., Simoes, S., Acker, C. M., Figueroa, H., et al. (2013). Small misfolded Tau species are internalized via bulk endocytosis and anterogradely and retrogradely transported in neurons. *The Journal of Biological Chemistry*, *288*(3), 1856–1870. http://dx.doi.org/10.1074/jbc.M112.394528.

Xia, P., Chen, H.-S. V., Zhang, D., & Lipton, S. A. (2010). Memantine preferentially blocks extrasynaptic over synaptic NMDA receptor currents in hippocampal autapses. *Journal of Neuroscience*, *30*(33), 11246–11250. http://dx.doi.org/10.1523/JNEUROSCI.2488-10.2010.

Xiao, J., Perry, G., Troncoso, J., & Monteiro, M. J. (1996). Alpha-calcium-calmodulin-dependent kinase II is associated with paired helical filaments of Alzheimer's disease. *Journal of Neuropathology and Experimental Neurology*, *55*(9), 954–963.

Yankner, B. A., Duffy, L. K., & Kirschner, D. A. (1990). Neurotrophic and neurotoxic effects of amyloid beta protein: reversal by tachykinin neuropeptides. *Science*, *250*(4978), 279–282.

Zaidi, T., Grundke-Iqbal, I., & Iqbal, K. (1994). Role of abnormally phosphorylated tau in the breakdown of microtubules in Alzheimer disease. *Proceedings of the National Academy of Sciences of the United States of America*, *91*(12), 5562–5566.

Zempel, H., Luedtke, J., Kumar, Y., Biernat, J., Dawson, H., Mandelkow, E., et al. (2013). Amyloid-β oligomers induce synaptic damage via Tau-dependent microtubule severing by TTLL6 and spastin. *The EMBO Journal*, *32*(22), 2920–2937. http://dx.doi.org/10.1038/emboj.2013.207.

Zhang, W., Arteaga, J., Cashion, D. K., Chen, G., Gangadharmath, U., Gomez, L. F., et al. (2012). A highly selective and specific PET tracer for imaging of tau pathologies. *Journal of Alzheimer's Disease*, *31*(3), 601–612. http://dx.doi.org/10.3233/JAD-2012-120712.

Zhou, J., Gennatas, E. D., Kramer, J. H., Miller, B. L., & Seeley, W. W. (2012). Predicting regional neurodegeneration from the healthy brain functional connectome. *Neuron*, *73*(6), 1216–1227. http://dx.doi.org/10.1016/j.neuron.2012.03.004.

Chapter 5

Vascular Dementia

D.G. Munoz[1], N. Weishaupt[2]
[1]*University of Toronto, Toronto, ON, Canada; [2]University of Western Ontario, London, ON, Canada*

INTRODUCTION: THE CHALLENGE OF VASCULAR DEMENTIA

Vascular dementia is essentially a pathological construct, *pathology* being understood in the broad sense of both lesions demonstrable under the microscope and physiopathological mechanisms. Few, if any, conditions affecting the brain have resulted in so much confusion for such a long time as this apparently simple concept. Some pathological substrates of dementia, as for example TAR DNA-binding protein-43 (TDP-43), have only recently been recognized, but once this critical threshold was crossed, clinical–pathological correlations rapidly followed (Neumann et al., 2006). In contrast, the cerebral lesions resulting from vascular injuries have been fairly well known since the early 20th century, but the clinical correlates of these lesions have been very difficult to establish. The fact that in a meta-analysis of the proportion of dementias resulting from vascular dementia based on pathological studies ranges from 0.03% to 85.2% (Jellinger, 2008) is a clear indication that we are far from establishing a firm basis of understanding the relationship between lesions and symptoms. Probably the main reason for this discrepancy is that vascular lesions are easy to identify, not only on the pathological examination of the brain, but since the development of computed tomography (CT) in the early second half of the 20th century, by diagnostic imaging methods. However, the histological lesions that define the other causes of dementia, characterized by deposits of amyloid, tau, alpha synuclein, TDP-43, or fused in sarcoma remain largely invisible to imaging methods, with a recent exception of positron imaging tomography for β-amyloid (Aβ) (O'Brien & Herholz, 2015).

RISK FACTORS FOR VASCULAR COGNITIVE IMPAIRMENT

Epidemiological studies indicate that age is the major risk factor for vascular dementia, as it is for Alzheimer's disease. There is a consistent increase in incidence and prevalence at least until age 90 years. A male predominance contrasts with the preferential female prevalence of Alzheimer's disease. As expected, all

The Cerebral Cortex in Neurodegenerative and Neuropsychiatric Disorders.
http://dx.doi.org/10.1016/B978-0-12-801942-9.00005-7

vascular risk factors, including peripheral atherosclerosis, midlife hypertension, midlife diabetes, fat-rich diet, elevated plasma cholesterol, obesity, smoking, and elevated plasma homocysteine increase the risk of vascular dementia.

Although it is as a risk factor for systemic atherosclerosis (Leblanc, Meschia, Stuss, & Hachinski, 2006), the apolipoprotein EE4 allele could be expected to be also a risk factor for vascular dementia; surprisingly it is not or minimally so (Treves et al., 1996), and neither is it for stroke (Abboud et al., 2008). Head trauma, a risk factor for Alzheimer's disease, does not seem to modify the risk of vascular dementia (Korczyn, Vakhapova, & Grinberg, 2012).

CORTICAL VASCULAR LESIONS OFTEN ASSOCIATED WITH DEMENTIA

Obviously, **infarcts** involving specific areas of the cerebral cortex or their associated subcortical regions may produce aphasia, agnosia, apraxia, or epileptic seizures. Of greater interest are general deficits associated with widespread subcortical damage, including white matter lesions. Signs and symptoms characteristic of this condition include the predominance of executive dysfunction over memory deficits (O'Brien et al., 2003; Roman & Royall, 1999) and the association with gait abnormalities, urinary incontinence, and parkinsonism (Koga et al., 2009; Roman, 2004).

Depression is a common neuropsychological disorder in this context (Roman, 2006). Neuropsychological tests tend to demonstrate slow reaction time, executive dysfunction, and alterations in emotion (Nordlund et al., 2007). Although these tests may show differences in the aggregate groups of vascular dementia versus patients with Alzheimer's disease, they have very limited utility in the diagnosis of individual patients. However, these neuropsychological tests and the presence of executive dysfunction emphasize the potential importance of the cerebral cortex in vascular dementia.

The course of vascular dementia is highly variable, but in contrast to the steady progression of Alzheimer's disease, a stepwise deterioration or long periods of stabilization are considered supportive of the diagnosis. There are several diagnostic criteria for vascular dementia, all of which require a syndromic diagnosis of dementia (Chui et al., 1992; Knopman, Rocca, Cha, Edland, & Kokmen, 2002; Roman et al., 1993). The different sets of criteria are not concordant. The term *vascular cognitive impairment* (Hachinski et al., 2006) is more inclusive, as it incorporates mild cognitive impairment of vascular etiology. This diagnosis has significant prognostic implications, because the risk of developing dementia is estimated at 50% over 5 years (Wentzel et al., 2001). The harmonization standards from the Canadian stroke network and the National Institute of Neurological Disorders and Stroke are a significant step in the right direction, recognizing that neuropathology cannot provide the gold standard in this condition (Hachinski, et al., 2006).

An interesting subset of vascular dementia is that of **poststroke dementia**, referring to a subgroup of previously cognitively normal patients who develop dementia after a stroke, usually in the first few months (Pendlebury & Rothwell, 2009; Selnes & Vinters, 2006; Sun, Tan, & Yu, 2014; Tatemichi et al., 1994). The incidence of poststroke dementia is estimated at 20% at 3 months and 33% at 5 years (Barba et al., 2000; Henon et al., 2001). A history of stroke approximately doubles the prevalence of dementia at a given age in the Framingham study (Ivan et al., 2004). This is a purely clinically defined group, and its pathological substrates have not been established, although there is an obvious association with large-vessel pathological disruption in most cases.

VASCULAR ALTERATIONS LEADING TO CEREBRAL DAMAGE

First it should be stated that ischemic injury can occur in the presence of a perfectly normal vascular tree in the event of cardiac arrest, strangulation, or hypoxia. In addition, emboli may arise from the heart, most commonly in relation to atrial fibrillation, but also from cardiac myxomas. However, in the vast majority of cases, pathosis affecting the blood vessels is considered to be the major factor associated with the development of disease.

The type of vascular lesion is intimately associated with the size of the vessel. Atherosclerosis affects large (elastic) and medium-sized (muscular) arteries. In relation to the brain, atherosclerotic plaques at the bifurcation of the carotid artery in the neck, the arteries of the circle of Willis, and the leptomeningeal arteries are most important. The lipid deposits form intimal plaques that result in progressive stenosis. Probably more important for our topic of discussion, hemorrhage and necrosis in the plaque can sometimes break through the endothelium and result in the formation of mural thrombi. This can occlude the vessel on the site, or detach and travel to a distant location creating an artery to artery embolus.

Small-vessel disease is a far more complex entity. It comprises three common size-related and overlapping nonspecific categories: small-vessel atherosclerosis, lipohyalinosis, and arteriolosclerosis, relating to vessels of decreasing diameter. In addition to rarer forms of vasculitis, there are diseases selectively affecting small blood vessels, of which cerebral amyloid angiopathy and cerebral autosomal dominant arteriopathy with subcortical infarcts and leukoencephalopathy (CADASIL) are the most common.

The microvasculature of the brain is different from that of other organs in their expression profile (Ohtsuki et al., 2014). This can be related to their participation in the blood–brain barrier, as well as autoregulation. In relation to the latter, endothelial cells release the gas hormone nitric oxide, which reduces contractile tone of smooth muscle cells, as well as the vasoconstrictor hormone endothelin 1. Endothelial cells have a further function as gatekeepers of inflammation, signaling leukocytes in the blood to attach and migrate through the barrier to reach the brain (Hainsworth, Oommen, & Bridges, 2015).

Small-vessel atherosclerosis affects arteries with a diameter of 200–800 μm, mostly represented by leptomeningeal arteries. Lipohyalinosis involves small arteries of 40–300 μm and is characterized by lipid deposits and disruption of the architecture (Lammie, 2002). Arteriolosclerosis involves small arteries and arterioles with outer diameters ranging from 40 to 150 μm and is characterized by replacement of smooth muscle with collagen fibers. In contrast to the loss of myocytes highlighted by immunostaining for smooth muscle actin, the endothelial layer, which can be labeled by cluster of differentiation (CD) 34, CD31, factor VIII, or glucose transporter 1, appears morphologically normal. Moreover, there is no upregulation of markers of endothelial activation, typically seen in response to noxious stimuli, such as intercellular adhesion molecule 1 or interleukin 6, but the potent anticoagulant thrombomodulin is upregulated, suggesting that thrombotic events are not part of the mechanism resulting in leukoaraiosis. There is indirect evidence of abnormal function in subcortical leukoencephalopathy. The degree of microvascular stenosis is determined by the sclerotic index, which is defined as (outer diameter minus inner diameter)/ outer diameter (Hainsworth et al., 2015).

Cerebral amyloid angiopathy is characterized by deposition of Aβ in the walls of small arteries, arterioles, and capillaries located in the cerebral and cerebellar cortices and the leptomeninges overlying them. This selectivity is somewhat surprising, in view of the much wider distribution of Aβ deposits in the neuropil. The affected vessels maintain a circular shape, suggesting rigidity. Splitting, leading to a so-called "double-barrel pattern," is often seen (Fig. 5.1). The prevalence in the population is 10% at age 60 years (Rotterdam Study, Poels et al., 2011). Many of the reports in the literature concerning cerebral amyloid angiopathy fail to incorporate any quantitative assessment and thus are near meaningless, because the density may vary from

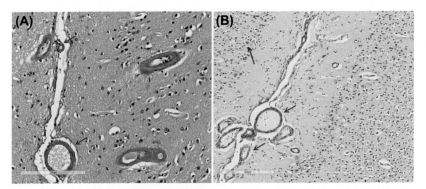

FIGURE 5.1 Cerebral amyloid angiopathy. (A) Hematoxylin and eosin (H&E) stained section of superficial cerebral cortex demonstrating deposits of eosinophilic amorphous material in cortical *(green arrows)* as well as leptomeningeal blood vessels *(blue arrows)*. Note the rigidity of the involved vessels demonstrated by the indentation created in the superficial cortex by the lower leptomeningeal artery. (B) Sections stained with Congo Red, showing the deposits in cortical and leptomeningeal arteries *(same color coding as A)*. In addition, Congo red stained the core of amyloid plaques *(red arrow)*.

a rare finding, as in many cases of Alzheimer's disease, to the overwhelming pathological condition of the brain. Amyloid angiopathy can be considered relevant (moderate to severe) in approximately one-fourth of patients with Alzheimer's disease.

CADASIL, which stands for *cerebral autosomal dominant arteriopathy with subcortical infarcts and leukoencephalopathy* (Tournier-Lasserve, Iba-Zizen, Romero, & Bousser, 1991), is a hereditary disease caused by mutations in the *Notch3* gene, located in chromosome 19 (Joutel et al., 1996). The accumulation of the mutated Notch3 protein on the surface of smooth muscle cells located in the walls of cerebral small blood vessels leads to their degeneration (Fig. 5.2). Patients experience stroke starting at an average age of 46 years, with a range of 30–76 years. In many cases, episodes of migraine precede the strokes by several years. The vessels affected are predominantly arterioles located in the leptomeninges, the white matter, the basal ganglia, the thalamus, and, to a lesser degree, the pons. The spinal cord is minimally involved. The infarcts seen in the brain are typically lacunar and predominantly involve the hemispheric white matter and basal

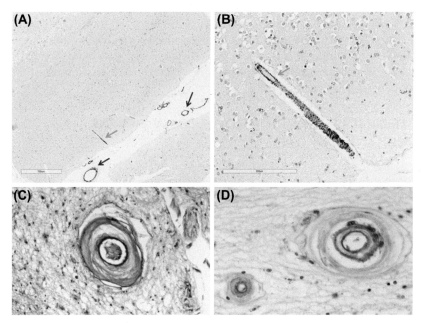

FIGURE 5.2   **CADASIL.** (A) and (B) Sections of cerebral cortex immunostained with an antibody to mutated *Notch3*. (A) Low-power image demonstrating the presence of the abnormal protein in leptomeningeal blood vessels *(red arrow)*, as well as penetrating cortical arteries *(green arrows)*. (B) High-power image showing deposits in capillaries *(yellow arrows)*, in addition to the penetrating arteries *(green arrows)*. (C) and (D) High-power, hematoxylin and eosin (H&E)–stained sections showing thickening of the wall accompanied by hyalinization and loss of the cellular elements in small arteries in the cortex (C) and white matter (D).

ganglia. In addition, the brain shows an extensive leukoencephalopathy and dilation of perivascular spaces, referred to as *status cribrosus*, affecting the basal ganglia, thalamus, and white matter at the cortical–subcortical junction.

Although a relatively rare condition, CADASIL is of great importance as a model of pure vascular dementia, a condition rarely seen in the elderly population (O'Sullivan, Barrick, Morris, Clark, & Markus, 2005; O'Sullivan et al., 2009; O'Sullivan, Singhal, Charlton, & Markus, 2004). An important example is the association of cognitive decline with cortical atrophy, in spite of the relative scarcity of cortical pathology in CADASIL (Peters et al., 2006). The substrate of the atrophy is widespread neuronal apoptosis, especially in layers 3 and 5. The apoptosis is not related to the rare cortical infarcts, but rather to the subcortical white matter degeneration (Viswanathan, Gray, Bousser, Baudrimont, & Chabriat, 2006). In addition, given the hereditary character of the disease, it has been possible to demonstrate white matter lesions many years before the development of symptoms. The lesions demonstrated on T2-weighted and fluid-attenuated inversion recovery sequences of magnetic resonance imaging (MRI) are similar to those of leukoaraiosis and Binswanger disease. However, patients with CADASIL typically show lesions in the external capsule, the anterior pole of the temporal lobe, and, in some cases, the corpus callosum. The hyperintensities in the anterior temporal pole are considered a radiological marker of CADASIL (O'Sullivan et al., 2001). Although very important as an example of a pure vascular dementia, the disease is rare enough to be of minimal significance as a public health problem.

CEREBRAL LESIONS RESULTING FROM VASCULAR MECHANISMS

Vascular lesions can be divided into three groups: infarcts, bleeds, and diffuse leukoencephalopathy. A proposed classification of pathological substrates of vascular dementia is shown in Table 5.1.

Infarcts

Infarcts can be classical large areas of necrosis involving the cortex and subcortical white matter, and may be located in the territory of one of the named cerebral arteries or in the watershed areas (Fig. 5.3). Cortical microinfarcts measure less than 2 mm in diameter and are usually vertically oriented. Lacunes are small, cavitated infarcts, 0.2–15 mm in diameter, located in subcortical structures, including the centrum semiovale, basal ganglia, thalamus, internal capsule, and basis pontis (Fig. 5.4). MRI demonstrates infarcts less than 3 mm in diameter in 20% of the population over the age of 65, with a prevalence 20 times greater than large infarct (Longstreth, Diehr, Beauchamp, & Manolio, 2001).

TABLE 5.1 Proposed Classification of Pathological Substrates of Vascular Dementia

I	Multiinfarct dementia (large infarct or several infarcts with more than 50 mL loss of tissue)
II	Small-vessel disease (small infarcts, microinfarcts, lacunes, microhemorrhages, white matter lesions)
III	Strategic infarcts
IV	Cerebral hypoperfusion (cortical laminar necrosis, border zone infarcts, hippocampal sclerosis)
V	Cerebral hemorrhage (lobar, deep, subarachnoid)
VI	Combined with Alzheimer's pathological findings

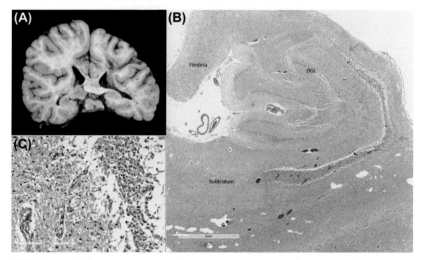

FIGURE 5.3 **Infarcts.** (A) Gross appearance of a large infarct in the left parietal lobe. The lesion is old and the cavity has collapsed. Note that the infarct has a roof formed by the remnants of the most superficial layers at the crest of the gyrus. (B) Infarct in the hippocampus, demonstrating cavitation restricted to the CA1 sector *(green arrows)* and to a lesser degree the CA4 sector. The dentate granular layer (DGL) is spared. (C) Microscopic appearance of an infarct, with macrophages filling the cavity on the right and gliosis developing in the adjacent neuropil on the left.

Hemorrhages

Large hemorrhages related to hypertension usually occur in the basal ganglia, thalamus, basis pontis, and cerebellum. The other major source of hemorrhages is cerebral amyloid angiopathy. Large hemorrhages related to this entity tend to be more superficially located, involving the cerebral cortex and subcortical structures, than hypertensive hemorrhages.

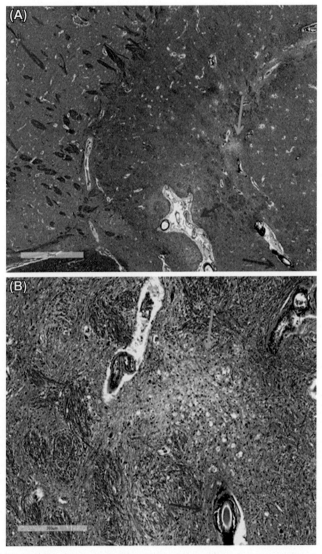

FIGURE 5.4   **Lacunae.** (A) A small infarct in the globus pallidus *(green arrows)*, not cavitated at this level. Also seen are commonly associated lesions, including expanded Virchow-Robin spaces, often mistaken for lacunae *(blue arrows)*, and calcified blood vessels *(red arrow)*. (B) High-power image of the region of infarct *(green arrows)*, demonstrating the loss of myelinated fibers and gliosis. At this magnification glial cells appear as *red dots*. The calcified blood vessels are labeled with a *red arrow*.

Diffuse Leukoencephalopathy

Diffuse leukoencephalopathy was first described by Binswanger (Roman, 1987). This severity of pathological condition is uncommon, but it was subsequently recognized that CT scans and, to a much better resolution, MRIs of the brain identify widespread subcortical white matter abnormalities, which were named *leukoaraiosis* by Hachinski, Potter, and Merskey (1987). Improvements in technology now show leukoaraiosis in up to 90% of elderly subjects. Furthermore, diffusion tensor MRI shows abnormalities extending beyond those seen in conventional MRI, and these abnormalities have a better correlation with executive dysfunction and presumably cortical degeneration than leukoaraiosis alone (O'Sullivan et al., 2004).

VASCULAR CONTRIBUTIONS TO COGNITIVE IMPAIRMENT AND DEMENTIA

A recent phase of our understanding of vascular dementia is based on the realization that whereas infarcts and hemorrhages are rarely the only cause of dementia, their interaction with Alzheimer's lesions, and possibly with other neurodegenerative diseases, greatly modifies the clinical expression of these conditions (Snowdon et al., 1997; Strozyk et al., 2010). In addition, late-onset Alzheimer's disease shares many risk factors with cerebral vascular disease and cardiovascular disease in general, including hypertension, hypercholesterolemia, overweight/obesity, tobacco use, lack of physical activity, unhealthy diet, and diabetes (Chaves et al., 2004; De Reuck et al., 2013; Gelber, Launer, & White, 2012; Hofman et al., 1997; Wolf, 2012). These two elements have contributed to the current concept of vascular contributions to cognitive impairment and dementia (Gorelick et al., 2011). The current challenge is to identify the specific mechanisms through which vascular risk factors and vascular abnormalities contribute to the development of dementia. At this point, the effect on the clinical expression is clear, although the mechanisms are not, whereas whether vascular mechanisms are involved in the development of neurodegenerative pathology in humans is a matter of vigorous debate.

The single most important contribution to our understanding of vascular dementia was started by the surprising finding of Snowdon in the Nun Study of Aging and Alzheimer's Disease that the presence of small infarcts, at a density no differing from that found in the brains of cognitively normal subjects, markedly amplified the effect of a moderate load of Alzheimer-type pathosis (Snowdon, et al., 1997). Dementia appeared at a much lower tangle density in patients with even a few lacunar infarcts. This finding was later documented in numerous populations. Of particular interest is the study of Esiri, Nagy, Smith, Barnetson, and Smith (1999) showing that the presence of vascular lesions has minimal or no impact on cognitive status in patients with either no Alzheimer's lesions or severe Alzheimer's pathosis, but deeply influences those with a moderate level of Alzheimer's type lesions, corresponding to Braak stages 3 and 4. From a population point of view, this observation is extremely important, because the most common finding in the brains of elderly demented people is a combination of Alzheimer's disease and vascular lesions (De Reuck, et al., 2013; Jellinger & Attems, 2007; Rahimi & Kovacs, 2014). It has also been known from multiple epidemiological studies that vascular risk factors are associated with dementia

(Gorelick, et al., 2011). This information was difficult to mesh with the scarcity of pure vascular dementia (Jellinger & Attems, 2010), but fits perfectly well with the observations concerning the modulatory effect of vascular lesions on the clinical expression of moderate Alzheimer's pathosis. Snowdon et al.'s discovery offers alternative interpretations of epidemiological data. For example, the well-known fact that poor formal education is a risk factor for dementia had been interpreted as indicative of education providing increased cognitive reserve, possibly by means of augmenting synaptic density. However, we have shown that the lower educational attainment is much more common in patients with Alzheimer's disease plus infarct than in those with pure Alzheimer's disease, in accordance with the known relationship of stroke with lower socioeconomic status (Del Ser, Hachinski, Merskey, & Munoz, 1999).

A constant stream of epidemiological studies indicates that vascular risk factors in midlife influence the probability of developing dementia in late life. The question is how they do it, and on this point there is a marked discrepancy between studies utilizing cell-based or animal-based experimental approaches and those basing their conclusions on observations in human brains.

Multiple studies have shown that ischemia (as well as other injuries) increases the production of amyloid precursor protein. Moreover, we have shown that when Aβ is injected in the brain in combination with experimentally induced ischemia, the deposition of Aβ in brain parenchyma is markedly increased (Amtul et al., 2015). Others have obtained similar results, utilizing a genetic mouse model of Alzheimer's disease in combination with ischemia (Whitehead et al., 2010). However, observations in the human brain do not show a topographical association between infarct and either plaques or tangles. This discrepancy may have been explained by showing that the effects of ischemia on amyloid deposition in the brain are transient (Garcia-Alloza et al., 2011). Furthermore, whereas statins appear to have an effect in reducing the incidence of dementia in epidemiological studies (Williams, 2015), an autopsy study found no effect on the load of senile plaques or neurofibrillary tangles (Arvanitakis et al., 2008). Such discrepancy is reminiscent of the effect of regular use of nonsteroidal antiinflammatory agents, which decreases the risk of Alzheimer's disease but not the load of plaque and tangles. A different mechanism of action is suggested in the case of nonsteroidal antiinflammatory agents, which reduce microglia activation, and thus neuroinflammation (Mackenzie & Munoz, 1998).

Neuroinflammation is a complex process that involves recruitment and activation of microglia and astroglia, termed *gliosis*, as well as the production of proinflammatory cytokines and oxidative radicals. Increased Iba1 signal, a commonly used immunolabel for microglia cells of all activation states, is consistently reported in animal models of vascular dementia (Hattori et al., 2015; Ramos-Rodriguez et al., 2016). Accumulation of Iba1-positive microglia is specifically found in cortical areas, in the hippocampus (Ramos-Rodriguez et al., 2016), in white matter tracts (Coltman et al., 2011; Hattori et al., 2015), and in close association with vascular lesions (Holland, Searcy, et al., 2015; Pannozzo et al., 2013). The fact that markers of neuroinflammation are so consistently observed points to an important role for inflammatory action in the disease process. However, few studies characterize inflammation in more detail beyond quantification of microglia or astroglia. Neuroinflammation can, depending on the activation state of inflammatory cells, both aid in the resolution of tissue damage or contribute to cell degeneration. Therefore it will be necessary to conduct further investigations into the time course and the molecular nature of inflammatory processes in experimental models of vascular dementia. Targeted antiinflammatory or immune-modulating treatments, as mentioned, may prove beneficial for delaying the progression of the disease.

POTENTIAL MECHANISMS OF INTERACTION BETWEEN VASCULAR CONDITIONS AND DEMENTIA

At this point the mechanism through which vascular lesions modulate the effect of Alzheimer's pathosis is not understood. It is possible, however, to speculate based on the understanding of the relationship between vascular flow and neuronal activity. Neurovascular coupling is the phenomenon by which blood flow to different parts of the brain is regulated in a second-to-second fashion in response to the metabolic needs of the tissue, as we all have become aware through familiarity with functional MRI. Such coupling, which depends on all of the interactions between neurons, astrocytes, and smooth muscle and endothelial cells in the microvasculature, is also involved in the regulation of the blood–brain barrier and immune surveillance (Lecrux & Hamel, 2011). An emerging hypothesis is that alterations of the neurovascular coupling resulting from such factors as systolic blood pressure variability could initiate or potentiate neurodegenerative processes, with or without deposition of Aβ. It is not proven that amyloid deposits represent a step in the process by which vascular risk factors push the brain toward dementia, but if it is, the relationship between neuronal activity and amyloid deposition would be an interesting link. Such a relationship is postulated to explain the reduction in amyloid production during sleep (Lucey & Holtzman, 2015). In turn, Aβ impairs cerebrovascular autoregulation, thus completing a vicious circle (Iadecola, 2004).

The best experimental evidence so far relates to cerebral amyloid angiopathy. Amyloid deposited in the brain parenchyma must cross the blood–brain barrier to enter the perivascular space, and then drain along it. Vascular pulsations are assumed to be the driving force, and stiffening of the arteries is expected to result in reduction in drainage. Such reduction will cause increased deposition in the vessel wall, which in turn would create a more rigid vessel and thus a feedforward process of reduced draining and increased deposition (Weller, Preston, Subash, & Carare, 2009). It has been possible to demonstrate experimentally that Aβ drains along arteries and capillaries but not veins, and that such drainage is impaired after conclusion of the feeding artery (Arbel-Ornath et al., 2013).

EXPERIMENTAL MODELS OF VASCULAR DEMENTIA

Vascular dementia encompasses a wide range of brain pathological states and underlying conditions. Likewise, there is no one animal model that replicates each and every aspect of vascular dementia. In contrast, a range of animal models has been developed, each addressing one underlying aspect of vascular dementia, such as ischemic lesions, hypertension, diabetes, or genetic vasculopathies (eg, CADASIL).

Mice are most commonly used for the simple reason that a wide range of transgenic and gene knockout mice are commercially available [eg, Notch3 (Joutel, 2011); LDLr −/− (Bink, Ritz, Aronica, van der Weerd, & Daemen, 2013); db/db (Ramos-Rodriguez et al., 2015)]. However, rat models are increasingly popular because rats are generally better suited for cognitive testing than mice, which is of utmost importance for translationally meaningful studies into vascular dementia. Primates offer substantially higher translational validity over rodents, not only because of their cognitive capabilities, but also because primates, like humans, have gyrencephalic cortices and a markedly higher white matter–to–gray matter ratio (Ventura-Antunes, Mota, & Herculano-Houzel, 2013; Zhang & Sejnowski, 2000). However, for ethical reasons, only a minority of experiments is conducted in nonhuman primates, with limited statistical power (Hainsworth, Brittain, & Khatun, 2012; Hainsworth & Markus, 2008; Jiwa, Garrard, & Hainsworth, 2010).

Ischemic Models

Vascular cognitive impairment is readily induced in rats by fully occluding both common carotid arteries (CCAs), termed *bilateral carotid artery occlusion (BCAO)*, or narrowing both CCAs with microcoils in rats or mice, termed *bilateral carotid artery stenosis (BCAS)* (Hattori et al., 2015). The BCAO model can be modified with the use of ameroid constrictor devices that allow a gradual occlusion of the CCAs, producing mainly white matter pathological changes and working memory deficits (Hattori et al., 2015; Kitamura et al., 2012). The chronic, global hypoperfusion induced by classic BCAO in the rat results in a progressive decline in spatial and recognition memory, which is accompanied by hippocampal degeneration, cholinergic dysfunction, and white matter pathosis (Pappas, de la Torre, Davidson, Keyes, & Fortin, 1996; Tanaka, Ogawa, Asanuma, Kondo, & Nomura, 1996). Progressive brain atrophy, vasculopathy, and ischemic lesions in the cortex have been observed in BCAS mouse models (Holland, Pannozzo, et al., 2015; Holland, Searcy, et al., 2015), accompanied by blood–brain barrier alterations and gliosis. Behaviorally, CCA stenosis in the mouse leads to working memory deficits measurable in maze tasks (Bink et al., 2013; Coltman et al., 2011; Holland, Searcy, et al., 2015). The degree of stenosis is an essential parameter, because a decrease in microcoil diameter of only 0.02 mm (to 0.016 mm) on only one CCA can significantly increase the severity of the model, resulting in unwanted deficits in vision and locomotion (Bink et al., 2013). When hypoperfusion was induced by BCAS in $APP_{Swe/Ind}$ transgenic mice, cortical Aβ levels and the number of apoptotic cells in the cortex were increased in comparison with controls, indicating an interaction of vascular pathosis with Aβ (Kitaguchi et al., 2009). Likewise, carrying the transgene and suffering hypoperfusion synergistically worsened learning performance, and cognitive performance was inversely correlated with cortical neuron density (Yamada et al., 2011). Supporting the notion of synergism between these two pathologies are findings from a comorbid rat model of elevated Aβ load and striatal ischemia, induced by stereotactical injections of Aβ25–35 fragment and the vasoconstrictor endothelin 1, respectively (Amtul et al., 2015). In the cortex of comorbid animals, more Aβ-containing cells and activated microglia were found than in either condition (Aβ-load or ischemia) alone (Amtul et al., 2015). Mechanistic explanations for this synergism are incomplete, but processes such as oxidative stress, inflammation, and blood–brain barrier breakdown are thought to be involved (Venkat, Chopp, & Chen, 2015). Further mechanistic investigations in comorbid animal models are needed, calling for a combination of Aβ load [via *APP* transgene or by injection of Aβ25–35 fragment (Whitehead, Hachinski, & Cechetto, 2005)] and stroke [such as by endothelin 1 injection (Nguemeni, Gomez-Smith, Jeffers, Schuch, & Corbett, 2015); photothrombosis (Schoknecht et al., 2014); injection of microspheres (Silasi, She, Boyd, Xue, & Murphy, 2015); or middle cerebral artery occlusion (Fluri, Schuhmann, & Kleinschnitz, 2015)].

Hypertensive Models

Chronic hypertension surgically induced in monkeys by coarctation of the aorta produces microinfarcts in white and gray matter, including cortical areas; impairs executive function; and leads to progressive memory decline (Kemper, Moss, Hollander, & Prusty, 1999; Kemper, Blatt, Killiany, & Moss, 2001). In rats, hypertension can be induced acutely by parenteral angiotensin delivery (Jiang et al., 2016) or by N(omega)nitro-L-arginine methyl ester treatment (Kobayashi, Hara, Watanabe, Higashi, & Matsuoka, 2000). Because vascular dementia studies are usually conducted over a long time, requiring a model of chronic hypertension, the spontaneously hypertensive rat stroke-prone (SHRSP) is a widely used model (Hainsworth et al., 2012). The SHRSP rat reproduces most key features of small vessel disease such as microinfarction, vasculopathy, diffuse white matter damage, and cognitive impairment (Hainsworth & Markus, 2008). Eighty percent of ischemic lesions in aged SHRSP rats are found in the cortex; most of the remaining lesions are typically located in the basal ganglia. A disadvantage for the study of vascular dementia is the fact that these rats suffer spontaneous microinfarcts in nonpredictable locations, which can result in neurological symptoms that are directly stroke-related, complicating the interpretation of cognitive function over time.

Diabetic Models

A commonly used model of type 1 diabetes in experimental animals is intravenous or intraperitoneal injection of streptozotocin (STZ), a broad-spectrum antibiotic. The substance selectively kills insulin-producing β cells in pancreatic islets, resulting in diabetic blood glucose levels within a few days after injection (Deeds et al., 2011). However, sensitivity to STZ varies among mouse strains, and males are generally more sensitive and therefore often used (Deeds et al., 2011). Type 2 diabetes can be modeled by knocking out the leptin receptor gene in db/db mice (Ramos-Rodriguez et al., 2013). Diabetic mouse models do not only develop a metabolic syndrome similar to the human condition; they also show cognitive impairment (Ramos-Rodriguez et al., 2013). Because diabetes is a risk factor for both vascular dementia and Alzheimer's disease, experimentally inducing diabetes in transgenic Alzheimer's disease mouse models has been widely used as a comorbid model to study the interaction between vascular pathological states and neurodegenerative disease. In a combined model of STZ-induced type I diabetes and Alzheimer's disease, a range of pathological synergisms have been found in the cortex. Thus an overall reduction in cortex size was slightly more severe in *APP/Psen1* mice treated with STZ, and levels of soluble Aβ40, Aβ42 and phosphorylated tau protein were higher in the combined condition (Ramos-Rodriguez et al., 2016). Likewise, the cortex suffered an increased burden of neuroinflammation and microhemorrhages in diabetic transgenic animals. This pathology translated into impairments in working and episodic memory, which were worst in the combined model. A similar pathological synergy was found in a combined model of Alzheimer's disease and type II diabetes [*APP/Psen1* transgenic mice crossed with db/db transgenic mice (Ramos-Rodriguez et al., 2015)]. An age-dependent cortical shrinkage was more severe in diabetic transgenic mice, and levels of phosphorylated tau and soluble Aβ40 and Aβ42 were likewise highest in the cortex of aged comorbid animals. The number of microglia was also significantly increased in comorbid models compared with nondiabetic *APP/Psen1* animals in some cortical regions. These consistent results strengthen the hypothesis of an interactive pathosis, especially regarding the cortex, and speak for diabetic models as useful experimental tools for the investigation of the mechanisms behind the observed pathogenic synergism.

CADASIL Models

CADASIL, as explained, is caused by a mutation in the *Notch3* gene. Because genetic manipulation in mice is widely used, several mouse lines carrying different *Notch3* mutations are available to model CADASIL preclinically. Transgenic mice exhibit impaired microvascular autoregulation (Lacombe, Oligo, Domenga, Tournier-Lasserve, & Joutel, 2005; Ruchoux et al., 2003). Studies of *Notch3* transgenic mice have largely concentrated on vasculopathology, with little evidence of brain lesions characteristic for the human condition (Skehan, Hutchinson, & MacErlaine, 1995) except for white matter pathosis (Cognat, Cleophax, Domenga-Denier, & Joutel, 2014; Joutel et al., 2010).

PREVENTION AND TREATMENT

Control of vascular risk factors has led to a precipitous decline in the incidence of stroke in Western countries. Possibly the importance of vascular contributions to dementia could be assessed by determining whether a similar decrease in the age-adjusted incidence of dementia has been observed. A recent paper (Matthews et al., 2013) suggests that such reduction may be taking place. It is clear, however, that the magnitude of the effect is much smaller than that observed in stroke, which is consistent with the fact that other factors contribute to the degenerative of aspect of dementia.

The translation of the basic science and epidemiological knowledge to practical results is of enormous social importance. The magnitude of the issue is based on three factors: the number of people surviving to old age, the very high prevalence of dementia in this population, and the long period of dependency. Thus it would be a major achievement if we were able to reduce the burden of dementia by treating the vascular risk factors even if by only 20%. Efficacious drug and nondrug treatments are available, in contrast to the situation in Alzheimer's disease. Epidemiological evidence indicates that the use of statin, but not other cholesterol-lowering drugs, is associated with a 61% reduction in the risk of Alzheimer's disease (Williams, 2015). Unfortunately, a study demonstrating that intervention is effective has not yet been published. Such is the challenge for our time.

Animal models of vascular dementia, specifically comorbid models, confirm both behaviorally and histologically that cortical pathological change plays a significant role. Cortical involvement translates into executive deficits in nonhuman primate models, and is reflected by working memory deficits in rodent models of vascular dementia. The cortex is also a site of interactive synergism between vascular pathology, amyloid pathology, and neuronal degeneration. Accumulation of microglia is consistently observed in models of vascular dementia, pointing to a potential mechanistic role of neuroinflammation in the pathological process. Further investigation into specific targets for immunomodulatory treatment and for therapeutic strategies that target synergistic mechanisms in comorbid conditions are needed to move these preclinical findings from bench to bedside.

REFERENCES

Abboud, S., Viiri, L. E., Lutjohann, D., Goebeler, S., Luoto, T., Friedrichs, S., et al. (2008). Associations of apolipoprotein E gene with ischemic stroke and intracranial atherosclerosis. *European Journal of Human Genetics*, *16*(8), 955–960.

Amtul, Z., Whitehead, S. N., Keeley, R. J., Bechberger, J., Fisher, A. L., McDonald, R. J., et al. (2015). Comorbid rat model of ischemia and beta-amyloid toxicity: striatal and cortical degeneration. *Brain Pathology*, *25*(1), 24–32.

Arbel-Ornath, M., Hudry, E., Eikermann-Haerter, K., Hou, S., Gregory, J. L., Zhao, L., et al. (2013). Interstitial fluid drainage is impaired in ischemic stroke and Alzheimer's disease mouse models. *Acta Neuropathologica*, *126*(3), 353–364.

Arvanitakis, Z., Schneider, J. A., Wilson, R. S., Bienias, J. L., Kelly, J. F., Evans, D. A., et al. (2008). Statins, incident Alzheimer disease, change in cognitive function, and neuropathology. *Neurology*, *70*(19 Pt 2), 1795–1802.

Barba, R., Martinez-Espinosa, S., Rodriguez-Garcia, E., Pondal, M., Vivancos, J., & Del Ser, T. (2000). Poststroke dementia: clinical features and risk factors. *Stroke, 31*(7), 1494–1501.

Bink, D. I., Ritz, K., Aronica, E., van der Weerd, L., & Daemen, M. J. (2013). Mouse models to study the effect of cardiovascular risk factors on brain structure and cognition. *Journal of Cerebral Blood Flow & Metabolism, 33*(11), 1666–1684.

Chaves, P. H., Kuller, L. H., O'Leary, D. H., Manolio, T. A., Newman, A. B., & Cardiovascular Health, S.. (2004). Subclinical cardiovascular disease in older adults: insights from the Cardiovascular Health Study. *American Journal of Geriatric Cardiology, 13*(3), 137–151.

Chui, H. C., Victoroff, J. I., Margolin, D., Jagust, W., Shankle, R., & Katzman, R. (1992). Criteria for the diagnosis of ischemic vascular dementia proposed by the state of California Alzheimer's disease diagnostic and treatment centers. *Neurology, 42*(3 Pt 1), 473–480.

Cognat, E., Cleophax, S., Domenga-Denier, V., & Joutel, A. (2014). Early white matter changes in CADASIL: evidence of segmental intramyelinic oedema in a pre-clinical mouse model. *Acta Neuropathologica Communications, 2*, 49.

Coltman, R., Spain, A., Tsenkina, Y., Fowler, J. H., Smith, J., Scullion, G., et al. (2011). Selective white matter pathology induces a specific impairment in spatial working memory. *Neurobiology of Aging, 32*(12), 2324.e7–2324.e12.

De Reuck, J., Deramecourt, V., Cordonnier, C., Leys, D., Pasquier, F., & Maurage, C. A. (2013). Prevalence of cerebrovascular lesions in patients with Lewy body dementia: a neuropathological study. *Clinical Neurology and Neurosurgery, 115*(7), 1094–1097.

Deeds, M. C., Anderson, J. M., Armstrong, A. S., Gastineau, D. A., Hiddinga, H. J., Jahangir, A., et al. (2011). Single dose streptozotocin-induced diabetes: considerations for study design in islet transplantation models. *Laboratory Animals, 45*(3), 131–140.

Del Ser, T., Hachinski, V., Merskey, H., & Munoz, D. G. (1999). An autopsy-verified study of the effect of education on degenerative dementia. *Brain, 122*(Pt 12), 2309–2319.

Esiri, M. M., Nagy, Z., Smith, M. Z., Barnetson, L., & Smith, A. D. (1999). Cerebrovascular disease and threshold for dementia in the early stages of Alzheimer's disease. *Lancet, 354*(9182), 919–920.

Fluri, F., Schuhmann, M. K., & Kleinschnitz, C. (2015). Animal models of ischemic stroke and their application in clinical research. *Drug Design, Development and Therapy [Electronic Resource], 9*, 3445–3454.

Garcia-Alloza, M., Gregory, J., Kuchibhotla, K. V., Fine, S., Wei, Y., Ayata, C., et al. (2011). Cerebrovascular lesions induce transient beta-amyloid deposition. *Brain, 134*(Pt 12), 3697–3707.

Gelber, R. P., Launer, L. J., & White, L. R. (2012). The Honolulu-Asia Aging Study: epidemiologic and neuropathologic research on cognitive impairment. *Current Alzheimer Research, 9*(6), 664–672.

Gorelick, P. B., Scuteri, A., Black, S. E., Decarli, C., Greenberg, S. M., Iadecola, C., et al. (2011). Vascular contributions to cognitive impairment and dementia: a statement for healthcare professionals from the American Heart Association/American Stroke Association. *Stroke, 42*(9), 2672–2713.

Hachinski, V., Iadecola, C., Petersen, R. C., Breteler, M. M., Nyenhuis, D. L., Black, S. E., et al. (2006). National Institute of neurological disorders and stroke-Canadian stroke network vascular cognitive impairment harmonization standards. *Stroke, 37*(9), 2220–2241.

Hachinski, V. C., Potter, P., & Merskey, H. (1987). Leuko-araiosis. *Archives of Neurology, 44*(1), 21–23.

Hainsworth, A. H., Brittain, J. F., & Khatun, H. (2012). Pre-clinical models of human cerebral small vessel disease: utility for clinical application. *Journal of the Neurological Sciences, 322*(1–2), 237–240.

Hainsworth, A. H., & Markus, H. S. (2008). Do in vivo experimental models reflect human cerebral small vessel disease? A systematic review. *Journal of Cerebral Blood Flow & Metabolism*, *28*(12), 1877–1891.

Hainsworth, A. H., Oommen, A. T., & Bridges, L. R. (2015). Endothelial cells and human cerebral small vessel disease. *Brain Pathology*, *25*(1), 44–50.

Hattori, Y., Enmi, J., Kitamura, A., Yamamoto, Y., Saito, S., Takahashi, Y., et al. (2015). A novel mouse model of subcortical infarcts with dementia. *The Journal of Neuroscience*, *35*(9), 3915–3928.

Henon, H., Durieu, I., Guerouaou, D., Lebert, F., Pasquier, F., & Leys, D. (2001). Poststroke dementia: incidence and relationship to prestroke cognitive decline. *Neurology*, *57*(7), 1216–1222.

Hofman, A., Ott, A., Breteler, M. M., Bots, M. L., Slooter, A. J., van Harskamp, F., et al. (1997). Atherosclerosis, apolipoprotein E, and prevalence of dementia and Alzheimer's disease in the Rotterdam Study. *Lancet*, *349*(9046), 151–154.

Holland, P. R., Pannozzo, M. A., Bastin, M. E., McNeilly, A. D., Ferguson, K. J., Caughey, S., et al. (2015). Hypertension fails to disrupt white matter integrity in young or aged Fisher (F44) Cyp1a1Ren2 transgenic rats. *Journal of Cerebral Blood Flow & Metabolism*, *35*(2), 188–192.

Holland, P. R., Searcy, J. L., Salvadores, N., Scullion, G., Chen, G., Lawson, G., et al. (2015). Gliovascular disruption and cognitive deficits in a mouse model with features of small vessel disease. *Journal of Cerebral Blood Flow & Metabolism*, *35*(6), 1005–1014.

Iadecola, C. (2004). Neurovascular regulation in the normal brain and in Alzheimer's disease. *Nature Reviews. Neuroscience*, *5*(5), 347–360.

Ivan, C. S., Seshadri, S., Beiser, A., Au, R., Kase, C. S., Kelly-Hayes, M., et al. (2004). Dementia after stroke: the Framingham study. *Stroke*, *35*(6), 1264–1268.

Jellinger, K. A. (2008). The pathology of "vascular dementia": a critical update. *Journal of Alzheimer's Disease*, *14*(1), 107–123.

Jellinger, K. A., & Attems, J. (2007). Neuropathological evaluation of mixed dementia. *Journal of the Neurological Sciences*, *257*(1–2), 80–87.

Jellinger, K. A., & Attems, J. (2010). Is there pure vascular dementia in old age? *Journal of the Neurological Sciences*, *299*(1–2), 150–154.

Jiang, D., Tokashiki, M., Hayashi, H., Kawagoe, Y., Kuwasako, K., Kitamura, K., et al. (2016). Augmented blood pressure variability in hypertension induced by angiotensin II in rats. *American Journal of Hypertension*, *29*(2), 163–169.

Jiwa, N. S., Garrard, P., & Hainsworth, A. H. (2010). Experimental models of vascular dementia and vascular cognitive impairment: a systematic review. *Journal of Neurochemistry*, *115*(4), 814–828.

Joutel, A. (2011). Pathogenesis of CADASIL: transgenic and knock-out mice to probe function and dysfunction of the mutated gene, *Notch3,* in the cerebrovasculature. *Bioessays*, *33*(1), 73–80.

Joutel, A., Corpechot, C., Ducros, A., Vahedi, K., Chabriat, H., Mouton, P., et al. (1996). *Notch3* mutations in CADASIL, a hereditary adult-onset condition causing stroke and dementia. *Nature*, *383*(6602), 707–710.

Joutel, A., Monet-Lepretre, M., Gosele, C., Baron-Menguy, C., Hammes, A., Schmidt, S., et al. (2010). Cerebrovascular dysfunction and microcirculation rarefaction precede white matter lesions in a mouse genetic model of cerebral ischemic small vessel disease. *The Journal of Clinical Investigation*, *120*(2), 433–445.

Kemper, T., Moss, M. B., Hollander, W., & Prusty, S. (1999). Microinfarction as a result of hypertension in a primate model of cerebrovascular disease. *Acta Neuropathologica*, *98*(3), 295–303.

Kemper, T. L., Blatt, G. J., Killiany, R. J., & Moss, M. B. (2001). Neuropathology of progressive cognitive decline in chronically hypertensive rhesus monkeys. *Acta Neuropathologica*, *101*(2), 145–153.

Kitaguchi, H., Tomimoto, H., Ihara, M., Shibata, M., Uemura, K., Kalaria, R. N., et al. (2009). Chronic cerebral hypoperfusion accelerates amyloid beta deposition in APPSwInd transgenic mice. *Brain Research, 1294*, 202–210.

Kitamura, A., Fujita, Y., Oishi, N., Kalaria, R. N., Washida, K., Maki, T., et al. (2012). Selective white matter abnormalities in a novel rat model of vascular dementia. *Neurobiology of Aging, 33*(5), 1012.e25–1012.e35.

Knopman, D. S., Rocca, W. A., Cha, R. H., Edland, S. D., & Kokmen, E. (2002). Incidence of vascular dementia in Rochester, Minn, 1985-1989. *Archives of Neurology, 59*(10), 1605–1610.

Kobayashi, N., Hara, K., Watanabe, S., Higashi, T., & Matsuoka, H. (2000). Effect of imidapril on myocardial remodeling in L-NAME-induced hypertensive rats is associated with gene expression of NOS and ACE mRNA. *American Journal of Hypertension, 13*(2), 199–207.

Koga, H., Takashima, Y., Murakawa, R., Uchino, A., Yuzuriha, T., & Yao, H. (2009). Cognitive consequences of multiple lacunes and leukoaraiosis as vascular cognitive impairment in community-dwelling elderly individuals. *Journal of Stroke and Cerebrovascular Diseases, 18*(1), 32–37.

Korczyn, A. D., Vakhapova, V., & Grinberg, L. T. (2012). Vascular dementia. *Journal of the Neurological Sciences, 322*(1–2), 2–10.

Lacombe, P., Oligo, C., Domenga, V., Tournier-Lasserve, E., & Joutel, A. (2005). Impaired cerebral vasoreactivity in a transgenic mouse model of cerebral autosomal dominant arteriopathy with subcortical infarcts and leukoencephalopathy arteriopathy. *Stroke, 36*(5), 1053–1058.

Lammie, G. A. (2002). Hypertensive cerebral small vessel disease and stroke. *Brain Pathology, 12*(3), 358–370.

Leblanc, G. G., Meschia, J. F., Stuss, D. T., & Hachinski, V. (2006). Genetics of vascular cognitive impairment: the opportunity and the challenges. *Stroke, 37*(1), 248–255.

Lecrux, C., & Hamel, E. (2011). The neurovascular unit in brain function and disease. *Acta Physiologica, 203*(1), 47–59.

Longstreth, W. T., Jr., Diehr, P., Beauchamp, N. J., & Manolio, T. A. (2001). Patterns on cranial magnetic resonance imaging in elderly people and vascular disease outcomes. *Archives of Neurology, 58*(12), 2074.

Lucey, B. P., & Holtzman, D. M. (2015). How amyloid, sleep and memory connect. *Nature Neuroscience, 18*(7), 933–934.

Mackenzie, I. R., & Munoz, D. G. (1998). Nonsteroidal anti-inflammatory drug use and Alzheimer-type pathology in aging. *Neurology, 50*(4), 986–990.

Matthews, F. E., Arthur, A., Barnes, L. E., Bond, J., Jagger, C., Robinson, L., et al. (2013). A two-decade comparison of prevalence of dementia in individuals aged 65 years and older from three geographical areas of England: results of the Cognitive Function and Ageing Study I and II. *Lancet, 382*(9902), 1405–1412.

Neumann, M., Sampathu, D. M., Kwong, L. K., Truax, A. C., Micsenyi, M. C., Chou, T. T., et al. (2006). Ubiquitinated TDP-43 in frontotemporal lobar degeneration and amyotrophic lateral sclerosis. *Science, 314*(5796), 130–133.

Nguemeni, C., Gomez-Smith, M., Jeffers, M. S., Schuch, C. P., & Corbett, D. (2015). Time course of neuronal death following endothelin-1 induced focal ischemia in rats. *Journal of Neuroscience Methods, 242*, 72–76.

Nordlund, A., Rolstad, S., Klang, O., Lind, K., Hansen, S., & Wallin, A. (2007). Cognitive profiles of mild cognitive impairment with and without vascular disease. *Neuropsychology, 21*(6), 706–712.

O'Brien, J. T., Erkinjuntti, T., Reisberg, B., Roman, G., Sawada, T., Pantoni, L., et al. (2003). Vascular cognitive impairment. *Lancet Neurology, 2*(2), 89–98.

O'Brien, J. T., & Herholz, K. (2015). Amyloid imaging for dementia in clinical practice. *BMC Medicine, 13*, 163.

Ohtsuki, S., Hirayama, M., Ito, S., Uchida, Y., Tachikawa, M., & Terasaki, T. (2014). Quantitative targeted proteomics for understanding the blood–brain barrier: towards pharmacoproteomics. *Expert Review of Proteomics, 11*(3), 303–313.

O'Sullivan, M., Barrick, T. R., Morris, R. G., Clark, C. A., & Markus, H. S. (2005). Damage within a network of white matter regions underlies executive dysfunction in CADASIL. *Neurology, 65*(10), 1584–1590.

O'Sullivan, M., Jarosz, J. M., Martin, R. J., Deasy, N., Powell, J. F., & Markus, H. S. (2001). MRI hyperintensities of the temporal lobe and external capsule in patients with CADASIL. *Neurology, 56*(5), 628–634.

O'Sullivan, M., Ngo, E., Viswanathan, A., Jouvent, E., Gschwendtner, A., Saemann, P. G., et al. (2009). Hippocampal volume is an independent predictor of cognitive performance in CADASIL. *Neurobiology of Aging, 30*(6), 890–897.

O'Sullivan, M., Singhal, S., Charlton, R., & Markus, H. S. (2004). Diffusion tensor imaging of thalamus correlates with cognition in CADASIL without dementia. *Neurology, 62*(5), 702–707.

Pannozzo, M. A., Holland, P. R., Scullion, G., Talbot, R., Mullins, J. J., & Horsburgh, K. (2013). Controlled hypertension induces cerebrovascular and gene alterations in Cyp1a1-Ren2 transgenic rats. *Journal of the American Society of Hypertension, 7*(6), 411–419.

Pappas, B. A., de la Torre, J. C., Davidson, C. M., Keyes, M. T., & Fortin, T. (1996). Chronic reduction of cerebral blood flow in the adult rat: late-emerging CA1 cell loss and memory dysfunction. *Brain Research, 708*(1–2), 50–58.

Pendlebury, S. T., & Rothwell, P. M. (2009). Risk of recurrent stroke, other vascular events and dementia after transient ischaemic attack and stroke. *Cerebrovascular Diseases, 3*(27 Suppl.), 1–11.

Peters, N., Holtmannspotter, M., Opherk, C., Gschwendtner, A., Herzog, J., Samann, P., et al. (2006). Brain volume changes in CADASIL: a serial MRI study in pure subcortical ischemic vascular disease. *Neurology, 66*(10), 1517–1522.

Poels, M. M., Ikram, M. A., van der Lugt, A., Hofman, A., Krestin, G. P., Breteler, M. M., et al. (2011). Incidence of cerebral microbleeds in the general population: the Rotterdam Scan Study. *Stroke, 42*(3), 656–661.

Rahimi, J., & Kovacs, G. G. (2014). Prevalence of mixed pathologies in the aging brain. *Alzheimer's Research & Therapy, 6*(9), 82.

Ramos-Rodriguez, J. J., Infante-Garcia, C., Galindo-Gonzalez, L., Garcia-Molina, Y., Lechuga-Sancho, A., & Garcia-Alloza, M. (2016). Increased spontaneous central bleeding and cognition impairment in *APP/PS1* mice with poorly controlled diabetes mellitus. *Molecular Neurobiology, 53*(4), 2685–2697.

Ramos-Rodriguez, J. J., Jimenez-Palomares, M., Murillo-Carretero, M. I., Infante-Garcia, C., Berrocoso, E., Hernandez-Pacho, F., et al. (2015). Central vascular disease and exacerbated pathology in a mixed model of type 2 diabetes and Alzheimer's disease. *Psychoneuroendocrinology, 62*, 69–79.

Ramos-Rodriguez, J. J., Ortiz, O., Jimenez-Palomares, M., Kay, K. R., Berrocoso, E., Murillo-Carretero, M. I., et al. (2013). Differential central pathology and cognitive impairment in prediabetic and diabetic mice. *Psychoneuroendocrinology, 38*(11), 2462–2475.

Roman, G. C. (1987). Senile dementia of the Binswanger type: a vascular form of dementia in the elderly. *JAMA, 258*(13), 1782–1788.

Roman, G. C. (2004). Vascular dementia: advances in nosology, diagnosis, treatment and prevention. *Panminerva Medica, 46*(4), 207–215.

Roman, G. C. (2006). Vascular depression: an archetypal neuropsychiatric disorder. *Biological Psychiatry, 60*(12), 1306–1308.

Roman, G. C., & Royall, D. R. (1999). Executive control function: a rational basis for the diagnosis of vascular dementia. *Alzheimer Disease and Associated Disorders, 3*(13 Suppl.), S69–S80.

Roman, G. C., Tatemichi, T. K., Erkinjuntti, T., Cummings, J. L., Masdeu, J. C., Garcia, J. H., et al. (1993). Vascular dementia: diagnostic criteria for research studies. Report of the NINDS-AIREN International Workshop. *Neurology, 43*(2), 250–260.

Ruchoux, M. M., Domenga, V., Brulin, P., Maciazek, J., Limol, S., Tournier-Lasserve, E., et al. (2003). Transgenic mice expressing mutant *Notch3* develop vascular alterations characteristic of cerebral autosomal dominant arteriopathy with subcortical infarcts and leukoencephalopathy. *The American Journal of Pathology, 162*(1), 329–342.

Schoknecht, K., Prager, O., Vazana, U., Kamintsky, L., Harhausen, D., Zille, M., et al. (2014). Monitoring stroke progression: in vivo imaging of cortical perfusion, blood–brain barrier permeability and cellular damage in the rat photothrombosis model. *Journal of Cerebral Blood Flow & Metabolism, 34*(11), 1791–1801.

Selnes, O. A., & Vinters, H. V. (2006). Vascular cognitive impairment. *Nature Clinical Practice Neurology, 2*(10), 538–547.

Silasi, G., She, J., Boyd, J. D., Xue, S., & Murphy, T. H. (2015). A mouse model of small-vessel disease that produces brain-wide-identified microocclusions and regionally selective neuronal injury. *Journal of Cerebral Blood Flow & Metabolism, 35*(5), 734–738.

Skehan, S. J., Hutchinson, M., & MacErlaine, D. P. (1995). Cerebral autosomal dominant arteriopathy with subcortical infarcts and leukoencephalopathy: MR findings. *AJNR. American Journal of Neuroradiology, 16*(10), 2115–2119.

Snowdon, D. A., Greiner, L. H., Mortimer, J. A., Riley, K. P., Greiner, P. A., & Markesbery, W. R. (1997). Brain infarction and the clinical expression of Alzheimer disease. The Nun Study. *JAMA, 277*(10), 813–817.

Strozyk, D., Dickson, D. W., Lipton, R. B., Katz, M., Derby, C. A., Lee, S., et al. (2010). Contribution of vascular pathology to the clinical expression of dementia. *Neurobiology of Aging, 31*(10), 1710–1720.

Sun, J. H., Tan, L., & Yu, J. T. (2014). Post-stroke cognitive impairment: epidemiology, mechanisms and management. *Annals of Translational Medicine, 2*(8), 80.

Tanaka, K., Ogawa, N., Asanuma, M., Kondo, Y., & Nomura, M. (1996). Relationship between cholinergic dysfunction and discrimination learning disabilities in Wistar rats following chronic cerebral hypoperfusion. *Brain Research, 729*(1), 55–65.

Tatemichi, T. K., Desmond, D. W., Stern, Y., Paik, M., Sano, M., & Bagiella, E. (1994). Cognitive impairment after stroke: frequency, patterns, and relationship to functional abilities. *Journal of Neurology, Neurosurgery, & Psychiatry, 57*(2), 202–207.

Tournier-Lasserve, E., Iba-Zizen, M. T., Romero, N., & Bousser, M. G. (1991). Autosomal dominant syndrome with strokelike episodes and leukoencephalopathy. *Stroke, 22*(10), 1297–1302.

Treves, T. A., Bornstein, N. M., Chapman, J., Klimovitzki, S., Verchovsky, R., Asherov, A., et al. (1996). APOE-epsilon 4 in patients with Alzheimer disease and vascular dementia. *Alzheimer Disease and Associated Disorders, 10*(4), 189–191.

Venkat, P., Chopp, M., & Chen, J. (2015). Models and mechanisms of vascular dementia. *Experimental Neurology, 272*, 97–108.

Ventura-Antunes, L., Mota, B., & Herculano-Houzel, S. (2013). Different scaling of white matter volume, cortical connectivity, and gyrification across rodent and primate brains. *Frontiers in Neuroanatomy, 7*, 3.

Viswanathan, A., Gray, F., Bousser, M. G., Baudrimont, M., & Chabriat, H. (2006). Cortical neuronal apoptosis in CADASIL. *Stroke*, *37*(11), 2690–2695.

Weller, R. O., Preston, S. D., Subash, M., & Carare, R. O. (2009). Cerebral amyloid angiopathy in the aetiology and immunotherapy of Alzheimer disease. *Alzheimer's Research & Therapy*, *1*(2), 6.

Wentzel, C., Rockwood, K., MacKnight, C., Hachinski, V., Hogan, D. B., Feldman, H., et al. (2001). Progression of impairment in patients with vascular cognitive impairment without dementia. *Neurology*, *57*(4), 714–716.

Whitehead, S. N., Hachinski, V. C., & Cechetto, D. F. (2005). Interaction between a rat model of cerebral ischemia and beta-amyloid toxicity: inflammatory responses. *Stroke*, *36*(1), 107–112.

Whitehead, S. N., Massoni, E., Cheng, G., Hachinski, V. C., Cimino, M., Balduini, W., et al. (2010). Triflusal reduces cerebral ischemia induced inflammation in a combined mouse model of Alzheimer's disease and stroke. *Brain Research*, *1366*, 246–256.

Williams, P. T. (2015). Lower risk of Alzheimer's disease mortality with exercise, statin, and fruit intake. *Journal of Alzheimer's Disease*, *44*(4), 1121–1129.

Wolf, P. A. (2012). Contributions of the Framingham Heart Study to stroke and dementia epidemiologic research at 60 years. *Archives of Neurology*, *69*(5), 567–571.

Yamada, M., Ihara, M., Okamoto, Y., Maki, T., Washida, K., Kitamura, A., et al. (2011). The influence of chronic cerebral hypoperfusion on cognitive function and amyloid beta metabolism in APP overexpressing mice. *PLoS One*, *6*(1), e16567.

Zhang, K., & Sejnowski, T. J. (2000). A universal scaling law between gray matter and white matter of cerebral cortex. *Proceedings of the National Academy of Sciences of the United States of America*, *97*(10), 5621–5626.

Chapter 6

Frontotemporal Dementia

A.E. Arrant, E.D. Roberson
University of Alabama at Birmingham, Birmingham, AL, United States

INTRODUCTION

Frontotemporal dementia (FTD) is an umbrella term for a family of disorders characterized by degeneration of brain networks located primarily in the frontal and temporal lobes. FTD is one of the most common causes of early-onset dementia, with a prevalence similar to Alzheimer's disease (AD) in those under age 65 years (Ratnavalli, Brayne, Dawson, & Hodges, 2002). FTD strikes patients relatively early in life, with a median age of onset in the late 50s, and has a shorter survival time (median of 9–10 years) than AD (Borroni et al., 2010; Chiu et al., 2010; Rascovsky et al., 2011; Roberson et al., 2005; Rosso et al., 2003).

In this chapter, we discuss how degeneration of networks containing specific cortical regions contributes to the most common FTD syndromes. We also review how recent discoveries involving the most common genetic causes of FTD have provided insight into potential molecular mechanisms common to multiple FTD subtypes.

CLINICAL MANIFESTATIONS

Frontotemporal Dementia Clinical Syndromes

The classification and nomenclature of FTD clinical syndromes has evolved, and generally includes six subtypes: behavioral variant FTD (bvFTD), FTD with amyotrophic lateral sclerosis (FTD-ALS; see Chapter 9), semantic variant primary progressive aphasia (svPPA), nonfluent/agrammatic primary progressive aphasia (nfPPA), progressive supranuclear palsy (PSP), and corticobasal syndrome (CBS) (Gorno-Tempini et al., 2011; Rascovsky et al., 2011). The latter two disorders, PSP and CBS, have predominant extrapyramidal and subcortical pathology, so we will not focus on them here, in the context of cortical pathology.

Behavioral variant FTD is the most common FTD syndrome. Patients with bvFTD do not typically have predominant memory deficits, but develop personality and behavioral changes that include disinhibition, apathy, loss of empathy, repetitive behavior, and changes in food preference, often presenting as

The Cerebral Cortex in Neurodegenerative and Neuropsychiatric Disorders.
http://dx.doi.org/10.1016/B978-0-12-801942-9.00006-9

141

hyperphagia or an increased preference for sweet-tasting food (Neary, Snowden, Northen, & Goulding, 1988; Rascovsky et al., 2011). These behavioral changes are disruptive to the patients' work and social relationships, especially with family members.

There is an intriguing overlap between FTD and ALS, with as many as 40% of FTD patients showing signs of motor neuron dysfunction, and around 50% of ALS patients exhibiting FTD-like behavioral or cognitive changes (Burrell, Kiernan, Vucic, & Hodges, 2011; Lomen-Hoerth et al., 2003; Ringholz et al., 2005; Witgert et al., 2010). FTD and ALS also have overlapping genetics, pathology, and potential underlying mechanisms, as discussed in recent reviews (Ling, Polymenidou, & Cleveland, 2013; Thomas, Alegre-Abarrategui, & Wade-Martins, 2013).

Semantic variant PPA, also known as *semantic dementia*, is characterized by impairment of word comprehension and by anomia (Gorno-Tempini et al., 2011). Perhaps the earliest description of svPPA was provided by Arnold Pick in the 1890s, though there is not sufficient data to conclusively diagnose the patient from this report (Pick, 1892). Early descriptions of svPPA were provided by Warrington (1975) and Mesulam (1982). Patients with svPPA generally speak fluently but have problems with naming objects, and progress to loss of their semantic knowledge about those objects. Patients who have svPPA do not have prominent AD-like episodic memory impairments, but they often develop bvFTD-like behavioral changes (Gorno-Tempini et al., 2011).

Patients with nfPPA (formerly known as *progressive nonfluent aphasia*) have difficulty speaking, often with apraxia of speech (Gorno-Tempini et al., 2011). Speech from these patients is slow and effortful, with frequent pauses, grammatical errors, and incorrect sounds. In contrast to svPPA patients, word comprehension is not affected, although nfPPA patients may have problems understanding complex sentences. Patients with nfPPA have difficulty with the motor aspects of speech that may extend to related motor problems such as difficulty swallowing, and may later develop into broader motor deficits (Caso et al., 2014; Gorno-Tempini et al., 2011).

Frontotemporal Dementia Pathology

Just as with the heterogeneity of clinical syndromes in FTD, there are many patterns of pathology, which as a group are referred to as *frontotemporal lobar degeneration (FTLD)* (Majounie et al. 2012). Gross examination of brains from FTD patients reveals a decrease in brain weight and atrophy of the frontal and temporal lobes (Cairns et al., 2007; Englund et al., 1994). Microscopic examination of FTD brains shows microvacuolation, gliosis, and neuronal loss primarily in layers 2 and 3 of the cortex, although these signs of degeneration spread through all cortical layers in some cases (Fig. 6.1) (Cairns et al., 2007; Englund et al., 1994; Tanzi et al., 1987).

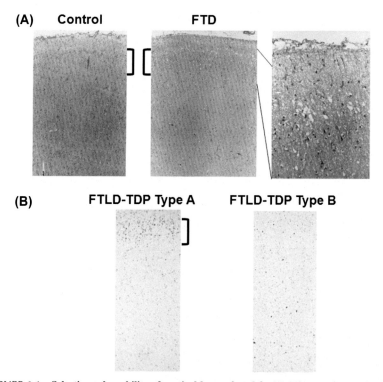

FIGURE 6.1   Selective vulnerability of cortical layers 2 and 3. (A) Microscopic examination of brains from patients with frontotemporal dementia (*FTD*) reveals degeneration of cortical layers 2 and 3 (*bracket*), with loss of neurons and microvacuolation, as seen in the higher magnification figure at *top right* (*Adapted with permission from Brun, A. (1987). Frontal lobe degeneration of non-Alzheimer type. I. Neuropathology.* Archives of Gerontology and Geriatrics, *6(3), 193–208.*) (B) Similarly, some subtypes of frontotemporal lobar degeneration (FTLD)-TDP pathology, particularly type A, are concentrated in cortical layers 2 and 3 (*bracket*), although other subtypes feature pathology throughout the cortex (FTLD-TDP type B). The brown aggregates in these images were immunostained for ubiquitin (*Adapted with permission from Sampathu, D.M., Neumann, M., Kwong, L.K., Chou, T.T., Micsenyi, M., Truax, A., et al. (2006). Pathological heterogeneity of frontotemporal lobar degeneration with ubiquitin-positive inclusions delineated by ubiquitin immunohistochemistry and novel monoclonal antibodies.* The American Journal of Pathology, *169(4), 1343–1352.* http://dx.doi.org/10.2353/ajpath.2006.060438.)

An intriguing aspect of neuronal loss in bvFTD is the selective early loss of von Economo neurons (VENs; see Chapter 1) and fork cells from the anterior cingulate and frontoinsular cortices (Fig. 6.2) (Kim et al., 2012; Santillo, Nilsson, & Englund, 2013; Seeley et al., 2006). VENs are large, bipolar neurons found only in the anterior cingulate and frontoinsular cortices of humans and a few other species (Allman et al., 2010). VENs are located mostly in layer 5, and loss of these neurons exceeds that of other neurons in layer 2/3 and layer 5 in patients with FTD (Kim et al., 2012; Santillo & Englund, 2014). Similarly, Fork cells are only found in the frontoinsular cortex, and are located in layer 5

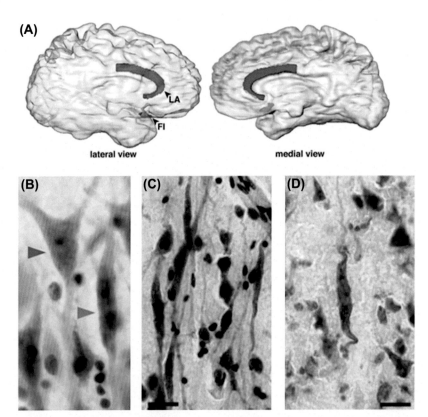

FIGURE 6.2 **Early loss of von Economo neurons (VENs) and fork cells in behavioral variant frontotemporal dementia (bvFTD).** (A) VENs and fork cells are found uniquely in the anterior cingulate and frontoinsular areas, regions selectively vulnerable in FTD. (*Adapted with permission from Allman, J. M., Tetreault, N. A., Hakeem, A. Y., Manaye, K. F., Semendeferi, K., Erwin, J. M., et al. (2011). The von Economo neurons in the frontoinsular and anterior cingulate cortex.* Annals of the New York Academy of Sciences, *1225, 59–71.* http://dx.doi.org/10.1111/j.1749-6632.2011.06011.x.) (B) VENs and fork cells are large projection neurons with unique morphology (*blue arrow,* fork cell; *pink arrow,* VEN) (*Adapted with permission from Kim, E.J., Sidhu, M., Gaus, S.E., Huang, E.J., Hof, P.R., Miller, B.L., et al. (2012). Selective frontoinsular von Economo neuron and fork cell loss in early behavioral variant frontotemporal dementia.* Cerebral Cortex, *22(2), 251–259.* http://dx.doi.org/10.1093/cercor/bhr004). (C and D) Relative to a healthy control brain (C) bvFTD patients show loss of VENs (D) and fork cells. FI, frontoinsular cortex; LA, anterior limbic area (*C and D adapted with permission from Seeley, W.W., Carlin, D.A., Allman, J.M., Macedo, M.N., Bush, C., Miller, B.L., et al.. (2006). Early frontotemporal dementia targets neurons unique to apes and humans.* Annals of Neurology, *60(6), 660–667.* http://dx.doi.org/10.1002/ana.21055.)

(Seeley et al., 2012). The function of VENs and fork cells is poorly understood, but their selective, early loss in bvFTD suggests that they might be involved in the emotional and social deficits of bvFTD patients. This finding could have exciting implications for bvFTD therapy, because understanding the mechanism behind the selective vulnerability of these neurons could highlight new targets for treatment in the early stages of bvFTD.

Current classification of FTLD pathology includes four classes based on the proteins found in pathological aggregates. These classes are termed *FTLD-tau (containing the microtubule associated protein tau), FTLD-TDP (containing the RNA-binding protein TDP43), FTLD-FUS (containing the RNA-binding protein FUS),* and *FTLD-UPS (containing ubiquitinated aggregates negative for the other FTD-related proteins)* (Mackenzie et al., 2010). FTLD-tau and FTLD-TDP together comprise 85–90% of all FTLD cases (Mackenzie et al., 2010). FTLD-tau was the first identified class of FTLD pathology. Early studies of postmortem FTD brains noted the presence of protein aggregates in neurons and glia, some of which were immunoreactive for tau (Englund et al., 1994). FTLD-tau has been heavily studied, and includes eight subtypes, the most common of which are Pick disease, PSP, and corticobasal degeneration (Mackenzie et al., 2010). These classes of pathology all involve aggregates of hyperphosphorylated tau that differ in morphology and anatomical distribution, as well as the isoforms of tau contained in the aggregates (Komori, 1999). All types of FTLD-tau pathology are distinct from the neurofibrillary tangles characteristic of AD (Delacourte et al., 1996; Ksiezak-Reding et al., 1994; Sergeant et al., 1997; Sergeant, Wattez, & Delacourte, 1999). Whereas the role of tau pathological change in disease is unknown, recent data have led to the hypothesis that tau can spread in a "prion-like" manner through the brain, incorporating normal tau molecules into tau pathological states and producing progressive neurodegeneration (Frost, Jacks, & Diamond, 2009; Sanders et al., 2014).

After many years of classifying all tau-negative FTLD as "FTLD-U" because of the presence of ubiquitinated protein inclusions, it was discovered that the majority of tau-negative FTLD cases have protein aggregates immunoreactive for the RNA-binding protein TDP-43 (Neumann et al., 2006). FTLD-TDP is grouped into four subtypes that vary in the anatomic and subcellular localization of the TDP-43 aggregates (Mackenzie et al., 2006, 2011; Sampathu et al., 2006). It is thought that loss of TDP-43 function caused by aggregation may be a factor in neurodegeneration in FTLD-TDP. TDP-43 is an RNA-binding protein that regulates splicing of hundreds of targets and is often depleted from the nucleus in FTLD-TDP (Cenik et al., 2011; Neumann et al., 2006). Additionally, data from postmortem FTLD-TDP brains and cell culture experiments have led to suggestions that TDP-43 pathological states may spread in a similar prion-like manner to tau pathology (Irwin et al., 2013; Nonaka et al., 2013).

Of the remaining 10–15% of FTLD cases, the majority have aggregates immunoreactive for the RNA binding protein FUS, and are termed *FTLD-FUS* (Neumann, Rademakers, et al., 2009). Interestingly, these cases have not been linked to mutations in FUS (Neumann, Rademakers, et al., 2009). The final class of FTD pathology is termed *FTLD-UPS* because it features ubiquitinated inclusions that are negative for tau, TDP-43, and FUS (Mackenzie et al., 2010). To date, FTLD-UPS is only known to occur in cases caused by mutations in the gene *CHMP2B* (Skibinski et al., 2005).

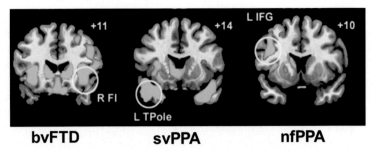

bvFTD   **svPPA**   **nfPPA**

FIGURE 6.3   **Distinct neuronal networks degenerate in each FTD syndrome.** Each FTD syndrome features degeneration of distinct neuronal networks. In behavioral variant frontotemporal dementia (*bvFTD*), the salience network degenerates, with the right frontoinsular cortex being a key brain region. Semantic variant primary progressive aphasia (*svPPA*) is characterized by temporal lobe degeneration, particularly the left temporal pole. The frontoinsular and perisylvian cortices are particularly affected in nonfluent/agrammatic primary progressive aphasia (*nfPPA*). *Adapted with permission from Seeley, W.W., Crawford, R.K., Zhou, J., Miller, B.L., & Greicius, M.D. (2009). Neurodegenerative diseases target large-scale human brain networks.* Neuron, *62(1), 42–52.* http://dx.doi.org/10.1016/j.neuron.2009.03.024; pii:S0896-6273(09)00249-9.

IMAGING STUDIES OF FRONTOTEMPORAL DEMENTIA

FTD has been the subject of many imaging studies using structural magnetic resonance imaging (MRI), ^{18}F-fluorodeoxyglucose positron emission tomography (FDG-PET), single photon emission computerized tomography (SPECT), and white matter imaging techniques. Functional MRI (fMRI) studies have also been used to identify the brain networks affected in each FTD subtype (Fig. 6.3). These studies have also identified associations between common FTD behavioral abnormalities and dysfunction in particular brain regions. Whereas the dysfunctional brain networks in FTD include a number of subcortical regions, degeneration (as measured by atrophy in MRI, hypoperfusion in SPECT, or hypometabolism in FDG-PET) of specific cortical regions appears to drive many of the behavioral and language deficits of FTD. In support of the importance of these changes for the clinical syndromes of patients with FTD, imaging studies of presymptomatic carriers of autosomal dominant genetic causes of FTD begin to show atrophy and reduced connectivity of relevant brain regions around 10–15 years before the appearance of FTD symptoms (Dopper et al., 2013; Ferrari et al., 2014).

Behavioral variant FTD is associated with degeneration of, and disruption of connectivity between, brain regions of the salience network (see Fig. 6.3) (Agosta et al., 2013; Boxer et al., 2011; Diehl et al., 2004; Rascovsky et al., 2011; Rosen et al., 2002; Seeley, Crawford, Zhou, Miller, & Greicius, 2009; Whitwell, Anderson, Scahill, Rossor, & Fox, 2004; Zhou et al., 2010). The salience network includes both cortical (insula, anterior cingulate cortex) and subcortical (putamen, amygdala, dorsomedial thalamus, hypothalamus) brain regions (Seeley et al., 2007). Imaging data collectively indicate that frontal and anterior temporal cortical degeneration and disrupted connectivity with

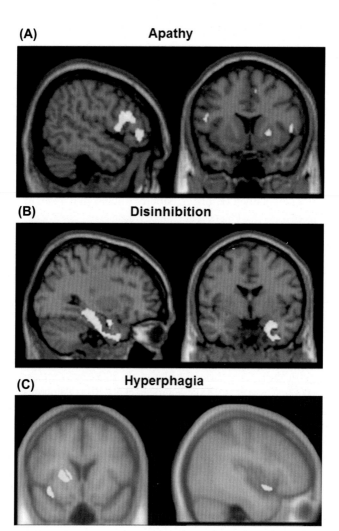

(A) Apathy

(B) Disinhibition

(C) Hyperphagia

FIGURE 6.4 **Abnormal behaviors in behavioral variant frontotemporal dementia (bvFTD) are associated with degeneration of specific cortical regions.** Whereas the salience network degenerates in bvFTD, certain abnormal behaviors are associated with degeneration of specific nodes of the salience network. Two common signs of bvFTD, apathy and disinhibition, are associated with degeneration of distinct brain regions. (A) Apathy is commonly associated with frontal cortical regions such as the orbitofrontal, anterior cingulate, and prefrontal cortices. (*Adapted with permission from Zamboni, G., Huey, E.D., Krueger, F., Nichelli, P.F., & Grafman, J. (2008). Apathy and disinhibition in frontotemporal dementia: insights into their neural correlates.* Neurology, *71(10), 736–742.* http://dx.doi.org/10.1212/01.wnl.0000324920.96835.95.) (B) Disinhibition is more associated with degeneration of temporal regions such as the insular cortex and subcortical regions such as the amygdala and nucleus accumbens. (*Adapted with permission from Zamboni, G., Huey, E.D., Krueger, F., Nichelli, P.F., & Grafman, J. (2008). Apathy and disinhibition in frontotemporal dementia: insights into their neural correlates.* Neurology, *71(10), 736–742.* http://dx.doi.org/10.1212/01.wnl.0000324920.96835.95.) (C) Dietary changes are another common sign of bvFTD, with hyperphagia being a common change. Hyperphagia in bvFTD is associated with degeneration of the right orbitofrontal and insular cortices (*Adapted with permission from Woolley, J.D., Gorno-Tempini, M.L., Seeley, W.W., Rankin, K., Lee, S.S., Matthews, B.R., et al. (2007). Binge eating is associated with right orbitofrontal-insular-striatal atrophy in frontotemporal dementia.* Neurology, *69(14), 1424–1433.* http://dx.doi.org/10.1212/01.wnl.0000277461.06713.23.)

subcortical regions underlies the abnormal behavior and personality changes of bvFTD. Within this broad network, dysfunction in particular brain regions is associated with some of the specific behavioral changes seen in bvFTD, namely apathy, disinhibition, and dietary changes (Fig. 6.4).

Apathy is most tightly correlated with degeneration of the frontal cortex (McMurtray et al., 2006). In particular, apathy ratings of patients correlate with dysfunction of the right orbitofrontal cortex, anterior cingulate cortex, and regions of the prefrontal cortex, as well as subcortical structures such as the right caudate and putamen (Eslinger, Moore, Antani, Anderson, & Grossman, 2012; Le Ber et al., 2006; Peters et al., 2006; Rosen et al., 2005; Zamboni, Huey, Krueger, Nichelli, & Grafman, 2008). In resting state fMRI, increased connectivity of the prefrontal cortex with the salience and executive networks is associated with increased apathy (Farb et al., 2013). This association is consistent with the importance of the executive network for behavioral inhibition (Smith, Tindell, Aldridge, & Berridge, 2009).

Disinhibition is strongly associated with dysfunction of brain networks in the temporal lobe, and is more weakly associated with frontal lobe dysfunction (McMurtray et al., 2006). Disinhibition scores correlate with dysfunction of the orbitofrontal cortex, as well as temporal brain regions such as the insular cortex, amygdala, and nucleus accumbens (Le Ber et al., 2006; McMurtray et al., 2006; Peters et al., 2006; Rosen et al., 2005; Schroeter et al., 2011; Zamboni et al., 2008). In resting state fMRI, disinhibition is correlated with impaired connectivity between the insular cortex and the rest of the salience network (Farb et al., 2013).

The two brain regions most commonly associated with dietary changes in FTD are the right insular cortex and the right orbitofrontal cortex (Schroeter et al., 2011; Whitwell et al., 2007; Woolley et al., 2007). These findings are consistent with the role of the insular cortex in interoception, including taste, and the orbitofrontal cortex in processing the enjoyment of rewarding stimuli such as sweet foods (Craig, 2009; Kringelbach, 2005; Maffei, Haley, & Fontanini, 2012).

Imaging studies of both PPA variants have revealed dysfunction in brain networks that overlap between the two variants and with bvFTD, but with important distinctions that result in the different clinical presentations. Patients with svPPA may develop dysfunction across the frontal and temporal lobes, but the characteristic lesion associated with svPPA is degeneration of the anterior temporal lobe, particularly the left temporal pole, a region important for semantic memory as well as for social behavior (Fig. 6.5) (Chan et al., 2001; Diehl et al., 2004; Drzezga et al., 2008; Galton et al., 2001; Gorno-Tempini et al., 2004, 2011; Grabowski, Cho, Vonsattel, Rebeck, & Greenberg, 2001; Mummery et al., 1999, 2000; Rabinovici et al., 2008; Rosen et al., 2002; Strand et al., 2007; Whitwell et al., 2004). In contrast, patients with nfPPA have dysfunction of the left frontoinsular cortex and the cortex around the Sylvian fissure, which include areas critical for language processing (Caso et al., 2014; Cruchaga et al., 2009; Gorno-Tempini et al., 2004, 2011; Nestor et al., 2003; Price, 2000; Rabinovici et al., 2008; Seeley et al., 2009; Whitwell et al., 2004).

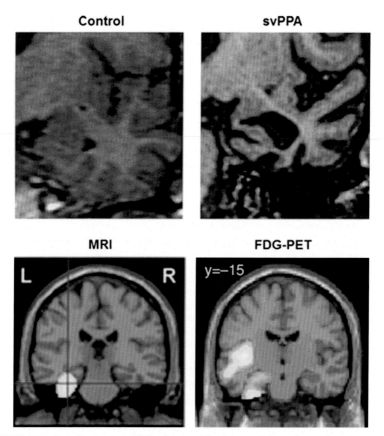

FIGURE 6.5   Anterior temporal lobe degeneration in semantic variant primary progressive aphasia (*svPPA*) correlates with deficits in semantic tasks. There is severe degeneration of the left temporal pole and other anterior temporal regions in svPPA (Top, *adapted with permission from Chan D., Fox N. C., Scahill R. I., Crum W. R., Whitwell J. L., Leschziner G., et al. (2001). Patterns of temporal lobe atrophy in semantic dementia and Alzheimer's disease. Annals of* Neurology, *49(4), 433–442.*) The degree of degeneration of these areas is associated with deficits in semantic tasks as shown by either by magnetic resonance imaging (MRI) (Bottom left, *adapted with permission from Williams, G.B., Nestor, P.J., & Hodges, J.R. (2005). Neural correlates of semantic and behavioral deficits in frontotemporal dementia.* Neuroimage, *24(4), 1042–1051.* http://dx.doi.org/10.1016/j.neuroimage.2004.10.023), or 18F-fluorodeoxyglucose positron emission tomography (FDG-PEG) (Bottom right, *adapted with permission from Mion, M., Patterson, K., Acosta-Cabronero, J., Pengas, G., Izquierdo-Garcia, D., Hong, Y. T., et al. (2010). What the left and right anterior fusiform gyri tell us about semantic memory.* Brain, *133(11), 3256–3268.* http://dx.doi.org/10.1093/brain/awq272.)

Multiple studies have also examined the association between the deficits in comprehension, speech, and language that occur in svPPA and nfPPA. As might be expected based on the degeneration of the anterior temporal lobe in svPPA, semantic deficits are associated with dysfunction of the anterior temporal lobe (San Pedro, Deutsch, Liu, & Mountz, 2000; Williams, Nestor, &

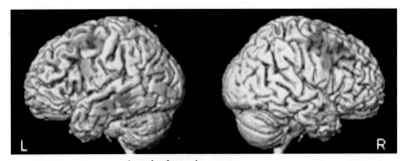

Apraxia of speech
nfPPA with apraxia of speech
PPA-not otherwise specified

FIGURE 6.6   Nonfluent/agrammatic primary progressive aphasia *(nfPPA)* **language deficits associated with degeneration of distinct brain regions.** The association of agrammatism and apraxia of speech with degeneration of distinct brain regions is emphasized by comparing regions of atrophy in patients with nfPPA and apraxia of speech *(green)* or with apraxia of speech only *(red)*. Apraxia of speech is associated with degeneration of premotor and supplementary motor cortices, whereas nfPPA patients also show the perisylvian degeneration that is associated with agrammatism. In this study, patients with aphasia that did not meet the criteria for nfPPA or semantic variant primary progressive aphasia (svPPA) *(blue,* PPA not otherwise specified) show a broader pattern of atrophy in both the frontal and temporal lobes. *Adapted with permission from Josephs, K.A., Duffy, J.R., Strand, E.A., Whitwell, J.L., Layton, K.F., Parisi, J.E., et al. (2006). Clinicopathological and imaging correlates of progressive aphasia and apraxia of speech. Brain, 129(Pt 6), 1385–1398.*

Hodges, 2005). Some studies have refined this association to the left inferior temporal gyrus and the anterior fusiform gyrus, although there is also a weaker association of semantic deficits with dysfunction of these regions in the right hemisphere (Mion et al., 2010; Mummery et al., 1999; Williams et al., 2005). A more recent study of svPPA patients revealed dysfunction across a network of brain regions, including regions of the anterior temporal lobe (temporal pole, amygdala, and anterior hippocampus) and the ventromedial frontal lobe (La Joie et al., 2014).

Although nfPPA involves both agrammatism and apraxia of speech, these two syndromes may occur separately in some patients (Josephs et al., 2012). Comparison of these patients has revealed distinct patterns of neurodegeneration that underlie each syndrome (Fig. 6.6). Apraxia of speech is associated with dysfunction of the left premotor and supplementary motor cortices (Josephs et al., 2006, 2010; Whitwell et al., 2013). In contrast, agrammatism is associated with dysfunction of a broader network of regions in the frontal and temporal lobes that includes perisylvian cortical regions, the insular cortex, and the Broca area (Josephs et al., 2006, 2010; Whitwell et al., 2013).

Collectively, imaging studies comparing the FTD syndromes, as well as those investigating signs and symptoms within each syndrome, reveal a robust association between the clinical presentation of a patient and the cortical regions most affected by the disease. The fact that atrophy and reduced connectivity can be observed a decade before symptom onset in dominantly inherited FTD cases further strengthens this association. Imaging data are much more strongly correlated with the clinical syndrome than is postmortem pathology. As we discuss in the following section, there is some association of causal genetic mutations with the clinical syndrome, but these associations are again weaker than those with imaging data.

FRONTOTEMPORAL DEMENTIA GENETICS

FTD has both sporadic and dominantly inherited forms, but genetics play a major role in FTD, given that around 40% of cases are familial and around 25% are dominantly inherited (Chow, Miller, Hayashi, & Geschwind, 1999; Goldman et al., 2005; Ratnavalli et al., 2002; Rohrer et al., 2009; Seelaar et al., 2008; Stevens et al., 1998). Dominantly inherited FTD is caused by mutations in seven known genes with diverse functions. By far the three most common genetic causes of FTD are mutations in the genes for the microtubule-associated protein tau *(MAPT),* the secreted growth factor progranulin *(GRN),* and the recently discovered gene *C9ORF72* (Boeve et al., 2012; Mahoney et al., 2012; Rademakers, Neumann, & Mackenzie, 2012). Reports on the incidence of each of these mutations are variable, with *C9ORF72* mutations (5–12% of all FTD, 10–35% of familial FTD) being more common than *MAPT* or *GRN* mutations (1–10% of all FTD, 5–25% of familial FTD) (Beck et al., 2008; Boeve et al., 2012; Cruts et al., 2006; DeJesus-Hernandez et al., 2011; Dobson-Stone et al., 2013; Gass et al., 2006; Gijselinck, Van Broeckhoven, & Cruts, 2008; Mahoney et al., 2012; Majounie et al., 2012; Pickering-Brown et al., 2008; Rademakers, Cruts, & van Broeckhoven, 2004; Seelaar et al., 2008; Sha et al., 2012; Snowden et al., 2012; Van Langenhove et al., 2013). Much less common FTD-related mutations include those in the RNA binding proteins TDP-43 *(TARDBP)* and FUS, the endosomal sorting complex required for transport (ESCRT-III) component *CHMP2B*, and the AAA-adenosine triphosphatase (ATPase) valosin containing protein *(VCP)* (Benajiba et al., 2009; Broustal et al., 2010; Skibinski et al., 2005; Synofzik et al., 2014; Van Langenhove et al., 2010; Watts et al., 2004).

The FTD-related mutation in *C9ORF72* is hexanucleotide repeat expansion of GGGGCC in a noncoding region of the gene (DeJesus-Hernandez et al., 2011; Renton et al., 2011). The expansion also causes ALS and FTD-ALS (see Chapter 9 and DeJesus-Hernandez et al., 2011; Renton et al., 2011). Healthy individuals typically have fewer than 20–30 GGGGCC repeats, whereas those with FTD and ALS are associated with having 700–1600 repeats (DeJesus-Hernandez et al., 2011). Experimental models have shown toxicity beginning around 30 repeats, with more repeats producing greater toxicity; greater numbers of repeats are also associated with shorter survival times in patients (van Blitterswijk et al., 2013; Lee et al., 2013; Mizielinska et al., 2014; Xu et al., 2013). *C9ORF72* expansions typically cause FTLD-TDP, and the GGGGCC repeats produce RNA foci that accumulate in neurons of the frontal cortex and spinal cord (Boeve et al., 2012; Boxer et al., 2011; DeJesus-Hernandez et al.,

2011; Mahoney et al., 2012; Simon-Sanchez et al., 2012; Snowden et al., 2012). The GGGGCC repeat RNA also undergoes an unusual form of translation referred to as *repeat-associated non-ATG (RAN) translation* to form a total of five distinct dipeptide repeat proteins [repeats of (GA), glycine–proline (GP), glycine–arginine (GR), proline–alanine (PA), and proline–arginine (PR)] that accumulate in the frontal, temporal, and motor cortices (Ash et al., 2013; Gendron et al., 2013; Mori et al., 2013; Zu et al., 2013). Patients with *C9ORF72* expansions most commonly develop bvFTD, but may also have with svPPA or nfPPA (Boeve et al., 2012; Mahoney et al., 2012; Simon-Sanchez et al., 2012; Snowden et al., 2012; Van Langenhove et al., 2013). The normal function of *C9ORF72* is poorly understood, as it received little study before identification as a major cause of FTD and ALS. However, available data suggest a role for *C9ORF72* in endosomal trafficking (Farg et al., 2014). This is intriguing given the association of mutations in other FTD-related genes with deficits in endosomal trafficking and protein degradation, such as *GRN*, *CHMP2B*, and *VCP*.

Mutations in the tau gene *(MAPT)* were the first genetic cause of FTD to be discovered. These *MAPT* mutations cause FTD with parkinsonism linked to chromosome 17 (FTDP-17), and at least 44 FTDP-17–associated *MAPT* mutations have now been identified (Hutton et al., 1998; Poorkaj et al., 1998; Rademakers et al., 2004, 2012; Spillantini et al., 1998). All FTD-related *MAPT* mutations are associated with FTLD-tau (Mackenzie et al., 2010). Patients with *MAPT* mutations most commonly exhibit bvFTD, although *MAPT* mutations may also cause PPA (generally nfPPA), CBS, and PSP (Higgins, Litvan, Pho, Li, & Nee, 1998; Pickering-Brown et al., 2008; Rohrer et al., 2009, 2011; Van Langenhove et al., 2013). Tau is a microtubule-associated protein with six isoforms expressed in the adult brain, composed of either three or four microtubule-binding domains (3R or 4R tau), and the inclusion of 0, 1, or 2 repeats near the N-terminus of the protein (Goedert, Spillantini, Potier, Ulrich, & Crowther, 1989). FTD-related *MAPT* mutations may interfere with the microtubule binding activity of tau, increase the propensity for phosphorylation and aggregation, or interfere with splicing of *MAPT* RNA (Goedert & Jakes, 2005; Rademakers et al., 2004).

Mutations in *GRN* were identified as a major genetic cause of FTD in 2006 (Baker et al., 2006; Cruts et al., 2006; Gass et al., 2006). All FTD-related *GRN* mutations are loss-of-function mutations. They occur throughout the entire gene and disrupt progranulin function through a variety of mechanisms, the most common of which is nonsense-mediated decay (Baker et al., 2006; Cruts et al., 2006; Gass et al., 2006; Shankaran et al., 2008; Wang et al., 2010). *GRN* mutations are associated with FTLD-TDP that is most severe in layer 2 of the cortex (Mackenzie et al., 2010, 2011). *GRN* mutations most commonly cause bvFTD, but commonly cause PPA variants as well (Beck et al., 2008; Kelley et al., 2009; Pickering-Brown et al., 2008; Rohrer et al., 2011). Progranulin is a secreted glycoprotein that acts as a growth factor and has antiinflammatory effects, and loss of either of these functions could play a role in FTD pathogenesis (Bateman & Bennett, 2009).

EXPERIMENTAL MODELS

To date, all experimental models of FTD have focused on the genetic causes of the disease. Both in vitro and in vivo approaches have been used, including cell lines, primary neuronal culture, and induced pluripotent stem cell (iPSC)–derived neurons in vitro, and in vivo use of animal models such as the fruit fly *Drosophila*, the nematode *Caenorhabditis elegans*, zebrafish, and mice. Given the recent discovery of most FTD-related genes, many of these models have been developed since 2010, and are beginning to provide insight into the mechanisms underlying both inherited and sporadic FTD. In the following sections, we will focus on models of FTD based on the common *C9ORF72*, *MAPT*, and *GRN* mutations, but exciting discoveries are also being made with models of FTD with *VCP* and *CHMP2B* mutations.

C9ORF72

With the discovery in 2011 that a repeat expansion in *C9ORF72* causes FTD, a major question has been the mechanism by which the expansion causes neuronal dysfunction and disease. Three potential mechanisms include loss of function resulting from reduced expression of C9ORF72, toxicity of the GGGGCC repeat RNA, or toxicity of the dipeptide repeat (DPR) proteins that are produced by RAN translation of the repeat RNA. The loss-of-function hypothesis came from observations that *C9ORF72* mRNA levels were reduced in individuals with the repeat expansion (Ciura et al., 2013; DeJesus-Hernandez et al., 2011; Renton et al., 2011). There is some experimental support for this hypothesis, as knockdown of *C9ORF72* impairs endocytosis in neuroblastoma cells and causes motor deficits in zebrafish (Ciura et al., 2013; Farg et al., 2014). However, knockdown of *C9ORF72* does not have adverse effects in mice and methylation of the *C9ORF72* gene reduces expression and appears to have protective effects in humans carrying the repeat expansion (Day & Roberson, 2015; Lagier-Tourenne et al., 2013). Thus most recent studies have focused on toxicity of the GGGGCC repeat RNA and DPR proteins.

There is evidence for toxicity of both GGGGCC repeat RNA and DPR proteins produced by the *C9ORF72* repeat expansion, and recent data suggest that they may interact. One potential mechanism for toxicity of GGGGCC repeat RNA is binding and sequestration of RNA binding proteins. A study expressing 38–72 GGGGCC repeats in neuroblastoma cells or zebrafish embryos found RNA foci that colocalized with RNA binding proteins; the cells with RNA foci also expressed apoptotic markers (Lee et al., 2013). Similarly, expression of 30 GGGGCC repeats in *Drosophila* eye caused binding of the RNA-binding protein Pur α to the repeat RNA, and overexpression of Pur α prevented eye degeneration (Xu et al., 2013). However, investigation of iPSC-derived neurons from *C9ORF72* expansion carriers revealed the presence of RNA foci without sequestration of RNA binding proteins (Almeida et al., 2013). The GGGGCC RNA may also bind to other types of proteins. A study using cell lines, as well as lymphocytes and iPSC-derived motor neurons from patients with the *C9ORF72* repeat expansion, revealed binding of the repeat RNA to the nucleolar protein nucleolin, with resulting nucleolar dysfunction (Haeusler et al., 2014).

Work with the *C9ORF72* RAN DPRs indicates potentially different mechanisms of toxicity for different DPR proteins. Studies of GA DPR proteins in cell lines and primary neurons indicates toxicity through interference with proteosomal activity, with subsequent impairment of dendritic branching and activation of apoptosis (May et al., 2014; Zhang et al., 2014). In further support for the importance of impaired protein degradation in DPR toxicity, primary neurons transfected with GGGGCC repeat constructs and iPSC-derived neurons from *C9ORF72* expansion carriers form p62-positive aggregates, a sign of autophagy dysfunction, similar to those in *C9ORF72* FTD and ALS patients (Almeida et al., 2013; May et al., 2014). Furthermore, iPSC-derived neurons containing the *C9ORF72* repeat expansion are more sensitive to toxicity from autophagy inhibitors (Almeida et al., 2013). There is also abundant evidence for toxicity of arginine-containing DPR peptides, particularly PR DPRs (Mizielinska et al., 2014; Wen et al., 2014; Zu et al., 2013). In contrast to poly-GA DPRs, the poly-PR and poly-GR DPRs may be toxic through interference with nucleolar function (Tao et al., 2015; Wen et al., 2014). The arginine-containing DPRs form aggregates in the nucleoli, with subsequent formation of stress granules in the cells (Tao et al., 2015; Wen et al., 2014).

Multiple studies have now investigated the comparative toxicity of GGGGCC repeat RNA and DPR proteins by designing expression constructs of GGGGCC RNA that are not translated into protein ("RNA only" constructs) and other constructs that express the DPR proteins without the GGGGCC RNA sequence. Both unmodified GGGGCC repeats and arginine-containing DPR peptides from non-GGGGCC sequences produced eye degeneration in *Drosophila*, but the RNA-only repeats did not, suggesting that the DPR peptides may be the more toxic species (Mizielinska et al., 2014). However, there may be synergistic toxic effects between the GGGGCC repeat RNA and DPR peptides. In a separate study, both the GGGGCC RNA-only repeats and PR DPR peptides were toxic to rat primary cortical neurons, but coexpression of an RNA-only construct with a 50-repeat poly-PR peptide produced much greater toxicity than either construct alone (Wen et al., 2014).

Taken together, experimental models have produced evidence that both the GGGGCC repeat RNA and the DPR proteins produced by RAN translation may contribute to development of FTD and ALS in patients carrying the *C9ORF72* repeat expansion. As such, strategies targeting the repeat RNA for degradation may be a promising therapeutic approach (Lagier-Tourenne et al., 2013; Su et al., 2014).

Tau (*MAPT*)

Due to its involvement in AD, FTD, and other disorders, there has been long-standing interest in modeling tau-mediated neurodegeneration. Tau has been heavily studied in both in vitro and in vivo models, so we will focus primarily on in vivo studies, which have tested the effects of expressing both wild-type and mutant human tau in animal models. Interestingly, expression of wild-type human tau produces adverse effects in some circumstances. In *Drosophila*, several studies have found that expressing wild-type human tau is somewhat toxic as measured by eye degeneration, reduced lifespan, or deformation of mushroom bodies (Jackson et al., 2002; Karsten et al., 2006; Kosmidis, Grammenoudi, Papanikolopoulou, & Skoulakis, 2010; Wittmann et al., 2001). Transgenic expression of wild-type tau in mice has produced variable results, with some studies reporting relatively minor adverse effects and others reporting tau hyperphosphorylation and aggregation, with neuronal axonopathy (Andorfer et al., 2003; Brion, Tremp, & Octave, 1999; Gotz et al., 1995; Spittaels et al., 1999).

The effects of FTD-related mutant tau in animal models are more severe than those of wild-type tau. The FTD-related mutations P301L, R406W, and V337M all produce similar toxic effects as wild-type human tau in *Drosophila*, with greater toxicity of mutant tau than wild-type tau (Karsten et al., 2006; Kosmidis et al., 2010; Wittmann et al., 2001). Multiple transgenic mouse lines have been developed that express the P301L, P301S, R406W, and V337M mutations. Most of these models develop cortical and hippocampal tau pathology that resembles aspects of that seen in FTD (Götz, Chen, Barmettler, & Nitsch, 2001; Ikeda et al., 2005; Lewis et al., 2000; Ramsden et al., 2005; Tanemura et al., 2001; Yoshiyama et al., 2007). Several of the P301L, P301S, and R406W models also develop cortical and hippocampal neuronal loss, with associated motor and memory deficits (Ikeda et al., 2005; Lewis et al., 2000; Ramsden et al., 2005; Yoshiyama et al., 2007). Similarly, expression of P301L tau in zebrafish causes tau hyperphosphorylation and aggregation, neuronal death, and motor deficits (Paquet et al., 2009).

Interestingly, several of these models dissociate tau pathology from functional deficits. The PS19 line of mice expressing the P301S mutation develops synapse loss and microgliosis before significant accumulation of tau pathology (Yoshiyama et al., 2007). Another V337M-expressing line does not develop tau aggregates, but nonetheless develops repetitive grooming behavior that may model the compulsive, repetitive behavior seen in FTD (Warmus et al., 2014). This repetitive behavior is caused by synaptic dysfunction in the insular cortex and ventral striatum (Warmus et al., 2014). The relationship between tau pathology and functional deficits has also been studied by using inducible transgenes to express mutant forms of tau in mice. This approach has been used to control expression of P301L tau or the "proaggregant" ΔK280 mutant tau, both of which cause tau pathology, loss of neurons and synapses, and impaired performance on memory tasks (Mocanu et al., 2008; SantaCruz et al., 2005; Sydow et al., 2011). In both mouse lines, switching off expression of mutant tau successfully reduced levels of mutant tau and rescued neuron/synapse loss and memory deficits (Mocanu et al., 2008; SantaCruz et al., 2005; Sydow et al., 2011). Tau pathology was not improved by reducing mutant tau expression, indicating that tau pathology is not sufficient to cause neuronal loss and memory deficits in these mouse lines and suggesting that soluble mutant tau may be responsible for these deleterious effects (Mocanu et al., 2008; SantaCruz et al., 2005; Sydow et al., 2011).

In summary, animal models of FTD-related tau mutations have shown that most of the mutations produce FTD-like tau pathological conditions with aggregates of hyperphosphorylated tau, as well as synaptic dysfunction, neuron loss, and behavioral deficits. However, multiple studies show some degree of dissociation between tau pathology and functional deficits, indicating that the tau aggregates may not be the toxic species in these models. Instead, soluble mutant tau may disrupt synaptic function through as yet undescribed mechanisms.

Progranulin (*GRN*)

Because all FTD-related *GRN* mutations are loss-of-function mutations, experimental models of FTD-*GRN* have used various strategies to produce partial or complete progranulin deficiency. Knocking down progranulin expression with small interfering RNA (siRNA) or short hairpin RNA (shRNA) in cell lines or primary neurons reduces cell survival and increases sensitivity to cellular stressors, with similar results in primary neurons from $Grn^{-/-}$ mice (Gao et al., 2010; Guo, Tapia, Bamji, Cynader, & Jia, 2010; Kleinberger et al., 2010; Ryan et al., 2009). Similarly, iPSC-derived neurons from FTD patients with loss-of-function *GRN* mutations are progranulin-deficient and are more sensitive to various stressors (Almeida et al., 2012). Primary $Grn^{-/-}$ neurons or neurons treated with progranulin siRNA have impaired dendritic outgrowth, which can be rescued by adding progranulin to the culture medium (Gass et al., 2012). Adding progranulin to the culture medium also improves survival and neurite outgrowth of primary motor neurons and cortical neurons even without progranulin knockdown (De Muynck et al., 2013; Van Damme et al., 2008). These effects are consistent with progranulin's function as a secreted growth factor in other cell types, and indicate that progranulin has neurotrophic effects (Bateman & Bennett, 2009). In vivo studies with zebrafish are consistent with these data and show that progranulin knockdown impairs axon growth in motor neurons, whereas progranulin overexpression increases axon growth (Chitramuthu, Baranowski, Kay, Bateman, & Bennett, 2010; De Muynck et al., 2013; Laird et al., 2010).

Several mouse lines have been generated to model FTD with *GRN* mutations, and mice with both partial ($Grn^{+/-}$) and complete ($Grn^{-/-}$) progranulin deficiency have been proposed as appropriate models. By 6–8 months of age, both $Grn^{+/-}$ and $Grn^{-/-}$ mice develop deficits in sociability, social dominance, and fear conditioning that resemble social withdrawal and emotional blunting in bvFTD (Filiano et al., 2013; Ghoshal, Dearborn, Wozniak, & Cairns, 2012; Kayasuga et al., 2007; Yin, Dumont, et al., 2010). When exposed to a novel, social environment, $Grn^{+/-}$ and $Grn^{-/-}$ mice exhibit reduced activation of the central amygdala that may indicate amygdala dysfunction (Filiano et al., 2013). As with certain tau mouse models, these functional deficits are dissociated from FTD-like pathology, because $Grn^{+/-}$ mice have not been reported to develop

TDP-43 aggregates, neuronal loss, or gliosis in any brain region (Filiano et al., 2013).

In contrast to $Grn^{+/-}$ mice, $Grn^{-/-}$ mice develop progressive gliosis, inflammation, and lipofuscinosis in multiple brain regions, particularly in the ventral posteromedial and posterolateral nuclei of the thalamus (Ahmed et al., 2010; Filiano et al., 2013; Gotzl et al., 2014; Tanaka, Chambers, Matsuwaki, Yamanouchi, & Nishihara, 2014; Wils et al., 2012; Yin, Dumont, et al., 2010). Some studies also report an increase in TDP-43 phosphorylation and aggregation in $Grn^{-/-}$ mice 20 months of age and older (Gotzl et al., 2014; Tanaka et al., 2014). $Grn^{-/-}$ mice have a hyperactive inflammatory response that results in increased susceptibility to inflammatory injury, which is likely caused by loss of microglial progranulin (Iguchi et al., 2013; Martens et al., 2012; Yin, Banerjee, et al., 2010). However, a major caveat for the use of $Grn^{-/-}$ mice as a model of FTD-GRN is the presence of lipofuscinosis. Accelerated accumulation of lipofuscin is characteristic of neuronal ceroid lipofuscinosis, a lysosomal storage disorder that has been reported in individuals homozygous for loss-of-function *GRN* mutations (Canafoglia et al., 2014; Smith et al., 2012). Thus it appears that in humans and mice, partial or complete progranulin haploinsufficiency produces two distinct disorders.

THERAPEUTIC APPROACHES

There are currently no disease-modifying treatments for FTD, although some drugs are used to manage FTD symptoms. Selective serotonin reuptake inhibitors may be useful in alleviating some of the abnormal behaviors of bvFTD, and atypical antipsychotics are also used in some cases (Huey, Putnam, & Grafman, 2006; Nardell & Tampi, 2014). However, the need for effective FTD treatments is great. As described, experimental models of FTD and genetic studies of FTD patients have highlighted promising targets for therapies for both sporadic and inherited FTD.

Therapies of General Relevance

One promising new target for FTD therapy is glutamate receptor dysfunction. Two recent studies using genetic mouse models of FTD support targeting glutamate receptor function. In one study, repetitive behaviors in a V337M tau mouse model were associated with synaptic dysfunction in the insular cortex and ventral striatum, and were corrected by the N-methyl-D-aspartate (NMDA) receptor agonist D-cycloserine (Warmus et al., 2014). NMDA agonists have not been tested in patients with FTD, but there is some evidence that NMDA antagonists may have detrimental effects. Despite promising initial case studies, trials of the NMDA antagonist memantine for FTD therapy have shown either no improvement or detrimental effects (Boxer et al., 2013; Diehl-Schmid, Forstl, Perneczky, Pohl, & Kurz, 2008; Swanberg, 2007; Vercelletto et al., 2011). Given these results, NMDA agonists may be useful for FTD treatment.

In another study using a mouse model of FTD from *CHMP2B* mutations, deficits in social behavior were associated with elevated expression of the α-amino-3-hydroxy-5-methyl-4-isoxazolepropionic acid (AMPA) subunit GluA2 in the medial prefrontal cortex, and were corrected by knocking down GluA2 or by treatment with an AMPA receptor antagonist (Gascon & Gao, 2014). Importantly, this study also showed elevated levels of GluA2 and GluA4 in the brains of patients with sporadic FTD or FTD-*GRN* (Gascon & Gao, 2014). It is therefore possible that drugs targeting glutamate receptors might improve FTD symptoms by correcting synaptic dysfunction underlying the disease.

There is also considerable interest in antiinflammatory therapies for FTD. Treatment of the PS19 mouse model of P301S tau mutations with the immunosuppressant drug FK506 improves survival and tau pathosis (Yoshiyama et al., 2007). In progranulin-deficient mice, loss of microglial progranulin increases susceptibility to inflammatory injury, which could be a potential mechanism in development of FTD-*GRN* (Martens et al., 2012). Furthermore, a recent genome-wide association study (GWAS) of FTD revealed immune system–related genes as a major FTD-associated pathway, particularly *TREM2*, a receptor involved in the immune response of myeloid cells, including microglia (Ferrari et al., 2014). Homozygous mutations in *TREM2* cause polycystic lipomembranous osteodysplasia with sclerosing leukoencephalopathy, in which patients develop dementia and bone cysts (Paloneva et al., 2002). However, several families with homozygous mutations have been found who developed an FTD-like dementia with no bone abnormalities (Chouery et al., 2008; Giraldo et al., 2013; Guerreiro, Bilgic, et al., 2013; Guerreiro, Lohmann, et al., 2013; Le Ber et al., 2014). Additionally, heterozygous mutations have been associated with sporadic FTD in several studies (Borroni et al., 2014; Cuyvers et al., 2014; Ruiz et al., 2014; Thelen et al., 2014). These genetic and experimental model studies suggest that inflammation may be an important underlying process in FTD.

Finally, targeting autophagy and lysosomal dysfunction may be a promising target for FTD therapy. Many of the FTD-related genes are directly or indirectly involved in endosomal or lysosomal function or protein degradation, including *GRN*, *CHMP2B*, *VCP*, and possibly *C9ORF72* (Farg et al., 2014; Skibinski et al., 2005; Smith et al., 2012; Watts et al., 2004). Recent GWAS data indicate that genes related to lysosomal function are another major FTD-associated pathway (Ferrari et al., 2014). There is also evidence that stimulating autophagy corrects deficits in transgenic mice expressing TDP-43 (Wang et al., 2012). These mice develop TDP-43 pathology, neurodegeneration, and memory deficits, all of which could be improved by treatment with rapamycin (Wang et al., 2012).

Therapies for Frontotemporal Dementia Genetic Subtypes

In addition to targeting deficits common to multiple FTD subtypes, strategies have also been in development to directly target some of the genetic causes of FTD. Promising therapeutic strategies are under development for each of the three most common genetic subtypes of FTD.

Experimental models of FTD resulting from *C9ORF72* mutations have suggested that the GGGGCC repeat expansion causes toxicity primarily through GGGGCC repeat RNA foci and RAN DPR proteins. As such, one potential therapeutic approach is to directly target the GGGGCC repeat RNA in an attempt to degrade the repeat RNA and prevent RAN translation into DPR proteins. Antisense oligonucleotides to *C9ORF72* eliminate the sense RNA foci in fibroblasts from *C9ORF72* expansion carriers (Lagier-Tourenne et al., 2013). Antisense oligonucleotides are also effective at reducing *c9orf72* in mouse brains and do not cause toxicity, making this a promising approach for *C9ORF72*-FTD (Lagier-Tourenne et al., 2013). Small molecules that bind the GGGGCC repeats have been developed, and prevent formation of RNA foci and RAN translation in cells expressing the *C9ORF72* repeat expansion or in fibroblast-derived neurons from patients carrying the *C9ORF72* expansion (Su et al., 2014).

Many therapeutic approaches have been tested in tau FTD models, but one of the most well-studied and promising approaches is tau reduction. Tau reduction has been tested in mouse models using immunotherapy, drugs, and antisense oligonucleotides, but the most thoroughly tested approach has been tau immunotherapy. Many studies with lines of mice carrying various FTD-related tau mutations show that either active immunization with tau peptides or passive immunization with tau antibodies results in improvement of tau pathology and motor function (Asuni, Boutajangout, Quartermain, & Sigurdsson, 2007; Bi, Ittner, Ke, Gotz, & Ittner, 2011; Boutajangout, Ingadottir, Davies, & Sigurdsson, 2011; Castillo-Carranza et al., 2014; Chai et al., 2011; Ittner et al., 2015; Yanamandra et al., 2013). Immunizing mice before or after the onset of behavioral deficits and pathological changes may improve both measures (Asuni et al., 2007; Bi et al., 2011; Boutajangout et al., 2011; Chai et al., 2011). However, as was suggested previously, in tau mouse models, reducing soluble tau may be more important than reducing aggregated tau (SantaCruz et al., 2005; Sydow et al., 2011; Warmus et al., 2014; Yoshiyama et al., 2007). An antibody directed at tau oligomers improves motor and memory deficits in the JNPL3 line of P301L tau mice without improving tau pathology (Castillo-Carranza et al., 2014). Similar results are seen with pharmacological reduction of tau using methylene blue. High doses of methylene blue reduce soluble tau levels and improve cognitive deficits in the rTg4510 line of P301L tau-expressing mice without improving tau pathology (O'Leary et al., 2010).

FTD-*GRN* may be the most straightforward of the inherited forms of FTD to target, because all FTD-related *GRN* mutations are loss-of-function mutations that cause haploinsufficiency. Therefore restoring progranulin to normal levels is a logical strategy to prevent or treat FTD in *GRN* mutation carriers. Based on data from primary neurons or iPSC-derived neurons, gene therapy with viral vectors may be an effective strategy to increase progranulin levels (Almeida et al., 2012; Gass et al., 2012). However, development of pharmacological approaches to increase progranulin levels is also underway. Progranulin expression is increased by histone deacetylase inhibitors in vitro, and this approach may be useful to boost progranulin expression from the wild-type allele of FTD-*GRN* patients (Cenik et al., 2011). Inhibition of progranulin degradation with alkalizing compounds or inhibitors of vacuolar ATPase also boosts progranulin levels in vitro (Capell et al., 2011). Finally, interfering with progranulin uptake into cells may be an effective approach. Sortilin regulates progranulin uptake into cells, and small molecule inhibitors of progranulin–sortilin binding increase extracellular progranulin levels, with modest increases in intracellular progranulin (Hu et al., 2010; Lee et al., 2014).

FUTURE DIRECTIONS

Major strides have been made in the last decade in understanding FTD from clinical, anatomical, and molecular perspectives. Clinical criteria for diagnosing the various FTD syndromes have been refined and improved. The brain networks underlying these syndromes and specific behavioral changes within each syndrome are now better understood, thanks to a variety of imaging techniques. Before the 2004 discovery that *VCP* mutations cause FTD (Watts et al., 2004), the only known genetic cause of FTD was tau (*MAPT*) mutations (Watts et al., 2004). Since that time, many additional FTD-related genes have been discovered. Similarly, FTD pathology was classified only as FTLD-tau or FTLD-U before the discovery that most FTLD-U cases are immunoreactive for TDP-43 or FUS (Neumann et al., 2006; Neumann, Tolnay, & Mackenzie, 2009). These genetic and pathological discoveries have provided new insights into the molecular mechanisms of FTD that are being leveraged to make new animal models and design new therapies. These discoveries have also opened up new avenues of research that will hopefully soon be addressed.

From a clinical perspective, development of disease-modifying treatments for FTD is a research question of the highest priority. Given the genetic, pathological, and clinical heterogeneity of FTD, it is unlikely that a single treatment that will be effective across the FTD spectrum. However, use of genetic animal models and iPSC-derived neurons from FTD patients will be helpful in validating approaches across genetic and pathological FTD subtypes. As new treatments come online, it will also be important to develop tests to determine whether a patient is a candidate for that particular treatment. Identification of early biomarkers for FTD will also be an important goal, as this would allow intervention before extensive cortical neuronal loss occurs. Imaging may be a helpful tool for this purpose, given the discovery of brain network dysfunction in FTD and findings of preclinical connectivity deficits in the anterior cingulate and frontoinsular cortices of FTD-related mutation carriers (Dopper et al., 2013, 2014; Seeley et al., 2009; Zhou et al., 2010).

Evidence from the studies described in this chapter highlights the central role of the cerebral cortex in FTD. Pathological studies have revealed early degeneration of cortical layers 2 and 3 in the frontal and temporal cortices, and the VENs and fork cells of layer 5 of the anterior cingulate and frontoinsular cortices are lost early in the disease. The cortical regions most affected in a patient correlate tightly with that patient's clinical syndrome, and even the severity of specific signs and symptoms that patient experiences. However, it must be noted that these cortical regions are parts of networks that degenerate in FTD. These networks include subcortical brain regions such as the striatum and amygdala that also degenerate in FTD and play an important role in the disease process. Ongoing and future studies of the functional and molecular changes in these networks in FTD will hopefully lead to the development of disease modifying treatments for this devastating disorder.

REFERENCES

Agosta, F., Sala, S., Valsasina, P., Meani, A., Canu, E., Magnani, G., et al. (2013). Brain network connectivity assessed using graph theory in frontotemporal dementia. *Neurology, 81*(2), 134–143. http://dx.doi.org/10.1212/WNL.0b013e31829a33f8.

Ahmed, Z., Sheng, H., Xu, Y. F., Lin, W. L., Innes, A. E., Gass, J., & Lewis, J. (2010). Accelerated lipofuscinosis and ubiquitination in granulin knockout mice suggest a role for progranulin in successful aging. *The American Journal of Pathology, 177*(1), 311–324. http://dx.doi.org/10.2353/ajpath.2010.090915 pii:ajpath.2010.090915.

Allman, J. M., Tetreault, N. A., Hakeem, A. Y., Manaye, K. F., Semendeferi, K., Erwin, J. M., et al. (2010). The von Economo neurons in frontoinsular and anterior cingulate cortex in great apes and humans. *Brain Structure and Function, 214*(5–6), 495–517. http://dx.doi.org/10.1007/s00429-010-0254-0.

Allman, J. M., Tetreault, N. A., Hakeem, A. Y., Manaye, K. F., Semendeferi, K., Erwin, J. M., et al. (2011). The von Economo neurons in the frontoinsular and anterior cingulate cortex. Annals of the New York Academy of Sciences, *1225*,59–371. http://dx.doi.org/10.1111/j.1749-6632.2011.06011.x.

Almeida, S., Gascon, E., Tran, H., Chou, H. J., Gendron, T. F., Degroot, S., et al. (2013). Modeling key pathological features of frontotemporal dementia with *C9ORF72* repeat expansion in iPSC-derived human neurons. *Acta Neuropathologica, 126*(3), 385–399. http://dx.doi.org/10.1007/s00401-013-1149-y.

Almeida, S., Zhang, Z., Coppola, G., Mao, W., Futai, K., Karydas, A., et al. (2012). Induced pluripotent stem cell models of progranulin-deficient frontotemporal dementia uncover specific reversible neuronal defects. *Cell Reports, 2*(4), 789–798. http://dx.doi.org/10.1016/j.celrep.2012.09.007.

Andorfer, C., Kress, Y., Espinoza, M., de Silva, R., Tucker, K. L., Barde, Y.-A., et al. (2003). Hyperphosphorylation and aggregation of tau in mice expressing normal human tau isoforms. *Journal of Neurochemistry, 86*(3), 582–590.

Ash, P. E., Bieniek, K. F., Gendron, T. F., Caulfield, T., Lin, W. L., Dejesus-Hernandez, M., et al. (2013). Unconventional translation of *C9ORF72* GGGGCC expansion generates insoluble polypeptides specific to c9FTD/ALS. *Neuron, 77*(4), 639–646. http://dx.doi.org/10.1016/j.neuron.2013.02.004 pii:S0896-6273(13)00135-9.

Asuni, A. A., Boutajangout, A., Quartermain, D., & Sigurdsson, E. M. (2007). Immunotherapy targeting pathological tau conformers in a tangle mouse model reduces brain pathology with associated functional improvements. *The Journal of Neuroscience, 27*(34), 9115–9129. http://dx.doi.org/10.1523/JNEUROSCI.2361-07.2007 pii:27/34/9115.

Baker, M., Mackenzie, I. R., Pickering-Brown, S. M., Gass, J., Rademakers, R., Lindholm, C., et al. (2006). Mutations in progranulin cause tau-negative frontotemporal dementia linked to chromosome 17. *Nature, 442*(7105), 916–919.

Bateman, A., & Bennett, H. P. (2009). The granulin gene family: from cancer to dementia. *Bioessays*, *31*(11), 1245–1254. http://dx.doi.org/10.1002/bies.200900086.

Beck, J., Rohrer, J. D., Campbell, T., Isaacs, A., Morrison, K. E., Goodall, E. F., et al. (2008). A distinct clinical, neuropsychological and radiological phenotype is associated with progranulin gene mutations in a large UK series. *Brain*, *131*(Pt 3), 706–720. http://dx.doi.org/10.1093/brain/awm320.

Benajiba, L., Le Ber, I., Camuzat, A., Lacoste, M., Thomas-Anterion, C., Couratier, P., & French Clinical Genetic Research Network on Frontotemporal Lobar Degeneration/Frontotemporal Lobar Degeneration with Motoneuron Disease (2009). *TARDBP* mutations in motoneuron disease with frontotemporal lobar degeneration. *Annals of Neurology*, *65*(4), 470–473. http://dx.doi.org/10.1002/ana.21612.

Bi, M., Ittner, A., Ke, Y. D., Gotz, J., & Ittner, L. M. (2011). Tau-targeted immunization impedes progression of neurofibrillary histopathology in aged P301L tau transgenic mice. *PLoS One*, *6*(12), e26860. http://dx.doi.org/10.1371/journal.pone.0026860 pii:PONE-D-11-15839.

van Blitterswijk, M., DeJesus-Hernandez, M., Niemantsverdriet, E., Murray, M. E., Heckman, M. G., Diehl, N. N., et al. (2013). Association between repeat sizes and clinical and pathological characteristics in carriers of *C9ORF72* repeat expansions (Xpansize-72): a cross-sectional cohort study. *Lancet Neurology*, *12*(10), 978–988. http://dx.doi.org/10.1016/S1474-4422(13)70210-2.

Boeve, B. F., Boylan, K. B., Graff-Radford, N. R., Dejesus-Hernandez, M., Knopman, D. S., Pedraza, O., et al. (2012). Characterization of frontotemporal dementia and/or amyotrophic lateral sclerosis associated with the GGGGCC repeat expansion in *C9ORF72*. *Brain*, *135*(Pt 3), 765–783. http://dx.doi.org/10.1093/brain/aws004 pii:aws004.

Borroni, B., Alberici, A., Grassi, M., Turla, M., Zanetti, O., Bianchetti, A., et al. (2010). Is frontotemporal lobar degeneration a rare disorder? Evidence from a preliminary study in Brescia county, Italy. *Journal of Alzheimer's Disease*, *19*(1), 111–116. http://dx.doi.org/10.3233/JAD-2010-1208.

Borroni, B., Ferrari, F., Galimberti, D., Nacmias, B., Barone, C., Bagnoli, S., et al. (2014). Heterozygous *TREM2* mutations in frontotemporal dementia. *Neurobiology of Aging*, *35*(4), 934 e937–910. http://dx.doi.org/10.1016/j.neurobiolaging.2013.09.017.

Boutajangout, A., Ingadottir, J., Davies, P., & Sigurdsson, E. M. (2011). Passive immunization targeting pathological phospho-tau protein in a mouse model reduces functional decline and clears tau aggregates from the brain. *Journal of Neurochemistry*, *118*(4), 658–667. http://dx.doi.org/10.1111/j.1471-4159.2011.07337.x.

Boxer, A. L., Knopman, D. S., Kaufer, D. I., Grossman, M., Onyike, C., Graf-Radford, N., et al. (2013). Memantine in patients with frontotemporal lobar degeneration: a multicentre, randomised, double-blind, placebo-controlled trial. *Lancet Neurology*, *12*(2), 149–156. http://dx.doi.org/10.1016/S1474-4422(12)70320-4.

Boxer, A. L., Mackenzie, I. R., Boeve, B. F., Baker, M., Seeley, W. W., Crook, R., et al. (2011). Clinical, neuroimaging and neuropathological features of a new chromosome 9p-linked FTD-ALS family. *Journal of Neurology, Neurosurgery, and Psychiatry*, *82*(2), 196–203. http://dx.doi.org/10.1136/jnnp.2009.204081.

Brion, J. P., Tremp, G., & Octave, J. N. (1999). Transgenic expression of the shortest human tau affects its compartmentalization and its phosphorylation as in the pretangle stage of Alzheimer's disease. *The American Journal of Pathology*, *154*(1), 255–270. http://dx.doi.org/10.1016/S0002-9440(10)65272-8.

Broustal, O., Camuzat, A., Guillot-Noël, L., Guy, N., Millecamps, S., Deffond, D., & French Clinical and Genetic Research Network on FTD/FTD-MND (2010). FUS mutations in frontotemporal lobar degeneration with amyotrophic lateral sclerosis. *Journal of Alzheimer's Disease*, *22*(3), 765–769.

Brun, A. (1987). Frontal lobe degeneration of non-Alzheimer type. I. Neuropathology. *Archives of Gerontology and Geriatrics*, *6*(3), 193–208.

Burrell, J. R., Kiernan, M. C., Vucic, S., & Hodges, J. R. (2011). Motor neuron dysfunction in frontotemporal dementia. *Brain*, *134*(Pt 9), 2582–2594. http://dx.doi.org/10.1093/brain/awr195.

Cairns, N. J., Bigio, E. H., Mackenzie, I. R., Neumann, M., Lee, V. M., Hatanpaa, K. J., & Consortium for Frontotemporal Lobar Degeneration (2007). Neuropathologic diagnostic and nosologic criteria for frontotemporal lobar degeneration: consensus of the Consortium for Frontotemporal Lobar Degeneration. *Acta Neuropathologica, 114*(1), 5–22. http://dx.doi.org/10.1007/s00401-007-0237-2.

Canafoglia, L., Morbin, M., Scaioli, V., Pareyson, D., D'Incerti, L., Fugnanesi, V., et al. (2014). Recurrent generalized seizures, visual loss, and palinopsia as phenotypic features of neuronal ceroid lipofuscinosis due to progranulin gene mutation. *Epilepsia, 55*(6), e56–59. http://dx.doi.org/10.1111/epi.12632.

Capell, A., Liebscher, S., Fellerer, K., Brouwers, N., Willem, M., Lammich, S., et al. (2011). Rescue of progranulin deficiency associated with frontotemporal lobar degeneration by alkalizing reagents and inhibition of vacuolar ATPase. *The Journal of Neuroscience, 31*(5), 1885–1894. http://dx.doi.org/10.1523/JNEUROSCI.5757-10.2011.

Caso, F., Mandelli, M. L., Henry, M., Gesierich, B., Bettcher, B. M., Ogar, J., et al. (2014). In vivo signatures of nonfluent/agrammatic primary progressive aphasia caused by FTLD pathology. *Neurology, 82*(3), 239–247. http://dx.doi.org/10.1212/WNL.0000000000000031.

Castillo-Carranza, D. L., Sengupta, U., Guerrero-Munoz, M. J., Lasagna-Reeves, C. A., Gerson, J. E., Singh, G., et al. (2014). Passive immunization with tau oligomer monoclonal antibody reverses tauopathy phenotypes without affecting hyperphosphorylated neurofibrillary tangles. *The Journal of Neuroscience, 34*(12), 4260–4272. http://dx.doi.org/10.1523/JNEUROSCI.3192-13.2014.

Cenik, B., Sephton, C. F., Dewey, C. M., Xian, X., Wei, S., Yu, K., et al. (2011). Suberoylanilide hydroxamic acid (vorinostat) up-regulates progranulin transcription: rational therapeutic approach to frontotemporal dementia. *Journal of Biological Chemistry, 286*(18), 16101–16108. http://dx.doi.org/10.1074/jbc.M110.193433.

Chai, X., Wu, S., Murray, T. K., Kinley, R., Cella, C. V., Sims, H., et al. (2011). Passive immunization with anti-tau antibodies in two transgenic models: reduction of tau pathology and delay of disease progression. *Journal of Biological Chemistry, 286*(39), 34457–34467. http://dx.doi.org/10.1074/jbc.M111.229633 pii:M111.229633.

Chan, D., Fox, N. C., Scahill, R. I., Crum, W. R., Whitwell, J. L., Leschziner, G., et al. (2001). Patterns of temporal lobe atrophy in semantic dementia and Alzheimer's disease. *Annals of Neurology, 49*(4), 433–442.

Chitramuthu, B. P., Baranowski, D. C., Kay, D. G., Bateman, A., & Bennett, H. P. (2010). Progranulin modulates zebrafish motoneuron development in vivo and rescues truncation defects associated with knockdown of survival motor neuron 1. *Molecular Neurodegeneration Other Titles, 5*, 41. http://dx.doi.org/10.1186/1750-1326-5-41.

Chiu, W. Z., Kaat, L. D., Seelaar, H., Rosso, S. M., Boon, A. J., Kamphorst, W., et al. (2010). Survival in progressive supranuclear palsy and frontotemporal dementia. *Journal of Neurology, Neurosurgery, and Psychiatry, 81*(4), 441–445. http://dx.doi.org/10.1136/jnnp.2009.195719.

Chouery, E., Delague, V., Bergougnoux, A., Koussa, S., Serre, J. L., & Megarbane, A. (2008). Mutations in *TREM2* lead to pure early-onset dementia without bone cysts. *Human Mutation, 29*(9), E194–E204. http://dx.doi.org/10.1002/humu.20836.

Chow, T. W., Miller, B. L., Hayashi, V. N., & Geschwind, D. H. (1999). Inheritance of frontotemporal dementia. *Archives of Neurology, 56*(7), 817–822.

Ciura, S., Lattante, S., Le Ber, I., Latouche, M., Tostivint, H., Brice, A., et al. (2013). Loss of function of *C9orf72* causes motor deficits in a zebrafish model of amyotrophic lateral sclerosis. *Annals of Neurology.* http://dx.doi.org/10.1002/ana.23946.

Craig, A. D. (2009). How do you feel—now? The anterior insula and human awareness. *Nature Reviews. Neuroscience, 10*(1), 59–70. http://dx.doi.org/10.1038/nrn2555.

Cruchaga, C., Fernandez-Seara, M. A., Seijo-Martinez, M., Samaranch, L., Lorenzo, E., Hinrichs, A., et al. (2009). Cortical atrophy and language network reorganization associated with a novel progranulin mutation. *Cerebral Cortex, 19*(8), 1751–1760. http://dx.doi.org/10.1093/cercor/bhn202.

Cruts, M., Gijselinck, I., van der Zee, J., Engelborghs, S., Wils, H., Pirici, D., et al. (2006). Null mutations in progranulin cause ubiquitin-positive frontotemporal dementia linked to chromosome 17q21. *Nature, 442*(7105), 920–924.

Cuyvers, E., Bettens, K., Philtjens, S., Van Langenhove, T., Gijselinck, I., van der Zee, J., & consortium, B., et al. (2014). Investigating the role of rare heterozygous *TREM2* variants in Alzheimer's disease and frontotemporal dementia. *Neurobiology of Aging, 35*(3), 726 e711–729. http://dx.doi.org/10.1016/j.neurobiolaging.2013.09.009.

Day, J. J., & Roberson, E. D. (2015). DNA methylation slows effects of *C9orf72* mutations: an epigenetic brake on genetic inheritance. *Neurology, 84*(16), 1616–1617. http://dx.doi.org/10.1212/WNL.0000000000001504.

De Muynck, L., Herdewyn, S., Beel, S., Scheveneels, W., Van Den Bosch, L., Robberecht, W., et al. (2013). The neurotrophic properties of progranulin depend on the granulin E domain but do not require sortilin binding. *Neurobiology of Aging, 34*(11), 2541–2547. http://dx.doi.org/10.1016/j.neurobiolaging.2013.04.022.

DeJesus-Hernandez, M., Mackenzie, I. R., Boeve, B. F., Boxer, A. L., Baker, M., Rutherford, N. J., et al. (2011). Expanded GGGGCC hexanucleotide repeat in noncoding region of *C9ORF72* causes chromosome 9p-linked FTD and ALS. *Neuron, 72*(2), 245–256. http://dx.doi.org/10.1016/j.neuron.2011.09.011 pii:S0896-6273(11)00828-2.

Delacourte, A., Robitaille, Y., Sergeant, N., Buee, L., Hof, P. R., Wattez, A., et al. (1996). Specific pathological tau protein variants characterize Pick's disease. *Journal of Neuropathology and Experimental Neurology, 55*(2), 159–168.

Diehl, J., Grimmer, T., Drzezga, A., Riemenschneider, M., Forstl, H., & Kurz, A. (2004). Cerebral metabolic patterns at early stages of frontotemporal dementia and semantic dementia: a PET study. *Neurobiology of Aging, 25*(8), 1051–1056. http://dx.doi.org/10.1016/j.neurobiolaging.2003.10.007.

Diehl-Schmid, J., Forstl, H., Perneczky, R., Pohl, C., & Kurz, A. (2008). A 6-month, open-label study of memantine in patients with frontotemporal dementia. *International Journal of Geriatric Psychiatry, 23*(7), 754–759. http://dx.doi.org/10.1002/gps.1973.

Dobson-Stone, C., Hallupp, M., Loy, C. T., Thompson, E. M., Haan, E., Sue, C. M., et al. (2013). *C9ORF72* repeat expansion in Australian and Spanish frontotemporal dementia patients. *PLoS One, 8*(2), e56899. http://dx.doi.org/10.1371/journal.pone.0056899.

Dopper, E. G., Rombouts, S. A., Jiskoot, L. C., den Heijer, T., de Graaf, J. R., de Koning, I., et al. (2013). Structural and functional brain connectivity in presymptomatic familial frontotemporal dementia. *Neurology, 80*(9), 814–823. http://dx.doi.org/10.1212/WNL.0b013e31828407bc.

Dopper, E. G., Rombouts, S. A., Jiskoot, L. C., den Heijer, T., de Graaf, J. R., de Koning, I., et al. (2014). Structural and functional brain connectivity in presymptomatic familial frontotemporal dementia. *Neurology, 83*(2), e19–26. http://dx.doi.org/10.1212/WNL.0000000000000583.

Drzezga, A., Grimmer, T., Henriksen, G., Stangier, I., Perneczky, R., Diehl-Schmid, J., et al. (2008). Imaging of amyloid plaques and cerebral glucose metabolism in semantic dementia and Alzheimer's disease. *Neuroimage, 39*(2), 619–633. http://dx.doi.org/10.1016/j.neuroimage.2007.09.020.

Englund, B., Brun, A., Gustafson, L., Passant, U., Mann, D. M. A., Neary, D., et al. (1994). Clinical and neuropathological criteria for frontotemporal dementia: The Lund and Manchester Groups. *Journal of Neurology, Neurosurgery, and Psychiatry, 57*(4), 416–418.

Eslinger, P. J., Moore, P., Antani, S., Anderson, C., & Grossman, M. (2012). Apathy in frontotemporal dementia: behavioral and neuroimaging correlates. *Behavioural Neurology, 25*(2), 127–136. http://dx.doi.org/10.3233/BEN-2011-0351.

Farb, N. A., Grady, C. L., Strother, S., Tang-Wai, D. F., Masellis, M., Black, S., et al. (2013). Abnormal network connectivity in frontotemporal dementia: evidence for prefrontal isolation. *Cortex*, *49*(7), 1856–1873. http://dx.doi.org/10.1016/j.cortex.2012.09.008.

Farg, M. A., Sundaramoorthy, V., Sultana, J. M., Yang, S., Atkinson, R. A., Levina, V., et al. (2014). *C9ORF72*, implicated in amyotrophic lateral sclerosis and frontotemporal dementia, regulates endosomal trafficking. *Human Molecular Genetics*, *23*(13), 3579–3595. http://dx.doi.org/10.1093/hmg/ddu068.

Ferrari, R., Hernandez, D. G., Nalls, M. A., Rohrer, J. D., Ramasamy, A., Kwok, J. B., et al. (2014). Frontotemporal dementia and its subtypes: a genome-wide association study. *Lancet Neurology*, *13*(7), 686–699. http://dx.doi.org/10.1016/S1474-4422(14)70065-1.

Filiano, A. J., Martens, L. H., Young, A. H., Warmus, B. A., Zhou, P., Diaz-Ramirez, G., et al. (2013). Dissociation of frontotemporal dementia–related deficits and neuroinflammation in progranulin haploinsufficient mice. *The Journal of Neuroscience*, *33*(12), 5352–5361. http://dx.doi.org/10.1523/JNEUROSCI.6103-11.2013 pii:33/12/5352.

Frost, B., Jacks, R. L., & Diamond, M. I. (2009). Propagation of tau misfolding from the outside to the inside of a cell. *Journal of Biological Chemistry*, *284*(19), 12845–12852. http://dx.doi.org/10.1074/jbc.M808759200 pii:M808759200.

Galton, C. J., Patterson, K., Graham, K., Lambon-Ralph, M. A., Williams, G., Antoun, N., et al. (2001). Differing patterns of temporal atrophy in Alzheimer's disease and semantic dementia. *Neurology*, *57*(2), 216–225.

Gao, X., Joselin, A. P., Wang, L., Kar, A., Ray, P., Bateman, A., et al. (2010). Progranulin promotes neurite outgrowth and neuronal differentiation by regulating GSK-3beta. *Protein & Cell*, *1*(6), 552–562. http://dx.doi.org/10.1007/s13238-010-0067-1.

Gascon, E., & Gao, F. B. (2014). The emerging roles of microRNAs in the pathogenesis of frontotemporal dementia-amyotrophic lateral sclerosis (FTD-ALS) spectrum disorders. *Journal of Neurogenetics*, *28*(1–2), 30–40. http://dx.doi.org/10.3109/01677063.2013.876021.

Gass, J., Cannon, A., Mackenzie, I. R., Boeve, B., Baker, M., Adamson, J., et al. (2006). Mutations in progranulin are a major cause of ubiquitin-positive frontotemporal lobar degeneration. *Human Molecular Genetics*, *15*(20), 2988–3001. http://dx.doi.org/10.1093/hmg/ddl241 pii:ddl241.

Gass, J., Lee, W. C., Cook, C., Finch, N., Stetler, C., Jansen-West, K., et al. (2012). Progranulin regulates neuronal outgrowth independent of sortilin. *Molecular Neurodegeneration*, *7*(1), 33. http://dx.doi.org/10.1186/1750-1326-7-33 pii:1750-1326-7-33.

Gendron, T. F., Bieniek, K. F., Zhang, Y. J., Jansen-West, K., Ash, P. E., Caulfield, T., et al. (2013). Antisense transcripts of the expanded *C9ORF72* hexanucleotide repeat form nuclear RNA foci and undergo repeat-associated non-ATG translation in c9FTD/ALS. *Acta Neuropathologica*, *126*(6), 829–844. http://dx.doi.org/10.1007/s00401-013-1192-8.

Ghoshal, N., Dearborn, J. T., Wozniak, D. F., & Cairns, N. J. (2012). Core features of frontotemporal dementia recapitulated in progranulin knockout mice. *Neurobiology of Disease*, *45*(1), 395–408. http://dx.doi.org/10.1016/j.nbd.2011.08.029.

Gijselinck, I., Van Broeckhoven, C., & Cruts, M. (2008). Granulin mutations associated with frontotemporal lobar degeneration and related disorders: an update. *Human Mutation*, *29*(12), 1373–1386. http://dx.doi.org/10.1002/humu.20785.

Giraldo, M., Lopera, F., Siniard, A. L., Corneveaux, J. J., Schrauwen, I., Carvajal, J., et al. (2013). Variants in triggering receptor expressed on myeloid cells 2 are associated with both behavioral variant frontotemporal lobar degeneration and Alzheimer's disease. *Neurobiology of Aging*, *34*(8), 2077 e2011–2078. http://dx.doi.org/10.1016/j.neurobiolaging.2013.02.016.

Goedert, M., & Jakes, R. (2005). Mutations causing neurodegenerative tauopathies. *Biochimica et Biophysica Acta*, *1739*(2–3), 240–250.

Goedert, M., Spillantini, M. G., Potier, M. C., Ulrich, J., & Crowther, R. A. (1989). Cloning and sequencing of the cDNA encoding an isoform of microtubule-associated protein tau containing four tandem repeats: differential expression of tau protein mRNAs in human brain. *The EMBO Journal, 8*(2), 393–399.

Goldman, J. S., Farmer, J. M., Wood, E. M., Johnson, J. K., Boxer, A., Neuhaus, J., et al. (2005). Comparison of family histories in FTLD subtypes and related tauopathies. *Neurology, 65*(11), 1817–1819.

Gorno-Tempini, M. L., Dronkers, N. F., Rankin, K. P., Ogar, J. M., Phengrasamy, L., Rosen, H. J., et al. (2004). Cognition and anatomy in three variants of primary progressive aphasia. *Annals of Neurology, 55*(3), 335–346.

Gorno-Tempini, M. L., Hillis, A. E., Weintraub, S., Kertesz, A., Mendez, M., Cappa, S. F., et al. (2011). Classification of primary progressive aphasia and its variants. *Neurology, 76*(11), 1006–1014. http://dx.doi.org/10.1212/WNL.0b013e31821103e6.

Götz, J., Chen, F., Barmettler, R., & Nitsch, R. M. (2001). Tau filament formation in transgenic mice expressing P301L tau. *Journal of Biological Chemistry, 276*(1), 529–534. http://dx.doi.org/10.1074/jbc.M006531200 pii:M006531200.

Gotz, J., Probst, A., Spillantini, M. G., Schafer, T., Jakes, R., Burki, K., et al. (1995). Somatodendritic localization and hyperphosphorylation of tau protein in transgenic mice expressing the longest human brain tau isoform. *The EMBO Journal, 14*(7), 1304–1313.

Gotzl, J. K., Mori, K., Damme, M., Fellerer, K., Tahirovic, S., Kleinberger, G., et al. (2014). Common pathobiochemical hallmarks of progranulin-associated frontotemporal lobar degeneration and neuronal ceroid lipofuscinosis. *Acta Neuropathologica, 127*(6), 845–860. http://dx.doi.org/10.1007/s00401-014-1262-6.

Grabowski, T. J., Cho, H. S., Vonsattel, J. P. G., Rebeck, G. W., & Greenberg, S. M. (2001). Novel amyloid precursor protein mutation in an Iowa family with dementia and severe cerebral amyloid angiopathy. *Annals of Neurology, 49*(6), 697–705.

Guerreiro, R., Bilgic, B., Guven, G., Bras, J., Rohrer, J., Lohmann, E., et al. (2013). Novel compound heterozygous mutation in *TREM2* found in a Turkish frontotemporal dementia-like family. *Neurobiology of Aging, 34*(12), 2890 e2891–2895. http://dx.doi.org/10.1016/j.neurobiolaging.2013.06.005.

Guerreiro, R. J., Lohmann, E., Bras, J. M., Gibbs, J. R., Rohrer, J. D., Gurunlian, N., et al. (2013). Using exome sequencing to reveal mutations in *TREM2* presenting as a frontotemporal dementia-like syndrome without bone involvement. *JAMA Neurology, 70*(1), 78–84. http://dx.doi.org/10.1001/jamaneurol.2013.579 pii:1557588.

Guo, A., Tapia, L., Bamji, S. X., Cynader, M. S., & Jia, W. (2010). Progranulin deficiency leads to enhanced cell vulnerability and TDP-43 translocation in primary neuronal cultures. *Brain Research, 1366*, 1–8. http://dx.doi.org/10.1016/j.brainres.2010.09.099.

Haeusler, A. R., Donnelly, C. J., Periz, G., Simko, E. A., Shaw, P. G., Kim, M. S., et al. (2014). *C9orf72* nucleotide repeat structures initiate molecular cascades of disease. *Nature, 507*, 195–200. http://dx.doi.org/10.1038/nature13124 pii:nature13124.

Higgins, J. J., Litvan, I., Pho, L. T., Li, W., & Nee, L. E. (1998). Progressive supranuclear gaze palsy is in linkage disequilibrium with the tau and not the alpha-synuclein gene. *Neurology, 50*(1), 270–273.

Huey, E. D., Putnam, K. T., & Grafman, J. (2006). A systematic review of neurotransmitter deficits and treatments in frontotemporal dementia. *Neurology, 66*(1), 17–22.

Hu, F., Padukkavidana, T., Vægter, C. B., Brady, O. A., Zheng, Y., Mackenzie, I. R., et al. (2010). Sortilin-mediated endocytosis determines levels of the frontotemporal dementia protein, progranulin. *Neuron, 68*(4), 654–667. http://dx.doi.org/10.1016/j.neuron.2010.09.034 pii:S0896-6273(10)00776-2.

Hutton, M., Lendon, C. L., Rizzu, P., Baker, M., Froelich, S., Houlden, H., et al. (1998). Association of missense and 5′-splice-site mutations in tau with the inherited dementia FTDP-17. *Nature, 393*, 702–705.

Iguchi, Y., Katsuno, M., Niwa, J., Takagi, S., Ishigaki, S., Ikenaka, K., et al. (2013). Loss of TDP-43 causes age-dependent progressive motor neuron degeneration. *Brain, 136*(Pt 5), 1371–1382. http://dx.doi.org/10.1093/brain/awt029 pii:awt029.

Ikeda, M., Shoji, M., Kawarai, T., Kawarabayashi, T., Matsubara, E., Murakami, T., et al. (2005). Accumulation of filamentous tau in the cerebral cortex of human tau R406W transgenic mice. *The American Journal of Pathology, 166*(2), 521–531. http://dx.doi.org/10.1016/S0002-9440(10)62274-2.

Irwin, D. J., McMillan, C. T., Brettschneider, J., Libon, D. J., Powers, J., Rascovsky, K., et al. (2013). Cognitive decline and reduced survival in *C9orf72* expansion frontotemporal degeneration and amyotrophic lateral sclerosis. *Journal of Neurology, Neurosurgery, and Psychiatry, 84*(2), 163–169. http://dx.doi.org/10.1136/jnnp-2012-303507.

Ittner, A., Bertz, J., Suh, L. S., Stevens, C. H., Gotz, J., & Ittner, L. M. (2015). Tau-targeting passive immunization modulates aspects of pathology in tau transgenic mice. *Journal of Neurochemistry, 132*(1), 135–145. http://dx.doi.org/10.1111/jnc.12821.

Jackson, G. R., Wiedau-Pazos, M., Sang, T. K., Wagle, N., Brown, C. A., et al. (2002). Human wild-type tau interacts with wingless pathway components and produces neurofibrillary pathology in *Drosophila. Neuron, 34*(4), 509–519.

Josephs, K. A., Duffy, J. R., Fossett, T. R., Strand, E. A., Claassen, D. O., Whitwell, J. L., et al. (2010). Fluorodeoxyglucose F18 positron emission tomography in progressive apraxia of speech and primary progressive aphasia variants. *Archives of Neurology, 67*(5), 596–605. http://dx.doi.org/10.1001/archneurol.2010.78.

Josephs, K. A., Duffy, J. R., Strand, E. A., Machulda, M. M., Senjem, M. L., Master, A. V., et al. (2012). Characterizing a neurodegenerative syndrome: primary progressive apraxia of speech. *Brain, 135*(Pt 5), 1522–1536. http://dx.doi.org/10.1093/brain/aws032.

Josephs, K. A., Duffy, J. R., Strand, E. A., Whitwell, J. L., Layton, K. F., Parisi, J. E., et al. (2006). Clinicopathological and imaging correlates of progressive aphasia and apraxia of speech. *Brain, 129*(Pt 6), 1385–1398.

Karsten, S. L., Sang, T. K., Gehman, L. T., Chatterjee, S., Liu, J., Lawless, G. M., et al. (2006). A genomic screen for modifiers of tauopathy identifies puromycin-sensitive aminopeptidase as an inhibitor of tau-induced neurodegeneration. *Neuron, 51*(5), 549–560.

Kayasuga, Y., Chiba, S., Suzuki, M., Kikusui, T., Matsuwaki, T., Yamanouchi, K., et al. (2007). Alteration of behavioural phenotype in mice by targeted disruption of the progranulin gene. *Behavioural Brain Research, 185*(2), 110–118. http://dx.doi.org/10.1016/j.bbr.2007.07.020 pii:S0166-4328(07)00369-5.

Kelley, B. J., Haidar, W., Boeve, B. F., Baker, M., Graff-Radford, N. R., Krefft, T., et al. (2009). Prominent phenotypic variability associated with mutations in progranulin. *Neurobiology of Aging, 30*(5), 739–751. http://dx.doi.org/10.1016/j.neurobiolaging.2007.08.022.

Kim, E. J., Sidhu, M., Gaus, S. E., Huang, E. J., Hof, P. R., Miller, B. L., et al. (2012). Selective frontoinsular von Economo neuron and fork cell loss in early behavioral variant frontotemporal dementia. *Cerebral Cortex, 22*(2), 251–259. http://dx.doi.org/10.1093/cercor/bhr004.

Kleinberger, G., Wils, H., Ponsaerts, P., Joris, G., Timmermans, J. P., Van Broeckhoven, C., et al. (2010). Increased caspase activation and decreased TDP-43 solubility in progranulin knockout cortical cultures. *Journal of Neurochemistry, 115*(3), 735–747. http://dx.doi.org/10.1111/j.1471-4159.2010.06961.x pii:JNC6961.

Komori, T. (1999). Tau-positive glial inclusions in progressive supranuclear palsy, corticobasal degeneration and Pick's disease. *Brain Pathology, 9*(4), 663–679.

Kosmidis, S., Grammenoudi, S., Papanikolopoulou, K., & Skoulakis, E. M. (2010). Differential effects of Tau on the integrity and function of neurons essential for learning in *Drosophila. The Journal of Neuroscience, 30*(2), 464–477. http://dx.doi.org/10.1523/JNEUROSCI.1490-09.2010.

Kringelbach, M. L. (2005). The human orbitofrontal cortex: linking reward to hedonic experience. *Nature Reviews. Neuroscience, 6*(9), 691–702. http://dx.doi.org/10.1038/nrn1747.

Ksiezak-Reding, H., Morgan, K., Mattiace, L. A., Davies, P., Liu, W. K., Yen, S. H., et al. (1994). Ultrastructure and biochemical composition of paired helical filaments in corticobasal degeneration. *The American Journal of Pathology, 145*(6), 1496–1508.

LaJoie, R., Landeau, B., Perrotin, A., Bejanin, A., Egret, S., Pelerin, A., et al. (2014). Intrinsic connectivity identifies the hippocampus as a main crossroad between Alzheimer's and semantic dementia-targeted networks. *Neuron, 81*(6), 1417–1428. http://dx.doi.org/10.1016/j.neuron.2014.01.026.

Lagier-Tourenne, C., Baughn, M., Rigo, F., Sun, S., Liu, P., Li, H. R., et al. (2013). Targeted degradation of sense and antisense *C9orf72* RNA foci as therapy for ALS and frontotemporal degeneration. *Proceedings of the National Academy of Sciences of the United States of America, 110*(47), E4530–E4539. http://dx.doi.org/10.1073/pnas.1318835110 pii:1318835110.

Laird, A. S., Van Hoecke, A., De Muynck, L., Timmers, M., Van den Bosch, L., Van Damme, P., et al. (2010). Progranulin is neurotrophic in vivo and protects against a mutant TDP-43 induced axonopathy. *PLoS One, 5*(10), e13368. http://dx.doi.org/10.1371/journal.pone.0013368.

Le Ber, I., De Septenville, A., Guerreiro, R., Bras, J., Camuzat, A., Caroppo, P., et al. (2014). Homozygous *TREM2* mutation in a family with atypical frontotemporal dementia. *Neurobiology of Aging, 35*(10), 2419 e2423–2415. http://dx.doi.org/10.1016/j.neurobiolaging.2014.04.010.

Le Ber, I., Guedj, E., Gabelle, A., Verpillat, P., Volteau, M., Thomas-Anterion, C., et al. (2006). Demographic, neurological and behavioural characteristics and brain perfusion SPECT in frontal variant of frontotemporal dementia. *Brain, 129*(Pt 11), 3051–3065. http://dx.doi.org/10.1093/brain/awl288.

Lee, W. C., Almeida, S., Prudencio, M., Caulfield, T. R., Zhang, Y. J., Tay, W. M., et al. (2014). Targeted manipulation of the sortilin–progranulin axis rescues progranulin haploinsufficiency. *Human Molecular Genetics, 23*(6), 1467–1478. http://dx.doi.org/10.1093/hmg/ddt534.

Lee, Y. B., Chen, H. J., Peres, J. N., Gomez-Deza, J., Attig, J., Stalekar, M., et al. (2013). Hexanucleotide repeats in ALS/FTD form length-dependent RNA foci, sequester RNA binding proteins, and are neurotoxic. *Cell Reports, 5*(5), 1178–1186. http://dx.doi.org/10.1016/j.celrep.2013.10.049 pii:S2211-1247(13)00648-7.

Lewis, J., McGowan, E., Rockwood, J., Melrose, H., Nacharaju, P., Van Slegtenhorst, M., et al. (2000). Neurofibrillary tangles, amyotrophy and progressive motor disturbance in mice expressing mutant (P301L) tau protein. *Nature Genetics, 25*(4), 402–405.

Ling, S. C., Polymenidou, M., & Cleveland, D. W. (2013). Converging mechanisms in ALS and FTD: disrupted RNA and protein homeostasis. *Neuron, 79*(3), 416–438. http://dx.doi.org/10.1016/j.neuron.2013.07.033 pii:S0896-6273(13)00657-0.

Lomen-Hoerth, C., Murphy, J., Langmore, S., Kramer, J. H., Olney, R. K., & Miller, B. (2003). Are amyotrophic lateral sclerosis patients cognitively normal? *Neurology, 60*(7), 1094–1097.

Mackenzie, I. R., Baborie, A., Pickering-Brown, S., Du Plessis, D., Jaros, E., Perry, R. H., et al. (2006). Heterogeneity of ubiquitin pathology in frontotemporal lobar degeneration: classification and relation to clinical phenotype. *Acta Neuropathologica, 112*(5), 539–549. http://dx.doi.org/10.1007/s00401-006-0138-9.

Mackenzie, I. R., Neumann, M., Baborie, A., Sampathu, D. M., Du Plessis, D., Jaros, E., et al. (2011). A harmonized classification system for FTLD-TDP pathology. *Acta Neuropathologica, 122*(1), 111–113. http://dx.doi.org/10.1007/s00401-011-0845-8.

Mackenzie, I. R., Neumann, M., Bigio, E. H., Cairns, N. J., Alafuzoff, I., Kril, J., et al. (2010). Nomenclature and nosology for neuropathologic subtypes of frontotemporal lobar degeneration: an update. *Acta Neuropathologica, 119*(1), 1–4. http://dx.doi.org/10.1007/s00401-009-0612-2.

Maffei, A., Haley, M., & Fontanini, A. (2012). Neural processing of gustatory information in insular circuits. *Current Opinion in Neurobiology, 22*(4), 709–716. http://dx.doi.org/10.1016/j.conb.2012.04.001.

Mahoney, C. J., Beck, J., Rohrer, J. D., Lashley, T., Mok, K., Shakespeare, T., et al. (2012). Frontotemporal dementia with the *C9ORF72* hexanucleotide repeat expansion: clinical, neuroanatomical and neuropathological features. *Brain, 135*(Pt 3), 736–750. http://dx.doi.org/10.1093/brain/awr361.

Majounie, E., Renton, A. E., Mok, K., Dopper, E. G., Waite, A., Rollinson, S., et al. (2012). Frequency of the *C9orf72* hexanucleotide repeat expansion in patients with amyotrophic lateral sclerosis and frontotemporal dementia: a cross-sectional study. *Lancet Neurology, 11*(4), 323–330. http://dx.doi.org/10.1016/S1474-4422(12)70043-1.

Martens, L. H., Zhang, J., Barmada, S. J., Zhou, P., Kamiya, S., Sun, B., et al. (2012). Progranulin deficiency promotes neuroinflammation and neuron loss following toxin-induced injury. *Journal of Clinical Investigation, 122*(11), 3955–3959.

May, S., Hornburg, D., Schludi, M. H., Arzberger, T., Rentzsch, K., Schwenk, B. M., et al. (2014). *C9orf72* FTLD/ALS-associated Gly-Ala dipeptide repeat proteins cause neuronal toxicity and *Unc119* sequestration. *Acta Neuropathologica, 128*(4), 485–503. http://dx.doi.org/10.1007/s00401-014-1329-4.

McMurtray, A. M., Chen, A. K., Shapira, J. S., Chow, T. W., Mishkin, F., Miller, B. L., et al. (2006). Variations in regional SPECT hypoperfusion and clinical features in frontotemporal dementia. *Neurology, 66*(4), 517–522. http://dx.doi.org/10.1212/01.wnl.0000197983.39436.e7.

Mesulam, M. M. (1982). Slowly progressive aphasia without generalized dementia. *Annals of Neurology, 11*(6), 592–598. http://dx.doi.org/10.1002/ana.410110607.

Mion, M., Patterson, K., Acosta-Cabronero, J., Pengas, G., Izquierdo-Garcia, D., Hong, Y. T., et al. (2010). What the left and right anterior fusiform gyri tell us about semantic memory. *Brain, 133*(11), 3256–3268. http://dx.doi.org/10.1093/brain/awq272.

Mizielinska, S., Gronke, S., Niccoli, T., Ridler, C. E., Clayton, E. L., Devoy, A., et al. (2014). *C9orf72* repeat expansions cause neurodegeneration in *Drosophila* through arginine-rich proteins. *Science, 345*(6201), 1192–1194. http://dx.doi.org/10.1126/science.1256800.

Mocanu, M. M., Nissen, A., Eckermann, K., Khlistunova, I., Biernat, J., Drexler, D., et al. (2008). The potential for β-structure in the repeat domain of tau protein determines aggregation, synaptic decay, neuronal loss, and coassembly with endogenous tau in inducible mouse models of tauopathy. *The Journal of Neuroscience, 28*(3), 737–748. http://dx.doi.org/10.1523/JNEUROSCI.2824-07. 2008 pii:28/3/737.

Mori, K., Arzberger, T., Grasser, F. A., Gijselinck, I., May, S., Rentzsch, K., et al. (2013). Bidirectional transcripts of the expanded *C9orf72* hexanucleotide repeat are translated into aggregating dipeptide repeat proteins. *Acta Neuropathologica, 126*(6), 881–893. http://dx.doi.org/10.1007/s00401-013-1189-3.

Mummery, C. J., Patterson, K., Price, C. J., Ashburner, J., Frackowiak, R. S., & Hodges, J. R. (2000). A voxel-based morphometry study of semantic dementia: relationship between temporal lobe atrophy and semantic memory. *Annals of Neurology, 47*(1), 36–45.

Mummery, C. J., Patterson, K., Wise, R. J., Vandenberghe, R., Price, C. J., & Hodges, J. R. (1999). Disrupted temporal lobe connections in semantic dementia. *Brain, 122*(Pt 1), 61–73.

Nardell, M., & Tampi, R. R. (2014). Pharmacological treatments for frontotemporal dementias: a systematic review of randomized controlled trials. *American Journal of Alzheimer's Disease and Other Dementias, 29*(2), 123–132. http://dx.doi.org/10.1177/1533317513507375.

Neary, D., Snowden, J. S., Northen, B., & Goulding, P. (1988). Dementia of frontal lobe type. *Journal of Neurology, Neurosurgery, & Psychiatry, 51*(3), 353–361.

Nestor, P. J., Graham, N. L., Fryer, T. D., Williams, G. B., Patterson, K., & Hodges, J. R. (2003). Progressive non-fluent aphasia is associated with hypometabolism centred on the left anterior insula. *Brain, 126*(Pt 11), 2406–2418. http://dx.doi.org/10.1093/brain/awg240.

Neumann, M., Rademakers, R., Roeber, S., Baker, M., Kretzschmar, H. A., & Mackenzie, I. R. (2009). A new subtype of frontotemporal lobar degeneration with FUS pathology. *Brain, 132*(Pt 11), 2922–2931. http://dx.doi.org/10.1093/brain/awp214 pii:awp214.

Neumann, M., Sampathu, D. M., Kwong, L. K., Truax, A. C., Micsenyi, M. C., Chou, T. T., et al. (2006). Ubiquitinated TDP-43 in frontotemporal lobar degeneration and amyotrophic lateral sclerosis. *Science, 314*(5796), 130–133.

Neumann, M., Tolnay, M., & Mackenzie, I. R. (2009). The molecular basis of frontotemporal dementia. *Expert Reviews in Molecular Medicine, 11*, e23. http://dx.doi.org/10.1017/S1462399409001136 pii:S1462399409001136.

Nonaka, T., Masuda-Suzukake, M., Arai, T., Hasegawa, Y., Akatsu, H., Obi, T., et al. (2013). Prion-like properties of pathological TDP-43 aggregates from diseased brains. *Cell Reports, 4*(1), 124–134. http://dx.doi.org/10.1016/j.celrep.2013.06.007.

O'Leary, J. C., 3rd, Li, Q., Marinec, P., Blair, L. J., Congdon, E. E., Johnson, A. G., et al. (2010). Phenothiazine-mediated rescue of cognition in tau transgenic mice requires neuroprotection and reduced soluble tau burden. *Molecular Neurodegeneration, 5*, 45. http://dx.doi.org/10.1186/1750-1326-5-45 pii:1750-1326-5-45.

Paloneva, J., Manninen, T., Christman, G., Hovanes, K., Mandelin, J., Adolfsson, R., et al. (2002). Mutations in two genes encoding different subunits of a receptor signaling complex result in an identical disease phenotype. *American Journal of Human Genetics, 71*(3), 656–662. http://dx.doi.org/10.1086/342259.

Paquet, D., Bhat, R., Sydow, A., Mandelkow, E. M., Berg, S., Hellberg, S., et al. (2009). A zebrafish model of tauopathy allows in vivo imaging of neuronal cell death and drug evaluation. *Journal of Clinical Investigation, 119*(5), 1382–1395. http://dx.doi.org/10.1172/JCI37537.

Peters, F., Perani, D., Herholz, K., Holthoff, V., Beuthien-Baumann, B., et al. (2006). Orbitofrontal dysfunction related to both apathy and disinhibition in frontotemporal dementia. *Dementia and Geriatric Cognitive Disorders, 21*(5–6), 373–379. http://dx.doi.org/10.1159/000091898.

Pick, A. (1892). Über die Beziehungen der sinilen Hirnatrophie zur Aphasie. *Prager Medizinische Wochenschrift, 17*, 165–167.

Pickering-Brown, S. M., Rollinson, S., Du Plessis, D., Morrison, K. E., Varma, A., Richardson, A. M., et al. (2008). Frequency and clinical characteristics of progranulin mutation carriers in the Manchester frontotemporal lobar degeneration cohort: comparison with patients with MAPT and no known mutations. *Brain, 131*(Pt 3), 721–731. http://dx.doi.org/10.1093/brain/awm331.

Poorkaj, P., Bird, T. D., Wijsman, E., Nemens, E., Garruto, R. M., Anderson, L., et al. (1998). Tau is a candidate gene for chromosome 17 frontotemporal dementia. *Annals of Neurology, 43*(6), 815–825.

Price, C. J. (2000). The anatomy of language: contributions from functional neuroimaging. *Journal of Anatomy, 197*(Pt 3), 335–359.

Rabinovici, G. D., Jagust, W. J., Furst, A. J., Ogar, J. M., Racine, C. A., Mormino, E. C., et al. (2008). Abeta amyloid and glucose metabolism in three variants of primary progressive aphasia. *Annals of Neurology, 64*(4), 388–401. http://dx.doi.org/10.1002/ana.21451.

Rademakers, R., Cruts, M., & van Broeckhoven, C. (2004). The role of tau (*MAPT*) in frontotemporal dementia and related tauopathies. *Human Mutation, 24*(4), 277–295.

Rademakers, R., Neumann, M., & Mackenzie, I. R. (2012). Advances in understanding the molecular basis of frontotemporal dementia. *Nature Reviews. Neurology, 8*(8), 423–434. http://dx.doi.org/10.1038/nrneurol.2012.117.

Ramsden, M., Kotilinek, L., Forster, C., Paulson, J., McGowan, E., SantaCruz, K., et al. (2005). Age-dependent neurofibrillary tangle formation, neuron loss, and memory impairment in a mouse model of human tauopathy (P301L). *The Journal of Neuroscience, 25*(46), 10637–10647.

Rascovsky, K., Hodges, J. R., Knopman, D., Mendez, M. F., Kramer, J. H., Neuhaus, J., et al. (2011). Sensitivity of revised diagnostic criteria for the behavioural variant of frontotemporal dementia. *Brain, 134*, 2456–2477. http://dx.doi.org/10.1093/brain/awr179.

Ratnavalli, E., Brayne, C., Dawson, K., & Hodges, J. R. (2002). The prevalence of frontotemporal dementia. *Neurology, 58*(11), 1615–1621.

Renton, A. E., Majounie, E., Waite, A., Simón-Sánchez, J., Rollinson, S., Gibbs, J. R., et al. (2011). A hexanucleotide repeat expansion in *C9ORF72* is the cause of chromosome 9p21-linked ALS-FTD. *Neuron, 72*(2), 257–268. http://dx.doi.org/10.1016/j.neuron.2011.09.010 pii:S0896-6273(11)00797-5.

Ringholz, G. M., Appel, S. H., Bradshaw, M., Cooke, N. A., Mosnik, D. M., & Schulz, P. E. (2005). Prevalence and patterns of cognitive impairment in sporadic ALS. *Neurology, 65*(4), 586–590. http://dx.doi.org/10.1212/01.wnl.0000172911.39167.b6.

Roberson, E. D., Hesse, J. H., Rose, K. D., Slama, H., Johnson, J. K., Yaffe, K., et al. (2005). Frontotemporal dementia progresses to death faster than Alzheimer disease. *Neurology, 65*(5), 719–725.

Rohrer, J. D., Guerreiro, R., Vandrovcova, J., Uphill, J., Reiman, D., Beck, J., et al. (2009). The heritability and genetics of frontotemporal lobar degeneration. *Neurology, 73*(18), 1451–1456. http://dx.doi.org/10.1212/WNL.0b013e3181bf997a pii:73/18/1451.

Rohrer, J. D., Lashley, T., Schott, J. M., Warren, J. E., Mead, S., Isaacs, A. M., et al. (2011). Clinical and neuroanatomical signatures of tissue pathology in frontotemporal lobar degeneration. *Brain, 134*(Pt 9), 2565–2581. http://dx.doi.org/10.1093/brain/awr198.

Rosen, H. J., Allison, S. C., Schauer, G. F., Gorno-Tempini, M. L., Weiner, M. W., & Miller, B. L. (2005). Neuroanatomical correlates of behavioural disorders in dementia. *Brain, 128*(Pt 11), 2612–2625. http://dx.doi.org/10.1093/brain/awh628 pii:awh628.

Rosen, H. J., Gorno-Tempini, M. L., Goldman, W. P., Perry, R. J., Schuff, N., Weiner, M., et al. (2002). Patterns of brain atrophy in frontotemporal dementia and semantic dementia. *Neurology, 58*(2), 198–208.

Rosso, S. M., Donker Kaat, L., Baks, T., Joosse, M., de Koning, I., Pijnenburg, Y., et al. (2003). Frontotemporal dementia in The Netherlands: patient characteristics and prevalence estimates from a population-based study. *Brain, 126*(Pt 9), 2016–2022.

Ruiz, A., Dols-Icardo, O., Bullido, M. J., Pastor, P., Rodriguez-Rodriguez, E., & dementia genetic Spanish, c, et al. (2014). Assessing the role of the *TREM2* p.R47H variant as a risk factor for Alzheimer's disease and frontotemporal dementia. *Neurobiology of Aging, 35*(2), 444 e441–444. http://dx.doi.org/10.1016/j.neurobiolaging.2013.08.011.

Ryan, C. L., Baranowski, D. C., Chitramuthu, B. P., Malik, S., Li, Z., Cao, M., et al. (2009). Progranulin is expressed within motor neurons and promotes neuronal cell survival. *BMC Neuroscience, 10*, 130. http://dx.doi.org/10.1186/1471-2202-10-130 pii:1471-2202-10-130.

Sampathu, D. M., Neumann, M., Kwong, L. K., Chou, T. T., Micsenyi, M., Truax, A., et al. (2006). Pathological heterogeneity of frontotemporal lobar degeneration with ubiquitin-positive inclusions delineated by ubiquitin immunohistochemistry and novel monoclonal antibodies. *The American Journal of Pathology, 169*(4), 1343–1352. http://dx.doi.org/10.2353/ajpath.2006.060438.

San Pedro, E. C., Deutsch, G., Liu, H. G., & Mountz, J. M. (2000). Frontotemporal decreases in rCBF correlate with degree of dysnomia in primary progressive aphasia. *Journal of Nuclear Medicine, 41*(2), 228–233.

Sanders, D. W., Kaufman, S. K., DeVos, S. L., Sharma, A. M., Mirbaha, H., Li, A., et al. (2014). Distinct tau prion strains propagate in cells and mice and define different tauopathies. *Neuron, 82*(6), 1271–1288. http://dx.doi.org/10.1016/j.neuron.2014.04.047.

SantaCruz, K., Lewis, J., Spires, T., Paulson, J., Kotilinek, L., Ingelsson, M., et al. (2005). Tau suppression in a neurodegenerative mouse model improves memory function. *Science, 309*(5733), 476–481.

Santillo, A. F., & Englund, E. (2014). Greater loss of von Economo neurons than loss of layer II and III neurons in behavioral variant frontotemporal dementia. *American Journal of Neurodegenerative Disease*, *3*(2), 64–71.

Santillo, A. F., Nilsson, C., & Englund, E. (2013). Von Economo neurones are selectively targeted in frontotemporal dementia. *Neuropathology and Applied Neurobiology*, *39*(5), 572–579. http://dx.doi.org/10.1111/nan.12021.

Schroeter, M. L., Vogt, B., Frisch, S., Becker, G., Seese, A., Barthel, H., et al. (2011). Dissociating behavioral disorders in early dementia: an FDG-PET study. *Psychiatry Research*, *194*(3), 235–244. http://dx.doi.org/10.1016/j.pscychresns.2011.06.009.

Seelaar, H., Kamphorst, W., Rosso, S. M., Azmani, A., Masdjedi, R., de Koning, I., et al. (2008). Distinct genetic forms of frontotemporal dementia. *Neurology*, *71*(16), 1220–1226. http://dx.doi.org/10.1212/01.wnl.0000319702.37497.72 pii:01.wnl.0000319702.37497.72.

Seeley, W. W., Carlin, D. A., Allman, J. M., Macedo, M. N., Bush, C., Miller, B. L., et al. (2006). Early frontotemporal dementia targets neurons unique to apes and humans. *Annals of Neurology*, *60*(6), 660–667. http://dx.doi.org/10.1002/ana.21055.

Seeley, W. W., Crawford, R. K., Zhou, J., Miller, B. L., & Greicius, M. D. (2009). Neurodegenerative diseases target large-scale human brain networks. *Neuron*, *62*(1), 42–52. http://dx.doi.org/10.1016/j.neuron.2009.03.024 pii:S0896-6273(09)00249-9.

Seeley, W. W., Menon, V., Schatzberg, A. F., Keller, J., Glover, G. H., Kenna, H., et al. (2007). Dissociable intrinsic connectivity networks for salience processing and executive control. *The Journal of Neuroscience*, *27*(9), 2349–2356. http://dx.doi.org/10.1523/JNEUROSCI.5587-06.2007 pii:27/9/2349.

Seeley, W. W., Merkle, F. T., Gaus, S. E., Craig, A. D., Allman, J. M., & Hof, P. R. (2012). Distinctive neurons of the anterior cingulate and frontoinsular cortex: a historical perspective. *Cerebral Cortex*, *22*(2), 245–250. http://dx.doi.org/10.1093/cercor/bhr005.

Sergeant, N., David, J. P., Lefranc, D., Vermersch, P., Wattez, A., & Delacourte, A. (1997). Different distribution of phosphorylated tau protein isoforms in Alzheimer's and Pick's diseases. *FEBS Letters*, *412*(3), 578–582.

Sergeant, N., Wattez, A., & Delacourte, A. (1999). Neurofibrillary degeneration in progressive supranuclear palsy and corticobasal degeneration: tau pathologies with exclusively "exon 10" isoforms. *Journal of Neurochemistry*, *72*(3), 1243–1249.

Sha, S. J., Takada, L. T., Rankin, K. P., Yokoyama, J. S., Rutherford, N. J., Fong, J. C., et al. (2012). Frontotemporal dementia due to C9ORF72 mutations: clinical and imaging features. *Neurology*, *79*(10), 1002–1011. http://dx.doi.org/10.1212/WNL.0b013e318268452e.

Shankaran, S. S., Capell, A., Hruscha, A. T., Fellerer, K., Neumann, M., Schmid, B., et al. (2008). Missense mutations in the progranulin gene linked to frontotemporal lobar degeneration with ubiquitin-immunoreactive inclusions reduce progranulin production and secretion. *The Journal of Biological Chemistry*, *283*(3), 1744–1753. http://dx.doi.org/10.1074/jbc.M705115200 pii:M705115200.

Simon-Sanchez, J., Dopper, E. G., Cohn-Hokke, P. E., Hukema, R. K., Nicolaou, N., Seelaar, H., et al. (2012). The clinical and pathological phenotype of C9ORF72 hexanucleotide repeat expansions. *Brain*, *135*(Pt 3), 723–735. http://dx.doi.org/10.1093/brain/awr353.

Skibinski, G., Parkinson, N. J., Brown, J. M., Chakrabarti, L., Lloyd, S. L., Hummerich, H., et al. (2005). Mutations in the endosomal ESCRTIII-complex subunit *CHMP2B* in frontotemporal dementia. *Nature Genetics*, *37*(8), 806–808.

Smith, K. R., Damiano, J., Franceschetti, S., Carpenter, S., Canafoglia, L., Morbin, M., et al. (2012). Strikingly different clinicopathological phenotypes determined by progranulin-mutation dosage. *American Journal of Human Genetics*, *90*(6), 1102–1107. http://dx.doi.org/10.1016/j.ajhg.2012.04.021.

Smith, K. S., Tindell, A. J., Aldridge, J. W., & Berridge, K. C. (2009). Ventral pallidum roles in reward and motivation. *Behavioural Brain Research, 196*(2), 155–167. http://dx.doi.org/10.1016/j.bbr.2008.09.038 pii:S0166-4328(08)00539-1.

Snowden, J. S., Rollinson, S., Thompson, J. C., Harris, J. M., Stopford, C. L., Richardson, A. M., et al. (2012). Distinct clinical and pathological characteristics of frontotemporal dementia associated with *C9ORF72* mutations. *Brain, 135*(Pt 3), 693–708. http://dx.doi.org/10.1093/brain/awr355.

Spillantini, M. G., Murrell, J. R., Goedert, M., Farlow, M. R., Klug, A., & Ghetti, B. (1998). Mutation in the tau gene in familial multiple system tauopathy with presenile dementia. *Proceedings of the National Academy of Sciences of the United States of America, 95*(13), 7737–7741.

Spittaels, K., Van den Haute, C., Van Dorpe, J., Bruynseels, K., Vandezande, K., Laenen, I., et al. (1999). Prominent axonopathy in the brain and spinal cord of transgenic mice overexpressing four-repeat human tau protein. *The American Journal of Pathology, 155*(6), 2153–2165. http://dx.doi.org/10.1016/S0002-9440(10)65533-2.

Stevens, M., van Duijn, C. M., Kamphorst, W., de Knijff, P., Heutink, P., van Gool, W. A., et al. (1998). Familial aggregation in frontotemporal dementia. *Neurology, 50*(6), 1541–1545.

Strand, A. D., Aragaki, A. K., Baquet, Z. C., Hodges, A., Cunningham, P., Holmans, P., et al. (2007). Conservation of regional gene expression in mouse and human brain. *PLoS Genetics, 3*(4), e59. http://dx.doi.org/10.1371/journal.pgen.0030059 pii:06-PLGE-RA-0402R3.

Su, Z., Zhang, Y., Gendron, T. F., Bauer, P. O., Chew, J., Yang, W. Y., et al. (2014). Discovery of a biomarker and lead small molecules to target r(GGGGCC)-associated defects in c9FTD/ALS. *Neuron, 83*(5), 1043–1050. http://dx.doi.org/10.1016/j.neuron.2014.07.041.

Swanberg, M. M. (2007). Memantine for behavioral disturbances in frontotemporal dementia: a case series. *Alzheimer Disease and Associated Disorders, 21*(2), 164–166. http://dx.doi.org/10.1097/WAD.0b013e318047df5d.

Sydow, A., Van der Jeugd, A., Zheng, F., Ahmed, T., Balschun, D., Petrova, O., et al. (2011). Tau-induced defects in synaptic plasticity, learning, and memory are reversible in transgenic mice after switching off the toxic tau mutant. *The Journal of Neuroscience, 31*(7), 2511–2525. http://dx.doi.org/10.1523/JNEUROSCI.5245-10.2011 pii:31/7/2511.

Synofzik, M., Born, C., Rominger, A., Lummel, N., Schols, L., Biskup, S., et al. (2014). Targeted high-throughput sequencing identifies a *TARDBP* mutation as a cause of early-onset FTD without motor neuron disease. *Neurobiology of Aging, 35*(5), 1212 e1211–1215. http://dx.doi.org/10.1016/j.neurobiolaging.2013.10.092.

Tanaka, Y., Chambers, J. K., Matsuwaki, T., Yamanouchi, K., & Nishihara, M. (2014). Possible involvement of lysosomal dysfunction in pathological changes of the brain in aged progranulin-deficient mice. *Acta Neuropathologica Communications, 2*, 78. http://dx.doi.org/10.1186/s40478-014-0078-x.

Tanemura, K., Akagi, T., Murayama, M., Kikuchi, N., Murayama, O., Hashikawa, T., et al. (2001). Formation of filamentous tau aggregations in transgenic mice expressing V337M human tau. *Neurobiology of Disease, 8*(6), 1036–1045. http://dx.doi.org/10.1006/nbdi.2001.0439.

Tanzi, R. E., St George, H. P. H., Haines, J. L., Polinsky, R. J., Nee, L., Foncin, J. F., et al. (1987). The genetic defect in familial Alzheimer's disease is not tightly linked to the amyloid beta-protein gene. *Nature, 329*, 156–157.

Tao, Z., Wang, H., Xia, Q., Li, K., Li, K., Jiang, X., et al. (2015). Nucleolar stress and impaired stress granule formation contribute to *C9orf72* RAN translation-induced cytotoxicity. *Human Molecular Genetics.* http://dx.doi.org/10.1093/hmg/ddv005.

Thelen, M., Razquin, C., Hernandez, I., Gorostidi, A., Sanchez-Valle, R., Ortega-Cubero, S., et al. (2014). Investigation of the role of rare *TREM2* variants in frontotemporal dementia subtypes. *Neurobiology of Aging, 35*(11), 2657 e2613–2659. http://dx.doi.org/10.1016/j.neurobiolaging.2014.06.018.

Thomas, M., Alegre-Abarrategui, J., & Wade-Martins, R. (2013). RNA dysfunction and aggrephagy at the centre of an amyotrophic lateral sclerosis/frontotemporal dementia disease continuum. *Brain, 136*(Pt 5), 1345–1360. http://dx.doi.org/10.1093/brain/awt030 pii:awt030.

Van Damme, P., Van Hoecke, A., Lambrechts, D., Vanacker, P., Bogaert, E., van Swieten, J., et al. (2008). Progranulin functions as a neurotrophic factor to regulate neurite outgrowth and enhance neuronal survival. *Journal of Cell Biology, 181*(1), 37–41. http://dx.doi.org/10.1083/jcb.200712039 pii:jcb.200712039.

Van Langenhove, T., van der Zee, J., Gijselinck, I., Engelborghs, S., Vandenberghe, R., Vandenbulcke, M., et al. (2013). Distinct clinical characteristics of *C9orf72* expansion carriers compared with GRN, MAPT, and nonmutation carriers in a Flanders-Belgian FTLD cohort. *JAMA Neurology, 70*(3), 365–373. http://dx.doi.org/10.1001/2013.jamaneurol.181.

Van Langenhove, T., van der Zee, J., Sleegers, K., Engelborghs, S., Vandenberghe, R., Gijselinck, I., et al. (2010). Genetic contribution of *FUS* to frontotemporal lobar degeneration. *Neurology, 74*(5), 366–371. http://dx.doi.org/10.1212/WNL.0b013e3181ccc732 pii:74/5/366.

Vercelletto, M., Boutoleau-Bretonniere, C., Volteau, C., Puel, M., Auriacombe, S., Sarazin, M., & French research network on Frontotemporal, d (2011). Memantine in behavioral variant frontotemporal dementia: negative results. *Journal of Alzheimer's Disease, 23*(4), 749–759. http://dx.doi.org/10.3233/JAD-2010-101632.

Wang, I. F., Guo, B. S., Liu, Y. C., Wu, C. C., Yang, C. H., Tsai, K. J., et al. (2012). Autophagy activators rescue and alleviate pathogenesis of a mouse model with proteinopathies of the TAR DNA-binding protein 43. *Proceedings of the National Academy of Sciences of the United States of America, 109*(37), 15024–15029. http://dx.doi.org/10.1073/pnas.1206362109.

Wang, J., Van Damme, P., Cruchaga, C., Gitcho, M. A., Vidal, J. M., Seijo-Martinez, M., et al. (2010). Pathogenic cysteine mutations affect progranulin function and production of mature granulins. *Journal of Neurochemistry, 112*(5), 1305–1315. http://dx.doi.org/10.1111/j.1471-4159.2009.06546.x pii:JNC6546.

Warrington, E. K., et al. (1975). The selective impairment of semantic memory. Quarterly Journal of Experimental Psychology, 27(4), 635–657. http://dx.doi.org/10.1080/14640747508400525.

Warmus, B. A., Sekar, D., McCutchen, E., Schellenberg, G. D., Roberts, R., McMahon, L. L., et al. (2014). Tau-mediated NMDA receptor impairment underlies dysfunction of a selectively vulnerable network in a mouse model of frontotemporal dementia. *Journal of Neuroscience, 34*(49), 16482–16495. http://dx.doi.org/10.1523/JNEUROSCI.3418-14.2014.

Watts, G. D., Wymer, J., Kovach, M. J., Mehta, S. G., Mumm, S., Darvish, D., et al. (2004). Inclusion body myopathy associated with Paget disease of bone and frontotemporal dementia is caused by mutant valosin-containing protein. *Nature Genetics, 36*(4), 377–381.

Wen, X., Tan, W., Westergard, T., Krishnamurthy, K., Markandaiah, S. S., Shi, Y., et al. (2014). Antisense proline-arginine RAN dipeptides linked to *C9ORF72*-ALS/FTD form toxic nuclear aggregates that initiate in vitro and in vivo neuronal death. *Neuron, 84*(6), 1213–1225. http://dx.doi.org/10.1016/j.neuron.2014.12.010.

Whitwell, J. L., Anderson, V. M., Scahill, R. I., Rossor, M. N., & Fox, N. C. (2004). Longitudinal patterns of regional change on volumetric MRI in frontotemporal lobar degeneration. *Dementia and Geriatric Cognitive Disorders, 17*(4), 307–310. http://dx.doi.org/10.1159/000077160.

Whitwell, J. L., Duffy, J. R., Strand, E. A., Xia, R., Mandrekar, J., Machulda, M. M., et al. (2013). Distinct regional anatomic and functional correlates of neurodegenerative apraxia of speech and aphasia: an MRI and FDG-PET study. *Brain and Language, 125*(3), 245–252. http://dx.doi.org/10.1016/j.bandl.2013.02.005.

Whitwell, J. L., Sampson, E. L., Loy, C. T., Warren, J. E., Rossor, M. N., Fox, N. C., et al. (2007). VBM signatures of abnormal eating behaviours in frontotemporal lobar degeneration. *Neuroimage*, *35*(1), 207–213. http://dx.doi.org/10.1016/j.neuroimage.2006.12.006.

Williams, G. B., Nestor, P. J., & Hodges, J. R. (2005). Neural correlates of semantic and behavioural deficits in frontotemporal dementia. *Neuroimage*, *24*(4), 1042–1051. http://dx.doi.org/10.1016/j.neuroimage.2004.10.023.

Wils, H., Kleinberger, G., Pereson, S., Janssens, J., Capell, A., Van Dam, D., et al. (2012). Cellular ageing, increased mortality and FTLD-TDP-associated neuropathology in progranulin knockout mice. *The Journal of Pathology*, *228*(1), 67–76. http://dx.doi.org/10.1002/path.4043.

Witgert, M., Salamone, A. R., Strutt, A. M., Jawaid, A., Massman, P. J., Bradshaw, M., et al. (2010). Frontal-lobe mediated behavioral dysfunction in amyotrophic lateral sclerosis. *European Journal of Neurology*, *17*(1), 103–110. http://dx.doi.org/10.1111/j.1468-1331.2009.02801.x.

Wittmann, C. W., Wszolek, M. F., Shulman, J. M., Salvaterra, P. M., Lewis, J., Hutton, M., et al. (2001). Tauopathy in *Drosophila*: neurodegeneration without neurofibrillary tangles. *Science*, *293*(5530), 711–714.

Woolley, J. D., Gorno-Tempini, M. L., Seeley, W. W., Rankin, K., Lee, S. S., Matthews, B. R., et al. (2007). Binge eating is associated with right orbitofrontal-insular-striatal atrophy in frontotemporal dementia. *Neurology*, *69*(14), 1424–1433. http://dx.doi.org/10.1212/01.wnl.0000277461.06713.23.

Xu, Z., Poidevin, M., Li, X., Li, Y., Shu, L., Nelson, D. L., et al. (2013). Expanded GGGGCC repeat RNA associated with amyotrophic lateral sclerosis and frontotemporal dementia causes neurodegeneration. *Proceedings of the National Academy of Sciences of the United States of America*, *110*(19), 7778–7783. http://dx.doi.org/10.1073/pnas.1219643110 pii:1219643110.

Yanamandra, K., Kfoury, N., Jiang, H., Mahan, T. E., Ma, S., Maloney, S. E., et al. (2013). Anti-tau antibodies that block tau aggregate seeding in vitro markedly decrease pathology and improve cognition in vivo. *Neuron*, *80*(2), 402–414. http://dx.doi.org/10.1016/j.neuron.2013.07.046.

Yin, F., Banerjee, R., Thomas, B., Zhou, P., Qian, L., Jia, T., et al. (2010). Exaggerated inflammation, impaired host defense, and neuropathology in progranulin-deficient mice. *The Journal of Experimental Medicine*, *207*(1), 117–128. http://dx.doi.org/10.1084/jem.20091568 pii:jem.20091568.

Yin, F., Dumont, M., Banerjee, R., Ma, Y., Li, H., Lin, M. T., et al. (2010). Behavioral deficits and progressive neuropathology in progranulin-deficient mice: a mouse model of frontotemporal dementia. *FASEB Journal*, *24*(12), 4639–4647. http://dx.doi.org/10.1096/fj.10-161471.

Yoshiyama, Y., Higuchi, M., Zhang, B., Huang, S. M., Iwata, N., Saido, T. C., et al. (2007). Synapse loss and microglial activation precede tangles in a P301S tauopathy mouse model. *Neuron*, *53*(3), 337–351.

Zamboni, G., Huey, E. D., Krueger, F., Nichelli, P. F., & Grafman, J. (2008). Apathy and disinhibition in frontotemporal dementia: insights into their neural correlates. *Neurology*, *71*(10), 736–742. http://dx.doi.org/10.1212/01.wnl.0000324920.96835.95.

Zhang, Y. J., Jansen-West, K., Xu, Y. F., Gendron, T. F., Bieniek, K. F., Lin, W. L., et al. (2014). Aggregation-prone c9FTD/ALS poly(GA) RAN-translated proteins cause neurotoxicity by inducing ER stress. *Acta Neuropathologica*, *128*(4), 505–524. http://dx.doi.org/10.1007/s00401-014-1336-5.

Zhou, J., Greicius, M. D., Gennatas, E. D., Growdon, M. E., Jang, J. Y., Rabinovici, G. D., et al. (2010). Divergent network connectivity changes in behavioural variant frontotemporal dementia and Alzheimer's disease. *Brain*, *133*(Pt 5), 1352–1367. http://dx.doi.org/10.1093/brain/awq075 pii:awq075.

Zu, T., Liu, Y., Banez-Coronel, M., Reid, T., Pletnikova, O., Lewis, J., et al. (2013). RAN proteins and RNA foci from antisense transcripts in C9ORF72 ALS and frontotemporal dementia. *Proceedings of the National Academy of Sciences of the United States of America*, *110*(51), E4968–E4977. http://dx.doi.org/10.1073/pnas.1315438110.

Chapter 7

Parkinson's Disease and the Cerebral Cortex

D.F. Cechetto, M. Jog
University of Western Ontario, London, ON, Canada

INTRODUCTION

Parkinson's disease (PD) is a progressive neurodegenerative disease that is an age-related disorder, typically affecting middle-aged and elderly individuals. It is commonly associated with movement disorders such as tremor, rigidity, akinesia (poverty of movement), bradykinesia (slowness and impaired scaling of voluntary movement), and difficulty in walking and gait (Jankovic & Kapadia, 2001). However, there are additional behavioral symptoms that can occur in later stages of the disease. These can include various characteristics of dementia, depression, sleep and sensory disruption, and emotional issues. It is estimated that 6.3 million people have PD, of which there are approximately 1 million in the United States alone (Parkinson's Disease Foundation). It is a neurodegenerative disease that is second only to Alzheimer's disease for prevalence.

PATHOPHYSIOLOGY OF PARKINSON'S DISEASE

The motor symptoms of PD are primarily caused by the loss of dopaminergic neurons in the substantia nigra, *pars compacta* in the midbrain, although the cerebral cortex is intimately involved in all of the pathways associated with the dopamine input to the basal ganglia. In the early stages of PD, there is considerable dopamine loss in the dorsal part of the striatum with relatively little effect on dopamine levels in the ventral striatum (Bernheimer, Birkmayer, Hornykiewicz, Jellinger, & Seitelberger, 1973; Jellinger, 2001). As the disease progresses, there is, in addition, an extensive distribution of Lewy bodies (intraneuronal proteinaceous cytoplasmic inclusions), particularly in the neocortex (Jellinger, 2001). The typical treatment of PD involves administration of the dopamine prodrug levodopa. Unfortunately, the long-term use of levodopa for the treatment of PD eventually results in the development of motor complications in the vast majority of patients (Dauer & Przedborski, 2003). This has lead to a renewed interest in neurosurgical approaches such as deep brain stimulation to

The Cerebral Cortex in Neurodegenerative and Neuropsychiatric Disorders.
http://dx.doi.org/10.1016/B978-0-12-801942-9.00007-0

deal with the progressive deterioration in motor symptoms associated with PD. In particular, the technique of high-frequency stimulation of the subthalamic nucleus, a region of the brain involved in the pathways associated with control of movements, with implanted macroelectrodes is commonly used to continue to treat PD patients after chronic levodopa drug regimen results in motor fluctuations and dyskinesias (Benabid, Chabardes, Mitrofanis, & Pollak, 2009). As described in this section, the subthalamic nucleus represents a critical site for input from the motor cortex in the control of movements by the basal ganglia.

In healthy individuals, the dopamine neurons from the substantia nigra, *pars compacta* project to the striatum, releasing dopamine to modulate the direct and indirect striatopallidal pathways for the control of movement (Fig. 7.1). In particular, the initiation and strength of contraction are the elements of movement that are most modulated by the striatopallidal pathways. Multiple regions of the cerebral cortex including, in particular, the motor cortical regions and the prefrontal cortex, send a glutamatergic projection to the striatum (Mathai & Smith, 2011). In the direct striatopallidal pathway, the striatum sends an inhibitory γ-aminobutyric acid–transmitting (GABAergic) projection to the globus pallidus, *pars interna*.

The indirect striatopallidal pathway sends GABAergic projection neurons to the globus pallidus, *pars externa*, and an additional GABAergic projection to

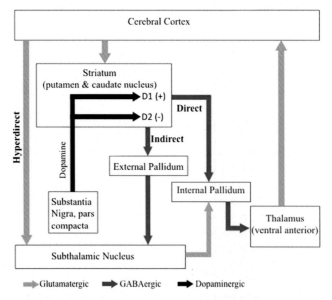

FIGURE 7.1 Schematic diagram of the pathways involved in basal ganglia control of motor function. The three direct, indirect, and hyperdirect pathways are shown with the dopamine input from the substantia nigra. The cerebral cortex has two major inputs to basal ganglia circuits through the striatum and the subthalamic nucleus. The primary feedback to the cortex is through the thalamus. *GABAergic*, γ-Aminobutyric acid–transmitting.

the subthalamic nucleus in the diencephalon. In what is termed the *hyperdirect pathway*, the subthalamic nucleus also receives a direct input from the cerebral cortex (Nambu, Tokuno, & Takada, 2002). The subthalamic nucleus then sends an excitatory glutamatergic projection to the globus pallidus, *pars interna* (Bevan, Atherton, & Baufreton, 2006).

It is the globus pallidus, *pars interna* that has an inhibitory GABAergic projection to the motor nuclei of the thalamus, in particular, the ventral anterior nucleus, which finally sends the excitatory or inhibitory feedback to the motor cortex via a glutamatergic projection (see Fig. 7.1). The overall effect of the combination of inhibitory and excitatory projections in these pathways is such that the direct striatopallidal pathway provides a feedforward excitatory input back to the motor cortex, whereas the indirect striatopallidal pathway provides a reduction in motor cortex activity when it is activated. This pathway can aid in the understanding of the mechanisms of deep brain stimulation and the role of the cerebral cortex. The mechanism of the effectiveness of deep brain stimulation can be related to the antidromic activation of cortical neurons projecting to the subthalamic nucleus that, in turn, negates the impact of input to the cortex from the thalamus (Santiello, Gale, Montgomery, & Sarma, 2010).

The dopaminergic projection from the substantia nigra, *pars compacta* terminates in the striatum. Although there are multiple dopamine receptor subtypes in the striatum, there are two that are of high interest regarding the way in which the basal ganglia control motor function and in particular, the deficits that occur in PD when the dopamine neurons are lost (Gerfen & Surmeier, 2011). The GABAergic projection neurons in the striatum have low-affinity dopaminergic D1 receptors, whereas the GABAergic projection neurons in the indirect striatopallidal pathway to the globus pallidus, *pars externa* express high-affinity dopamine D2 receptors (Gerfen & Surmeier, 2011). Dopamine activation of the D1 receptors in the direct pathway enhances the γ-aminobutyric acid (GABA) neuron excitability, while a reduction in excitability is seen at the dopamine D2 receptors in the indirect pathway. This organization has distinct changes in PD when there is loss of dopamine neurons in the substantia nigra, *pars compacta*. After chronic dopamine loss, the GABA projection neurons in the striatum undergo a reduction in excitability, while the striatal GABA neurons in the indirect pathway have an enhancement in excitability in response to input from the motor cortex. This effectively reduces the overall excitatory feedforward loop of the direct striatopallidal pathway and enhances the inhibitory feedback loop of the indirect striatopallidal pathway.

Thus it is clear that although PD is considered a disease directly affecting the basal ganglia, there is no doubt that there will be considerable impact on the function of the cerebral cortex. Multiple regions of the cortex project to the striatum, although the direct input to the subthalamic nucleus arises primarily from the frontal cortex (Nambu et al., 2002). The output neurons from the primary motor cortex to the striatum appear to send a bilateral projection and receive only a minor input from the basal ganglia thalamic relay nuclei (Pasquereau & Turner, 2011).

In fact, the thalamic input may terminate primarily on the pyramidal tractlike cortical neurons projecting to the subthalamic nucleus (Mathai & Smith, 2011). The other means by which the cerebral cortex becomes involved in PD is that as the disease progresses, there is a more widespread distribution of pathological components, including extensive deposit of Lewy bodies in the neocortex (Jellinger, 2001).

As described in later sections, there are three symptoms of PD for which the cerebral cortex has been implicated. These include the tremors associated with PD, other motor disturbances such as akinesia, and some of the cognitive disturbances, including dementia. Although each of these symptoms has been examined clinically in PD, the details of the mechanisms have been elaborated in animal models, including nonhuman primates, rats, and mice.

ANIMAL MODELS OF PARKINSON'S DISEASE

Animal models of PD have been particularly effective in delineating the mechanisms of this condition and have been particularly useful for understanding the role of cortical circuits in both motor and nonmotor dysfunction. The animal models have been considerably useful because they replicate relatively closely the specific pathophysiology and therefore the symptoms of PD. Animal models of PD primarily rely on the use of the selective monoaminergic toxin, 1-methyl-4-phenyl-1,2,3,6-tetrahydropyridine (MPTP). The ability of MPTP to reproduce PD symptoms was discovered in 1982 when intravenous-drug users making meperidine accidentally synthesized MPTP (Langston, Ballard, Tetrud, & Irwin, 1983). MPTP toxicity creates the critical neurological symptoms and a complete and selective loss of dopaminergic neurons in the substantia nigra, *pars compacta*. In both humans and nonhuman primates, MPTP creates all of the motor symptoms of PD, including tremor, rigidity, akinesia, bradykinesia, postural instability and gait disturbances (Dauer & Przedborski, 2003). Other elements that make MPTP a good model for PD include the fact that susceptibility to symptoms increases with age, levodopa is beneficial in the treatment of the model, and it causes the development of untreatable motor complications over the long term (Dauer & Przedborski, 2003; Ovadia, Zhang, & Gash, 1995; Rose et al., 1993). Furthermore, as described in more detail in Neurotransmitters and Gene Expression in the Cortex, changes in the cerebral cortex develop similar to those observed in PD in the clinical setting.

The selective loss of dopamine neurons in the substantia nigra appears to be a consistent feature of the MPTP models whether it is used in nonhuman primates or mice (Dauer & Przedborski, 2003), although there is some issue regarding the efficacy of dopamine loss in the rat (Cenci, Whishaw, & Schallert, 2002). It has been shown that MPTP causes degeneration of dopamine terminals in mice but not in rats, because of a higher capacity of vesicular sequestration of MPTP and possibly the ability of rat monoadrenergic neurons to survive impaired energy metabolism (Cenci, Whishaw, & Schallert, 2002; Sundström & Samuelsson, 1997).

MPTP, like other toxic models of PD described in the following paragraphs, appears to cause neurodegeneration via the generation of reactive oxygen species (Nicklas, Youngster, Kindt, & Heikkila, 1987). However, animals exposed to MPTP do not develop the loss of other monoaminergic neurons, such as the noradrenergic neurons in the locus coeruleus, and there is no clear evidence of the formation of Lewy bodies in the nonhuman primate models or in humans accidentally exposed to MPTP (Forno, 1996; Forno, DeLanney, Irwin, & Ricaurte, 1993; Forno, Langston, DeLanney, Irwin, & Ricaurte, 1986).

An additional monoaminergic neuron–selective model of PD includes the use of the toxin 6-hydroxydopamine (6-OHDA). 6-OHDA can enter neurons via monoamine transporters. Once in the cell, it is oxidized to toxic free radicals. It is not permeable to the blood–brain barrier and must be administered via stereotaxic surgery to the midbrain. It can be delivered by injection directly into the substantia nigra, the striatum, or the medial forebrain bundle (the dopaminergic pathway from the substantia nigra to the striatum), resulting in considerable loss of dopaminergic neurons in the substantia nigra, *pars compacta* (Dauer & Przedborski, 2003; Javoy, Sotelo, Herbet, & Agid, 1976; Jonsson, 1980). MPTP injected into the striatum or the medial forebrain bundle is taken up by dopamine axons or terminals and retrogradely transported to the dopamine cell body, resulting a slower degeneration of the neurons (Przedborski et al., 1995; Sauer & Oertel, 1994).

Other, more recently developed models include the use of the herbicide paraquat (N,N′-dimethyl-4,4′-bipyridinium) that has structural similarity to 1-methyl-4-phenylpyridinium (MPP+), the active ingredient of MPTP. Paraquat exposure can lead to an increased risk for PD (Liou et al., 1997). In addition, rotenone, an insecticide, binds at the same site as MPP+ and has very similar molecular and systemic effects as MPTP (Betarbet et al., 2000; Dauer & Przedborski, 2003).

TREMORS AND THE CEREBRAL CORTEX

Tremor, the involuntary shaking movement in a body part such as the hand or foot, especially the resting tremor often seen in PD, is one of the most obvious aspects of the condition. Some patients with PD develop a very prominent and often disabling tremor. Nevertheless, 10% of patients are without any tremor, 60% have tremor as their presenting symptom, and 30% will have tremor at some point in their course, although not prominently (Hoehn & Yahr, 1967). This finding contributes to the definition of two extreme types of PD, the akinetic-rigid and the tremor-dominant types (Burn et al., 2006; Jankovic et al., 1990; Lewis et al., 2005; Rajput, Pahwa, Pahwa, & Rajput, 1993; Zetusky, Jankovic, & Pirozzolo, 1985). Other types of PD include a gait predominant type and those that have all the symptoms within the first 5 years.

There are additional differences between tremors and other PD symptoms. The tremor does not necessarily show up on the same side as the rigidity and bradykinesia. It can be seen contralateral to the side most severely affected by the other symptoms (Helmich, Hallett, Deuschl, Toni, & Bloem, 2012). In addition, the tremor does not progress at the same rate as the other PD symptoms, including bradykinesia, rigidity, gait, and balance disturbances (Louis et al., 1999). Finally, the severity of the tremor is not related to the degree of severity of the other symptoms and levodopa treatment is less likely to improve the tremor (Fishman, 2008; Koller, Busenbark, & Miner, 1994; Louis et al., 2001). These findings suggest that tremor has a very different pathophysiology that can be related to significant changes in circuits that include the cerebral cortex.

Experimental models have been useful in understanding the mechanisms of the tremor seen in PD and in particular to demonstrate the role of the cerebral cortex. What is most intriguing is that in the MPTP primate model of PD, tremor is not always a consistent finding. In fact, it appears to be species-specific. For example, Vervet monkeys treated with MPTP developed prolonged episodes of low-frequency tremor (Heimer et al., 2006; Raz, Vaadia, & Bergman, 2000) and African Green monkeys developed a classic rest tremor (Rivlin-Etzion, Elias, Heimer, & Bergman, 2010; Rivlin-Etzion et al., 2008). On the other hand, macaques administered MPTP developed only short episodes of high-frequency action/postural tremor (Burns et al., 1983) and rhesus monkeys developed infrequent and brief episodes of high-frequency tremor. Thus the nonhuman primate models with MPTP treatment can represent some of the differences seen in PD patient subtypes with tremulous PD and nontremor PD (Ellens & Leventhal, 2013; Rivlin-Etzion, Elias, Heimer, & Bergman, 2010). What is relatively consistent is that all of these primate species develop akinesia, rigidity, and severe postural instability in spite of the differences seen in the expression of tremor. This supports the notion derived from clinical observations that tremor has a different pathophysiology from the other PD symptoms, and there is evidence that the mechanism is found in cortical dysfunction.

Experimental models have implicated the motor cortex in the generation of tremors in PD. Recording of neurons in the globus pallidus does not demonstrate a consistent and coherent correlation with tremor (Hurtado, Gray, Tamas, & Sigvardt, 1999; Raz et al., 2000). However, the activity of neurons in the posterior ventral lateral nucleus of the thalamus are synchronized with the tremor (Helmich et al., 2012; Zaidel, Arkadir, Israel, & Bergman, 2009). These results and those of others highly suggest that there is a cerebellar–thalamic–cortical network that is responsible for the tremor in animal models of PD. This electrophysiological evidence is supported by magnetoencephalography experiments (Timmermann et al., 2003). Other metabolic studies have indicated that the circuits responsible for tremor converge are in the motor cortex (Helmich et al., 2012).

There are several possible models to describe the basis of tremor in PD, although the most substantial model places a great emphasis on the motor cortex in the production of the tremor (Helmich et al., 2012). A combination of functional magnetic resonance imaging (MRI) and electromyography recordings during the scanning have shown that the amplitude of tremor-related activity is time-locked and localized to a circuit that includes the ventral lateral nucleus of the thalamus, the cerebellum, and the motor cortex, and that there is increased functional connectivity between the basal ganglia with this circuit in patients who have PD compared with normal controls (van Duinen, Zijdewind, Hoogduin, & Maurits, 2005; Helmich, Janssen, Oyen, Bloem, & Toni, 2011; van Rootselaar et al., 2008).

Thus the evidence indicates that there is a cerebellar–thalamic–cortical network generating the tremor, but that this network is influenced by the changes in the basal ganglia and, in fact, the loss of dopamine in the basal ganglia would serve as the initial mechanism to trigger this dysfunctional network. Helmich has developed what is termed the "dimmer-switch model" of tremor in PD (Helmich et al., 2011). The changes in neuronal activity in the basal ganglia circuit produces tremor-related activity in the cerebellar–thalamic–cortical circuit, and both of these circuits converge in the motor cortex that, in turn, produces the tremor (Helmich et al., 2012). In addition, this model explains how the cerebellum is impacted in the tremor-related activity through an excitatory output from the motor cortex to the ventral lateral thalamus that is strongly connected to the cerebellum (Helmich et al., 2012). It also explains why there is electrophysiological evidence for increased connectivity between the motor cortex and the basal ganglia (Rivlin-Etzion et al., 2008).

AKINESIA AND BRADYKINESIA AND THE CEREBRAL CORTEX

Oscillations in neuronal firing are observed in the brains of patients with PD and MPTP-treated monkeys (Heimer, Bar-Gad, Goldberg, & Bergman, 2002; Heimer et al., 2006; Nini, Feingold, Slovin, & Bergman, 1995; Weinberger et al., 2006). It has been suggested that these oscillations may underlie the tremor or other symptoms of the disease and that the cerebral cortex plays a significant role in the alterations of these oscillations. This premise was tested in an experiment in normal and MPTP-treated Vervet monkeys using both neuronal recording and electrical stimulation in the motor cortex and the globus pallidus to mimic the bursting oscillations in patients who have PD. The results indicated that in the animals not treated with MPTP, microstimulation does demonstrate a functional link between the motor cortex and the globus pallidus. However, after the administration of MPTP this functional link was greatly enhanced. In addition, an analysis of the frequency domains of the motor cortex and the globus pallidus and frequencies of microstimulation responsible for activation of muscles suggested that the tremor seen in PD is not caused by the 5–10 Hz bursts of activity. In fact, it is most likely that the oscillations in neuronal firing in PD in the basal ganglia, thalamus, and motor cortex are responsible more for the negative symptoms such as bradykinesia, akinesia, and gait and postural dysfunction (Ellens & Leventhal, 2013; Rivlin-Etzion et al., 2008).

Thus it appears that neuronal oscillations in the motor cortex resulting from the synchronized activity of groups of neurons may be particularly important in the movement disorder in PD. One element of these oscillations is the phenomenon in which high-frequency activity can be coupled to a specific phase of a low-frequency oscillation (de Hemptinne et al., 2013). This coupling of broadband and low-frequency oscillations is important for the ongoing normal functions of cerebral cortex (de Hemptinne et al., 2015). The execution of movements relies on a decoupling of the broadband and low-frequency oscillations (Suffczynski, Crone, & Franaszczuk, 2014). This phase coupling has been observed in the cortex in which broadband 50–200 Hz signals are coupled with low-frequency cycles from 5 to 30 Hz (Canolty et al., 2006; Cohen, 2008; Cohen, Elger, & Fell, 2009).

It has been demonstrated in the motor cortex of patients with PD that the coupling between the low-frequency (13–30 Hz) rhythms and the broadband (50–200 Hz) was enhanced compared with patients who have a different movement disorder or those without a movement disorder (de Hemptinne et al., 2013). These findings support the idea that alterations in neuronal oscillations in the cerebral cortex play a significant role in the akinesia, bradykinesia, and gait and postural dysfunction seen in PD (de Hemptinne et al., 2013).

Additional evidence for the importance of the enhanced coupling between broadband and low-frequency oscillations for the generation of movement disorders in PD comes from the use of deep brain stimulation. Deep brain stimulation is commonly used as a therapeutic approach to relieve the motor dysfunction in PD and other brain disorders, although the precise mechanism of action is not well understood. However, it has been demonstrated that deep brain stimulation can effectively decouple the broadband frequency from the low-frequency cycle in the motor cortex of PD patients. This was observed in both resting conditions and during a motor task. Furthermore the decoupling occurred on the same time line as the improvement of motor function associated with the deep brain stimulation (de Hemptinne et al., 2015).

COGNITIVE IMPAIRMENT AND THE CEREBRAL CORTEX

PD is more obviously considered a movement disorder. However, there are often symptoms related to cognitive dysfunction in a relatively large number of patients with PD. The incidence of cognitive disorders is in the range of 25–30% (Aarsland et al., 2001; Brown & Marsden, 1984). The symptoms can include working memory and visuospatial impairments, executive dysfunction, and neuropsychiatric disorders (Crucian & Okun, 2003; Emre, 2003; Levin et al., 1991; Owen, Iddon, Hodges, Summers, & Robbins, 1997). In the early stages of PD, especially before the commencement of treatment, relatively mild cognitive impairment can be observed in 15–20% of patients (Aarsland et al., 2009). Although some of these conditions may be more closely associated with subcortical structures such as the amygdala and hippocampus, there is evidence that the cerebral cortex is critically implicated.

The obvious cognitive dysfunction that is more directly related to the cerebral cortex is the decline in executive function. PD patients without dementia and disruption of the striatal circuits are most commonly associated with a decline in executive function. It has been indicated that this executive function disorder is caused by the direct connectivity that the prefrontal cortex has with the dorsolateral region of the caudate nucleus (Poston & Eidelberg, 2012). It is likely that the loss of dopamine in the dorsal striatum plays a significant role because there is a loss of the strong relationship in the circuits between the prefrontal cortex and the dorsal striatum in PD. Furthermore it has been shown that depletion of dopamine levels in the prefrontal cortex in PD leads to significant changes in executive function (Leblois, Boraud, Meissner, Bergman, & Hansel, 2006). Imaging studies have demonstrated that dopamine replacement therapy can restore the connectivity in these circuits to a normal state and improve the executive function deficits (Lewis et al., 2005; Wu et al., 2009).

The other cognitive impairment symptoms can also be shown to have a relationship to dysfunction in the cerebral cortex. In addition to early changes in executive function, working memory and visuospatial impairment are quite prominent in PD (Dalrymple-Alford et al., 2011). The distribution of Lewy bodies and amyloid has been implicated in these additional cognitive impairment symptoms. Lewy bodies can be observed in both the striatum and the cortex in PD (Tessa et al., 2008). Furthermore the distribution of amyloid has been well documented in dementia (see the chapters on Alzheimer's disease and vascular dementia), and amyloid deposition has been consistently shown to accompany Lewy body dementia. Some of this amyloid deposition appears to occur in the early stages in the striatum and then later in the cortex in PD. Support for this comes from the evidence that cognitive decline is associated with the progressive increase in amyloid deposition in PD (Gomperts et al., 2013; Edison et al., 2008).

Metabolic studies using 2-deoxyglucose have demonstrated that there is a disruption in metabolic activity in the motor cortex as well as the prefrontal cortex, although the motor cortex metabolic changes appear to occur earlier and are of a greater magnitude (Bezard, Crossman, Gross, & Brotchie, 2001; Bezard, Dovero, et al., 2001; Carbon et al., 2003; Eidelberg et al., 1994; Huang et al., 2007). However, the disruption in metabolic activity in the prefrontal cortex is likely related to the cognitive impairment observed in PD. These metabolic changes precede the nonmotor symptoms of PD such as depression, cognitive dysfunction, and apathy (Löhle, Storch, & Reichmann, 2009). Furthermore the metabolic changes occur in areas of the cortex that have considerable alterations in dopamine and serotonin neurotransmitter levels (Tadeisky et al., 2008).

NEUROTRANSMITTERS AND GENE EXPRESSION IN THE CORTEX

In the previous section it was indicated that there are metabolic changes observed in motor and nonmotor cortical regions and that these changes occur in regions of the cortex that also have neurotransmitter changes including levels of dopamine and serotonin. In patients with PD, a reduction in tyrosine hydroxylase–labeled fibers from 24% to 79% has been demonstrated, with considerable variability in the reduction in the various layers of the cortex (Gaspar, Duyckaerts, Alvarez, Javoy-Agid, & Berger, 1991). Tyrosine hydroxylase is the rate-limiting enzyme for catecholamine synthesis, including dopamine. In MPTP-treated nonprimate models of PD, a reduction in dopamine content and dopamine fibers has been demonstrated. In the MPTP models, there are regional differences in the reductions of dopamine levels and fibers (Jan et al., 2003; Pifl, Schingnitz, & Hornykiewicz, 1991). In a model of hemi-Parkinson's syndrome using unilateral injections of MPTP in the right carotid artery of rhesus monkeys, there is an ipsilateral reduction of tyrosine hydroxylase–containing fibers in motor and prefrontal cortices (Fan et al., 2014).

It is entirely expected that there will be considerable changes in cortical glutamate activity in PD. As discussed, the common motor deficits are directly related to alterations in the basal ganglia circuits associated with the primary motor, the premotor, and the supplementary motor cortices. As a result of the loss of dopamine neurons in the substantia nigra, *pars compacta*, leading to a decrease in dopamine input to the globus pallidus, there is a concomitant loss of activity in the circuit that includes the thalamus and the motor cortex. In the cerebral cortex, the majority of neurons are glutamatergic output neurons from the pyramidal neurons. Thus the output neurons to the striatum and subthalamic nucleus, as shown in Fig. 7.1, use glutamate as a neurotransmitter. The changes in the striatopallidal–thalamic–cortical circuit resulting from loss of dopamine input to the basal ganglia lead to a diminished glutamatergic output from the motor cortex to the striatum and subthalamic nucleus. This concept is supported by investigations that have demonstrated a decrease in cortical activation in MPTP-treated animals using 2-deoxyglucose imaging to measure metabolic changes, as well as electrophysiological recordings of cortical activation (Fan et al., 2014; Schwartzman & Alexander, 1985). MRI imaging approaches have indicated that there is a decrease in glutamate levels in the brains of patients with PD (Griffith, Okonkwo, O'Brien, & Hollander, 2008). A more direct demonstration of the impact of PD on the cortical glutamatergic system comes from the injections of MPTP into the right carotid artery of the rhesus monkey, leading to a significant decrease in basal glutamate levels localized in the ipsilateral motor cortex (Fan et al., 2014).

There is a delay in the onset of motor dysfunction in PD after the onset of the loss of dopaminergic innervation of the striatum. In fact, more than a 70% decrease in dopamine levels in the striatum is required to initiate disruption of movements (Bernheimer et al., 1973). This suggests mechanisms in the circuitry involved that compensate for the dopamine depletion and subsequent modulation of the basal ganglia pathways (Bezard & Gross, 1998; Zigmond, Abercrombie, Berger, Grace, & Stricker, 1990). As indicated, one of the means by which the brain compensates for the dopamine depletion may be the result of changes in the levels of glutamate in the pathways from the cortex to the striatum and subthalamic nucleus. This idea is supported by the demonstration that the cortical–basal ganglia–thalamic–cortical loop is involved in the compensatory mechanism (Bezard, Gross, & Brotchie, 2003). It is also supported by the demonstration that there are early changes in cortical metabolism as indicated by 2-deoxyglucose, MRI, and electrophysiological studies in MPTP-treated nonhuman primates (Griffith et al., 2008; Johnson, Vitek, & McIntyre, 2009; Schwartzman & Alexander, 1985).

Another potential mechanism to explain the delay in onset of PD symptoms may be related to gene changes observed in the cortex. In the prefrontal cortex there are early specific transcriptomic changes seen in a progressive MPTP model of PD (Storvik et al., 2010). The microarray analysis of these transcriptomic alterations indicated that they are not present at a later time in this progressive PD model. However, similar transcriptomic changes can be demonstrated in postmortem brain samples from PD patients (Storvik et al., 2010). The changes in gene expression were correlated with the PD progression, suggesting that they may be compensatory mechanisms or, as indicated, the transcriptomic changes may be related to the nonmotor symptoms of PD that are closely related to the function of the prefrontal cortex. Some of the more interesting gene changes were those related to long-term potentiation that were downregulated, whereas genes in ubiquitin-mediated proteolysis were upregulated (Storvik et al., 2010). A decrease in long-term potentiation activity and an increase in protein degradation would result in considerable impairment in the normal function of the prefrontal cortex, particularly in the early stages of PD.

CONCLUSION

PD is a progressive neurodegenerative condition that typically is thought of from the point of view of the pathophysiology in the basal ganglia caused by the loss of dopamine input from the substantia nigra. However, there is an increasing amount of evidence to indicate that most of the motor and behavioral deficits are the result of alterations in the cerebral cortex, in particular, areas related to motor control and the prefrontal cortex for the neuropsychiatric symptoms. There are some very good animal models for the study of the mechanisms of PD. Administration of MPTP to nonhuman primates is the model that most closely aligns with the symptoms of PD observed clinically. In addition, these models can also be effectively used to demonstrate therapeutic approaches because they respond well to levodopa administration and deep brain stimulation. Animal models and clinical data have indicated that the source of tremors in PD are very closely related to changes in activity in the cerebral cortex and its connections with the thalamus and cerebellum. The motor symptoms of bradykinesia, akinesia, and gait disturbances have been determined to be related to uncoupling of neuronal oscillations in motor regions of the cortex. Metabolic studies and the distribution of Lewy bodies have indicated considerable alterations in the prefrontal cortex, and these in turn have been determined to be involved in the behavioral changes seen in PD. This implication of the cerebral cortex in most of the complications of PD provides an opportunity to explore in more detail the critical mechanisms and molecules contributing to this progressive debilitating disease and suggests new approaches for therapeutic targets.

REFERENCES

Aarsland, D., Andersen, K., Larsen, J. P., Lolk, A., Nielsen, H., & Kragh-Sørensen, P. (2001). Risk of dementia in Parkinson's disease: a community-based, prospective study. *Neurology, 56*(6), 730–736.

Aarsland, D., Brønnick, K., Larsen, J. P., Tysnes, O. B., Alves, G., & Group, N. P. S. (2009). Cognitive impairment in incident, untreated Parkinson disease: the Norwegian ParkWest study. *Neurology, 72*(13), 1121–1126.

Benabid, A. L., Chabardes, S., Mitrofanis, J., & Pollak, P. (2009). Deep brain stimulation of the subthalamic nucleus for the treatment of Parkinson's disease. *Lancet Neurology, 8*(1), 67–81.

Bernheimer, H., Birkmayer, W., Hornykiewicz, O., Jellinger, K., & Seitelberger, F. (1973). Brain dopamine and the syndromes of Parkinson and Huntington: clinical, morphological and neurochemical correlations. *Journal of the Neurological Sciences, 20*(4), 415–455.

Betarbet, R., Sherer, T. B., MacKenzie, G., Garcia-Osuna, M., Panov, A. V., & Greenamyre, J. T. (2000). Chronic systemic pesticide exposure reproduces features of Parkinson's disease. *Nature Neuroscience, 3*(12), 1301–1306.

Bevan, M. D., Atherton, J. F., & Baufreton, J. (2006). Cellular principles underlying normal and pathological activity in the subthalamic nucleus. *Current Opinion in Neurobiology, 16*(6), 621–628. http://dx.doi.org/10.1016/j.conb.2006.10.003.

Bezard, E., Crossman, A. R., Gross, C. E., & Brotchie, J. M. (2001). Structures outside the basal ganglia may compensate for dopamine loss in the presymptomatic stages of Parkinson's disease. *FASEB Journal, 15*(6), 1092–1094.

Bezard, E., Dovero, S., Prunier, C., Ravenscroft, P., Chalon, S., Guilloteau, D., et al. (2001). Relationship between the appearance of symptoms and the level of nigrostriatal degeneration in a progressive 1-methyl-4-phenyl-1,2,3,6-tetrahydropyridine-lesioned macaque model of Parkinson's disease. *The Journal of Neuroscience, 21*(17), 6853–6861.

Bezard, E., & Gross, C. E. (1998). Compensatory mechanisms in experimental and human parkinsonism: towards a dynamic approach. *Progress in Neurobiology, 55*(2), 93–116.

Bezard, E., Gross, C. E., & Brotchie, J. M. (2003). Presymptomatic compensation in Parkinson's disease is not dopamine-mediated. *Trends in Neurosciences, 26*(4), 215–221.

Brown, R. G., & Marsden, C. D. (1984). How common is dementia in Parkinson's disease? *Lancet, 2*(8414), 1262–1265.

Burn, D. J., Rowan, E. N., Allan, L. M., Molloy, S., O'Brien, J. T., & McKeith, I. G. (2006). Motor subtype and cognitive decline in Parkinson's disease, Parkinson's disease with dementia, and dementia with Lewy bodies. *Journal of Neurology, Neurosurgery, & Psychiatry, 77*(5), 585–589.

Burns, R. S., Chiueh, C. C., Markey, S. P., Ebert, M. H., Jacobowitz, D. M., & Kopin, I. J. (1983). A primate model of parkinsonism: selective destruction of dopaminergic neurons in the *pars compacta* of the substantia nigra by N-methyl-4-phenyl-1,2,3,6-tetrahydropyridine. *Proceedings of the National Academy of Sciences of the United States of America, 80*(14), 4546–4550.

Canolty, R. T., Edwards, E., Dalal, S. S., Soltani, M., Nagarajan, S. S., Kirsch, H. E., et al. (2006). High gamma power is phase-locked to theta oscillations in human neocortex. *Science, 313*(5793), 1626–1628.

Carbon, M., Ghilardi, M. F., Feigin, A., Fukuda, M., Silvestri, G., Mentis, M. J., et al. (2003). Learning networks in health and Parkinson's disease: reproducibility and treatment effects. *Human Brain Mapping, 19*(3), 197–211.

Cenci, M. A., Whishaw, I. Q., & Schallert, T. (2002). Animal models of neurological deficits: how relevant is the rat? *Nature Reviews. Neuroscience, 3*(7), 574–579.

Cohen, M. X. (2008). Assessing transient cross-frequency coupling in EEG data. *Journal of Neuroscience Methods, 168*(2), 494–499.

Cohen, M. X., Axmacher, N., Lenartz, D., Elger, C. E., Sturm, V., & Schlaepfer, T. E. (2009). Good vibrations: cross-frequency coupling in the human nucleus accumbens during reward processing. *Journal of Cognitive Neuroscience, 21*(5), 875–889.

Cohen, M. X., Elger, C. E., & Fell, J. (2009). Oscillatory activity and phase-amplitude coupling in the human medial frontal cortex during decision making. *Journal of Cognitive Neuroscience, 21*(2), 390–402.

Crucian, G. P., & Okun, M. S. (2003). Visual-spatial ability in Parkinson's disease. *Frontiers in Bioscience, 8*, s992–997.

Dalrymple-Alford, J. C., Livingston, L., MacAskill, M. R., Graham, C., Melzer, T. R., Porter, R. J., et al. (2011). Characterizing mild cognitive impairment in Parkinson's disease. *Movement Disorders, 26*(4), 629–636.

Dauer, W., & Przedborski, S. (2003). Parkinson's disease: mechanisms and models. *Neuron, 39*(6), 889–909.

van Duinen, H., Zijdewind, I., Hoogduin, H., & Maurits, N. (2005). Surface EMG measurements during fMRI at 3T: accurate EMG recordings after artifact correction. *Neuroimage, 27*, 240–246.

Edison, P., Rowe, C. C., Rinne, J. O., Ng, S., Ahmed, I., Kemppainen, N., et al. (2008). Amyloid load in Parkinson's disease dementia and Lewy body dementia measured with [11C]PIB positron emission tomography. *Journal of Neurology, Neurosurgery, & Psychiatry, 79*(12), 1331–1338.

Eidelberg, D., Moeller, J. R., Dhawan, V., Spetsieris, P., Takikawa, S., Ishikawa, T., et al. (1994). The metabolic topography of parkinsonism. *Journal of Cerebral Blood Flow & Metabolism, 14*(5), 783–801.

Ellens, D. J., & Leventhal, D. K. (2013). Review: electrophysiology of basal ganglia and cortex in models of Parkinson disease. *Journal of Parkinson's Disease, 3*(3), 241–254.

Emre, M. (2003). Dementia associated with Parkinson's disease. *Lancet Neurology, 2*(4), 229–237.

Fan, X. T., Zhao, F., Ai, Y., Andersen, A., Hardy, P., Ling, F., et al. (2014). Cortical glutamate levels decrease in a non-human primate model of dopamine deficiency. *Brain Research, 1552*, 34–40.

Fishman, P. S. (2008). Paradoxical aspects of parkinsonian tremor. *Movement Disorders, 23*(2), 168–173.

Forno, L. S. (1996). Neuropathology of Parkinson's disease. *Journal of Neuropathology and Experimental Neurology, 55*(3), 259–272.

Forno, L. S., DeLanney, L. E., Irwin, I., & Langston, J. W. (1993). Similarities and differences between MPTP-induced parkinsonism and Parkinson's disease. Neuropathologic considerations. *Advances in Neurology, 60*, 600–608.

Forno, L. S., Langston, J. W., DeLanney, L. E., Irwin, I., & Ricaurte, G. A. (1986). Locus ceruleus lesions and eosinophilic inclusions in MPTP-treated monkeys. *Annals of Neurology*, *20*(4), 449–455.

Gaspar, P., Duyckaerts, C., Alvarez, C., Javoy-Agid, F., & Berger, B. (1991). Alterations of dopaminergic and noradrenergic innervations in motor cortex in Parkinson's disease. *Annals of Neurology*, *30*(3), 365–374.

Gerfen, C. R., & Surmeier, D. J. (2011). Modulation of striatal projection systems by dopamine. *Annual Review of Neuroscience*, *34*, 441–466.

Gomperts, S. N., Locascio, J. J., Rentz, D., Santarlasci, A., Marquie, M., Johnson, K. A., et al. (2013). Amyloid is linked to cognitive decline in patients with Parkinson disease without dementia. *Neurology*, *80*(1), 85–91.

Griffith, H. R., Okonkwo, O. C., O'Brien, T., & Hollander, J. A. (2008). Reduced brain glutamate in patients with Parkinson's disease. *NMR in Biomedicine*, *21*(4), 381–387.

Heimer, G., Bar-Gad, I., Goldberg, J. A., & Bergman, H. (2002). Dopamine replacement therapy reverses abnormal synchronization of pallidal neurons in the 1-methyl-4-phenyl-1,2,3, 6-tetrahydropyridine primate model of parkinsonism. *The Journal of Neuroscience*, *22*(18), 7850–7855.

Heimer, G., Rivlin-Etzion, M., Bar-Gad, I., Goldberg, J. A., Haber, S. N., & Bergman, H. (2006). Dopamine replacement therapy does not restore the full spectrum of normal pallidal activity in the 1-methyl-4-phenyl-1,2,3,6-tetra-hydropyridine primate model of Parkinsonism. *The Journal of Neuroscience*, *26*(31), 8101–8114.

Helmich, R. C., Hallett, M., Deuschl, G., Toni, I., & Bloem, B. R. (2012). Cerebral causes and consequences of parkinsonian resting tremor: a tale of two circuits? *Brain*, *135*(Pt 11), 3206–3226.

Helmich, R. C., Janssen, M. J., Oyen, W. J., Bloem, B. R., & Toni, I. (2011). Pallidal dysfunction drives a cerebellothalamic circuit into Parkinson tremor. *Annals of Neurology*, *69*(2), 269–281.

de Hemptinne, C., Ryapolova-Webb, E. S., Air, E. L., Garcia, P. A., Miller, K. J., Ojemann, J. G., et al. (2013). Exaggerated phase-amplitude coupling in the primary motor cortex in Parkinson disease. *Proceedings of the National Academy of Sciences of the United States of America*, *110*(12), 4780–4785.

de Hemptinne, C., Swann, N. C., Ostrem, J. L., Ryapolova-Webb, E. S., San Luciano, M., Galifianakis, N. B., et al. (2015). Therapeutic deep brain stimulation reduces cortical phase-amplitude coupling in Parkinson's disease. *Nature Neuroscience*, *18*(5), 779–786.

Hoehn, M. M., & Yahr, M. D. (1967). Parkinsonism: onset, progression and mortality. *Neurology*, *17*(5), 427–442.

Huang, C., Tang, C., Feigin, A., Lesser, M., Ma, Y., Pourfar, M., et al. (2007). Changes in network activity with the progression of Parkinson's disease. *Brain*, *130*(Pt 7), 1834–1846.

Hurtado, J. M., Gray, C. M., Tamas, L. B., & Sigvardt, K. A. (1999). Dynamics of tremor-related oscillations in the human globus pallidus: a single case study. *Proceedings of the National Academy of Sciences of the United States of America*, *96*(4), 1674–1679.

Jan, C., Pessiglione, M., Tremblay, L., Tandé, D., Hirsch, E. C., & François, C. (2003). Quantitative analysis of dopaminergic loss in relation to functional territories in MPTP-treated monkeys. *The European Journal of Neuroscience*, *18*(7), 2082–2086.

Jankovic, J., & Kapadia, A. S. (2001). Functional decline in Parkinson disease. *Archives of Neurology*, *58*(10), 1611–1615.

Jankovic, J., McDermott, M., Carter, J., Gauthier, S., Goetz, C., Golbe, L., et al. (1990). Variable expression of Parkinson's disease: a base-line analysis of the DATATOP cohort. The Parkinson Study Group. *Neurology*, *40*(10), 1529–1534.

Javoy, F., Sotelo, C., Herbet, A., & Agid, Y. (1976). Specificity of dopaminergic neuronal degeneration induced by intracerebral injection of 6-hydroxydopamine in the nigrostriatal dopamine system. *Brain Research, 102*(2), 201–215.

Jellinger, K. A. (2001). The pathology of Parkinson's disease. *Advances in Neurology, 86*, 55–72.

Johnson, M. D., Vitek, J. L., & McIntyre, C. C. (2009). Pallidal stimulation that improves parkinsonian motor symptoms also modulates neuronal firing patterns in primary motor cortex in the MPTP-treated monkey. *Experimental Neurology, 219*(1), 359–362.

Jonsson, G. (1980). Chemical neurotoxins as denervation tools in neurobiology. *Annual Review of Neuroscience, 3*, 169–187.

Koller, W. C., Busenbark, K., & Miner, K. (1994). The relationship of essential tremor to other movement disorders: report on 678 patients. Essential Tremor Study Group. *Annals of Neurology, 35*(6), 717–723.

Langston, J. W., Ballard, P., Tetrud, J. W., & Irwin, I. (1983). Chronic Parkinsonism in humans due to a product of meperidine-analog synthesis. *Science, 219*(4587), 979–980.

Leblois, A., Boraud, T., Meissner, W., Bergman, H., & Hansel, D. (2006). Competition between feedback loops underlies normal and pathological dynamics in the basal ganglia. *The Journal of Neuroscience, 26*(13), 3567–3583.

Levin, B. E., Llabre, M. M., Reisman, S., Weiner, W. J., Sanchez-Ramos, J., Singer, C., et al. (1991). Visuospatial impairment in Parkinson's disease. *Neurology, 41*(3), 365–369.

Lewis, S. J., Foltynie, T., Blackwell, A. D., Robbins, T. W., Owen, A. M., & Barker, R. A. (2005). Heterogeneity of Parkinson's disease in the early clinical stages using a data driven approach. *Journal of Neurology, Neurosurgery, & Psychiatry, 76*(3), 343–348.

Lewis, S. J., Slabosz, A., Robbins, T. W., Barker, R. A., & Owen, A. M. (2005). Dopaminergic basis for deficits in working memory but not attentional set-shifting in Parkinson's disease. *Neuropsychologia, 43*(6), 823–832.

Liou, H. H., Tsai, M. C., Chen, C. J., Jeng, J. S., Chang, Y. C., Chen, S. Y., et al. (1997). Environmental risk factors and Parkinson's disease: a case-control study in Taiwan. *Neurology, 48*(6), 1583–1588.

Löhle, M., Storch, A., & Reichmann, H. (2009). Beyond tremor and rigidity: non-motor features of Parkinson's disease. *Journal of Neural Transmission, 116*(11), 1483–1492.

Louis, E. D., Levy, G., Côte, L. J., Mejia, H., Fahn, S., & Marder, K. (2001). Clinical correlates of action tremor in Parkinson disease. *Archives of Neurology, 58*(10), 1630–1634.

Louis, E. D., Tang, M. X., Cote, L., Alfaro, B., Mejia, H., & Marder, K. (1999). Progression of parkinsonian signs in Parkinson disease. *Archives of Neurology, 56*(3), 334–337.

Mathai, A., & Smith, Y. (2011). The corticostriatal and corticosubthalamic pathways: two entries, one target. So what? *Frontiers in Systems Neuroscience, 5*, 64.

Nambu, A., Tokuno, H., & Takada, M. (2002). Functional significance of the cortico-subthalamo–pallidal 'hyperdirect' pathway. *Neuroscience Research, 43*(2), 111–117.

Nicklas, W. J., Youngster, S. K., Kindt, M. V., & Heikkila, R. E. (1987). MPTP, MPP+ and mitochondrial function. *Life Sciences, 40*(8), 721–729.

Nini, A., Feingold, A., Slovin, H., & Bergman, H. (1995). Neurons in the globus pallidus do not show correlated activity in the normal monkey, but phase-locked oscillations appear in the MPTP model of parkinsonism. *Journal of Neurophysiology, 74*(4), 1800–1805.

Ovadia, A., Zhang, Z., & Gash, D. M. (1995). Increased susceptibility to MPTP toxicity in middle-aged rhesus monkeys. *Neurobiology of Aging, 16*(6), 931–937.

Owen, A. M., Iddon, J. L., Hodges, J. R., Summers, B. A., & Robbins, T. W. (1997). Spatial and non-spatial working memory at different stages of Parkinson's disease. *Neuropsychologia, 35*(4), 519–532.

Parkinson's Disease Foundation http://www.pdf.org/en/parkinson_statistics.

Pasquereau, B., & Turner, R. S. (2011). Primary motor cortex of the parkinsonian monkey: differential effects on the spontaneous activity of pyramidal tract-type neurons. *Cerebral Cortex*, *21*(6), 1362–1378.

Pifl, C., Schingnitz, G., & Hornykiewicz, O. (1991). Effect of 1-methyl-4-phenyl-1,2,3,6-tetrahydropyridine on the regional distribution of brain monoamines in the rhesus monkey. *Neuroscience*, *44*(3), 591–605.

Poston, K. L., & Eidelberg, D. (2012). Functional brain networks and abnormal connectivity in the movement disorders. *Neuroimage*, *62*(4), 2261–2270.

Przedborski, S., Levivier, M., Jiang, H., Ferreira, M., Jackson-Lewis, V., Donaldson, D., et al. (1995). Dose-dependent lesions of the dopaminergic nigrostriatal pathway induced by intrastriatal injection of 6-hydroxydopamine. *Neuroscience*, *67*(3), 631–647.

Rajput, A. H., Pahwa, R., Pahwa, P., & Rajput, A. (1993). Prognostic significance of the onset mode in parkinsonism. *Neurology*, *43*(4), 829–830.

Raz, A., Vaadia, E., & Bergman, H. (2000). Firing patterns and correlations of spontaneous discharge of pallidal neurons in the normal and the tremulous 1-methyl-4-phenyl-1,2,3,6-tetrahydropyridine Vervet model of parkinsonism. *The Journal of Neuroscience*, *20*(22), 8559–8571.

Rivlin-Etzion, M., Elias, S., Heimer, G., & Bergman, H. (2010). Computational physiology of the basal ganglia in Parkinson's disease. *Progress in Brain Research*, *183*, 259–273.

Rivlin-Etzion, M., Marmor, O., Saban, G., Rosin, B., Haber, S. N., Vaadia, E., et al. (2008). Lowpass filter properties of basal ganglia cortical muscle loops in the normal and MPTP primate model of parkinsonism. *The Journal of Neuroscience*, *28*(3), 633–649.

Rose, S., Nomoto, M., Jackson, E. A., Gibb, W. R., Jaehnig, P., Jenner, P., et al. (1993). Age-related effects of 1-methyl-4-phenyl-1,2,3,6-tetrahydropyridine treatment of common marmosets. *European Journal of Pharmacology*, *230*(2), 177–185.

van Rootselaar, A. F., Maurits, N. M., Renken, R., Koelman, J. H., Hoogduin, J. M., Leenders, K. L., et al. (2008). Simultaneous EMG-functional MRI recordings can directly relate hyperkinetic movements to brain activity. *Human Brain Mapping*, *29*, 1430–1441.

Santaniello, S., Gale, J. T., Montgomery, E. B., & Sarma, S. V. (2010). Modeling the effects of deep brain stimulation on sensorimotor cortex in normal and MPTP conditions. *Conference Proceedings: Annual International Conference of the IEEE Engineering in Medicine and Biology Society. IEEE Engineering in Medicine and Biology Society. Annual Conference*, *2010*, 2081–2084.

Sauer, H., & Oertel, W. H. (1994). Progressive degeneration of nigrostriatal dopamine neurons following intrastriatal terminal lesions with 6-hydroxydopamine: a combined retrograde tracing and immunocytochemical study in the rat. *Neuroscience*, *59*(2), 401–415.

Schwartzman, R. J., & Alexander, G. M. (1985). Changes in the local cerebral metabolic rate for glucose in the 1-methyl-4-phenyl-1,2,3,6-tetrahydropyridine (MPTP) primate model of Parkinson's disease. *Brain Research*, *358*(1–2), 137–143.

Storvik, M., Arguel, M. J., Schmieder, S., Delerue-Audegond, A., Li, Q., Qin, C., et al. (2010). Genes regulated in MPTP-treated macaques and human Parkinson's disease suggest a common signature in prefrontal cortex. *Neurobiology of Disease*, *38*(3), 386–394.

Suffczynski, P., Crone, N. E., & Franaszczuk, P. J. (2014). Afferent inputs to cortical fast-spiking interneurons organize pyramidal cell network oscillations at high-gamma frequencies (60-200 Hz). *Journal of Neurophysiology*, *112*(11), 3001–3011.

Sundström, E., & Samuelsson, E. B. (1997). Comparison of key steps in 1-methyl-4-phenyl-1,2,3, 6-tetrahydropyridine (MPTP) neurotoxicity in rodents. *Pharmacology & Toxicology*, *81*(5), 226–231.

Tadaiesky, M. T., Dombrowski, P. A., Figueiredo, C. P., Cargnin-Ferreira, E., Da Cunha, C., & Takahashi, R. N. (2008). Emotional, cognitive and neurochemical alterations in a premotor stage model of Parkinson's disease. *Neuroscience, 156*(4), 830–840.

Tessa, C., Giannelli, M., Della Nave, R., Lucetti, C., Berti, C., Ginestroni, A., et al. (2008). A whole-brain analysis in de novo Parkinson disease. *AJNR. American Journal of Neuroradiology, 29*(4), 674–680.

Timmermann, L., Gross, J., Dirks, M., Volkmann, J., Freund, H. J., & Schnitzler, A. (2003). The cerebral oscillatory network of parkinsonian resting tremor. *Brain, 126*, 199–212.

Weinberger, M., Mahant, N., Hutchison, W. D., Lozano, A. M., Moro, E., Hodaie, M., et al. (2006). Beta oscillatory activity in the subthalamic nucleus and its relation to dopaminergic response in Parkinson's disease. *Journal of Neurophysiology, 96*(6), 3248–3256.

Wu, T., Wang, L., Chen, Y., Zhao, C., Li, K., & Chan, P. (2009). Changes of functional connectivity of the motor network in the resting state in Parkinson's disease. *Neuroscience Letters, 460*(1), 6–10.

Zaidel, A., Arkadir, D., Israel, Z., & Bergman, H. (2009). Akineto-rigid vs. tremor syndromes in Parkinsonism. *Current Opinion in Neurology, 22*(4), 387–393.

Zetusky, W. J., Jankovic, J., & Pirozzolo, F. J. (1985). The heterogeneity of Parkinson's disease: clinical and prognostic implications. *Neurology, 35*(4), 522–526.

Zigmond, M. J., Abercrombie, E. D., Berger, T. W., Grace, A. A., & Stricker, E. M. (1990). Compensations after lesions of central dopaminergic neurons: some clinical and basic implications. *Trends in Neurosciences, 13*(7), 290–296.

Chapter 8

Huntington Disease

E.H. Kim, N. Mehrabi, L.J. Tippett, H.J. Waldvogel, R.L.M. Faull
University of Auckland, Auckland, New Zealand

INTRODUCTION

Huntington disease (HD) is an autosomal-dominant neurodegenerative disorder characterized by progressive involuntary choreiform movements and cognitive and psychiatric symptoms (Nance, 1998). The disease received widespread recognition after a comprehensive description, "On Chorea" by George Huntington (1872). The genetic mutation is associated with an unstable expansion of CAG trinucleotide repeats in exon 1 of the *Huntingtin (HTT)* gene located on the short arm of human chromosome 4 (Huntington's Disease Collaborative Research Group, 1993). Normal individuals have between 6 and 35 CAG repeats, coding for a polyglutamine stretch at the N-terminus of the protein product called huntingtin (Htt), whereas individuals with 36–39 CAG repeats show variable, incomplete penetrance with respect to the HD phenotype. When the repeat length reaches >39, the disease is considered to be fully penetrant. Expansions of >57 are typically associated with juvenile-onset HD (Andrew et al., 1993). Currently there is no effective treatment for HD, and the disease will eventually lead to death 15–20 years after symptomatic onset.

The number of CAG repeats has been inversely correlated with the age of onset (Langbehn, Hayden, & Paulsen, 2010). However, there is no clear association with symptom variation (Claes et al., 1995). Thus the source of variability in symptom subtypes is unclear, and there is much interest in understanding the underlying pathological changes in HD brains that may account for symptom heterogeneity.

Evaluation of postmortem HD tissue reveals striking degeneration in the striatum and the cerebral cortex (Fig. 8.1), with striatal medium spiny neurons (MSNs) and cortical pyramidal neurons greatly affected (Vonsattel, Keller, & Ramirez, 2011; Waldvogel, Kim, Tippett, Vonsattel, & Faull, 2014). Accordingly, the extent of striatal degeneration is used as the basis of a 5-point grading system to indicate the severity of the disease (Vonsattel et al., 1985). The exact pathogenic mechanism by which mutant Htt causes degeneration of neurons is yet to be fully understood; however, abnormal

The Cerebral Cortex in Neurodegenerative and Neuropsychiatric Disorders.
http://dx.doi.org/10.1016/B978-0-12-801942-9.00008-2
195

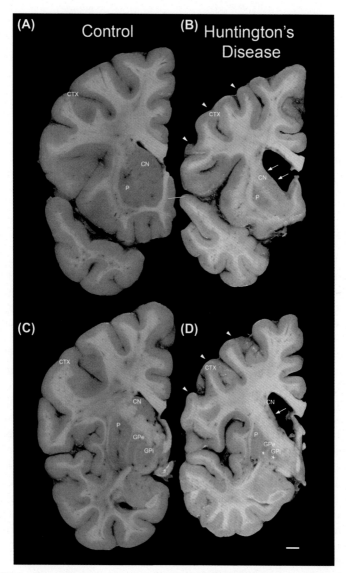

FIGURE 8.1 Neuropathology of Huntington disease (HD) showing coronal sections at two levels of the left hemisphere human brain. (A and C) A representative control case of a 35-year-old male. (B and D) a grade 3/4 HD case. (A and B) are at the level of the striatum and nucleus accumbens, and (C and D) are at the level of the globus pallidus. There is major shrinkage of the caudate nucleus and putamen *(arrows)*, as well as the globus pallidus *(asterisks)* and the cerebral cortex *(arrowhead)* in HD. *CN*, caudate nucleus; *CTX*, cerebral cortex; *GPe*, globus pallidus external segment; *GPi*, globus pallidus internal segment; *P*, putamen. (Scale bar = 1 cm.) *Adapted from Waldvogel, H. J., Kim, E. H., Tippett, L. J., Vonsattel, J. P., & Faull, R. L. (2014). The neuropathology of Huntington's disease. Current Topics in Behavioral Neurosciences.*

depositions of Htt fragments in the nuclei and cytoplasm of neurons, and the formation of protein aggregates have been postulated to initiate a pathogenic cascade leading to neuronal cell death (DiFiglia et al., 1997; Ross & Tabrizi, 2011).

Recent findings in functional neuroimaging and detailed neuropathological studies have shown an association between distinct patterns of degeneration in the striatum and cerebral cortex, and clinical heterogeneity in HD.

This is especially evident throughout the cerebral cortex, where neuroimaging studies have shown discrete patterns of cortical gray matter thinning, which were associated with variable cognitive and motor deficits (Rosas et al., 2008). In addition, extensive cortical pathological postmortem studies have demonstrated an association between the variable pattern of cell loss in the motor and cingulate cortices with dominant motor and mood symptom profiles of HD, respectively (Kim et al., 2014; Thu et al., 2010). These studies show that the different patterns of degeneration in the cerebral cortex may contribute significantly to the symptom heterogeneity in HD. Also, studies obtained from HD mouse models show dysfunctional signaling patterns between cortical pyramidal neurons and striatal MSNs before the appearance of HD behavioral phenotype and neuronal cell loss, suggesting early changes in the corticostriatal pathway in HD.

In summary, the current chapter outlines literature evaluating the structural and functional alterations in the cerebral cortex of HD, and how these alterations disrupt the corticocortical and corticostriatal systems, which may drive the characteristic HD manifestations.

CLINICAL FEATURES AND SYMPTOMS OF HUNTINGTON DISEASE

HD typically develops in midlife (adult-onset), and patients progressively display a clinical triad of motor, cognitive, and emotional disorders. The prevalence of clinically identified HD is highest among most European populations (5–7 per 100,000), and the rate is much lower in African and Asian populations (Harper, 1992; Pringsheim et al., 2012).

In the prediagnostic phase, many individuals show subtle changes of personality, increased forgetfulness, irritability, and clumsiness before the appearance of overt motor symptoms (Marder et al., 2000).

The clinical diagnosis of HD is usually based on distinct motor signs of chorea, incoordination, and slowed saccadic eye movements (Huntington Study Group, 1996). Most patients initially displaying chorea are progressively dominated by dystonia and rigidity at later stages of the disease (Mahant, McCusker, Byth, Graham, & Huntington Study Group, 2003). In addition, the patient's ability to speak and swallow is often affected, leaving the patient susceptible to aspiration pneumonia, a common cause of death.

The impairment of processing speed, short-term memory, attention, and executive functions (poor concentration and difficulties with multi-asking, organizing, and planning), and delay in the acquisition of new motor skills are examples of early HD cognitive defects (Stout et al., 2011). With disease progression, deterioration of verbal skills such as speech and comprehension, and difficulty in visuospatial functioning become evident (Lawrence, Watkins, Sahakian, Hodges, & Robbins, 2000).

HD is also associated with psychiatric deficits. However, unlike motor and cognitive decline, psychiatric symptoms do not exhibit a gradual progression with disease course. There is a wide range of associated neuropsychiatric complications including apathy, agitation, dysphoria, labile mood, and depression (Duff et al., 2007).

Although there is currently no cure, timely assessment and symptom management are of key importance in a range of treatment strategies. Thus it is important to have a clear understanding of the pathophysiology in brain regions responsible for specific functional roles that may underpin the characteristic clinical expression observed in HD.

CEREBRAL CORTEX IN HUNTINGTON DISEASE: POSTMORTEM STUDIES

The major degeneration of the cerebral cortex and the striatum of the basal ganglia (see Fig. 8.1), especially at advanced stages of the disease, is the prominent neuropathological feature of HD (Vonsattel et al., 2011; Waldvogel et al., 2014). However, it is now increasingly becoming clear that HD is a "polytypic process," where a limited number of structures may fail to fully characterize the extent of the disease course and/or the symptom variability in HD.

The earliest accounts of cortical neuropathological features were described by several authors including Bruyn (1968), Dunlap (1927), Lange (1981), and Tellez-Nagel, Johnson, and Terry (1974). Subsequently the evidence of global cortical atrophy was observed by de la Monte, Vonsattel, Richardson Jr (1988), with 30% of mean brain weight reduction (21–29% reduction in the cerebral cortex and 29–34% loss in the white matter). The findings of cortical atrophy were further supported by Halliday et al. (1998), with a reduction of cortical volume (19%) in all brain lobes, except relative sparing of the medial temporal lobe. The amount of cortical volume loss correlated with the degree of striatal atrophy, suggesting that the disease processes in the striatum and cortex were related.

More detailed investigations of cellular changes in HD brains have found changes in neuronal and glial cell size and density, dystrophic neurites, and neuronal cell loss in the cortex (see Table 8.1). The neurodegeneration of the HD cortex has been shown to be area- and laminar-specific, with a significant loss of pyramidal projection neurons in layers 3, 5, and 6. This was observed in the superior frontal cortex, with a 30–34% reduction of pyramidal neurons in layers

TABLE 8.1 Cortical Cellular Changes Observed in Key Postmortem Huntington Disease Studies

Region	Cellular Changes (% Cell Loss)	HD Cases (N)	Relation to Symptom Profile	References
Pyramidal Neurons				
Frontal Lobe				
Superior frontal cortex	↓ 30% pyramidal neurons in layers 3, 5	11 cases		Cudkowicz and Kowall (1990a)
Prefrontal cortex	↓ 31–71% pyramidal neurons in layer 5 and ↓ 35–57% in layer 6; ↓ neuronal size and density in layers 3, 5, and 6, and relative increase in glial cell density and size	–		Hedreen et al. (1991); Rajkowska et al. (1998); Selemon et al. (2004); Sotrel et al. (1991)
Motor regions (BA 4 and 6)	↓ 42–49% total neurons; ↓ 41% pyramidal neurons	5 cases		Macdonald and Halliday (2002)
Primary motor cortex (BA 4)	↓ 24% total neurons; ↓ 27% pyramidal neurons	12 cases	Loss of pyramidal neurons (↓ 45%) in motor-symptom–dominant HD cases	Thu et al. (2010)
Superior frontal cortex (BA 8)	↓ 42% total neurons; ↓ 34% pyramidal neurons	14 cases	Loss of pyramidal neurons (↓ 52%) in motor-symptom–dominant HD cases	Nana et al. (2014)
Parietal Lobe				
Angular gyrus	↓ 45% pyramidal neurons in layers 3 and 5	6 cases		Macdonald et al. (1997)
Primary somatosensory cortex (BA 3)	↓ 27% total neurons; ↓ 27% pyramidal neurons	14 cases	Loss of pyramidal neurons (↓ 38%) in motor-symptom–dominant HD cases	Nana et al. (2014)

Continued

TABLE 8.1 Cortical Cellular Changes Observed in Key Postmortem Huntington Disease Studies—cont'd

Region	Cellular Changes (% Cell Loss)	HD Cases (N)	Relation to Symptom Profile	References
Superior parietal cortex (BA 7)	↓ 36% total neurons; ↓ 30% pyramidal neurons	14 cases	Loss of pyramidal neurons (↓ 30–36%) in motor- and mood-dominant HD cases	Nana et al. (2014)
Occipital Lobe				
Primary visual cortex (BA 17)	↓ 12% total neurons; no pyramidal neuron loss	14 cases	No significant correlation to HD symptomatology	Nana et al. (2014)
Secondary visual cortex (BA 18)	↓ 27% total neurons; ↓ 41% pyramidal neurons	14 cases	Loss of pyramidal neurons (↓ 33–51%) in motor- and mood-dominant HD cases	Nana et al. (2014)
Temporal Lobe				
Middle temporal cortex (BA 21)	↓ 27% total neurons; ↓ 33% pyramidal neurons	14 cases	Loss of pyramidal neurons (↓ 38–40%) in motor- and mood-dominant HD cases	Nana et al. (2014)
Limbic/Medial Lobe				
Cingulate gyrus	↓ pyramidal neurons layers 3 and 5	11 cases		Cudkowicz and Kowall (1990a)
Anterior cingulate cortex (BA 24)	↓ 36% total neurons; ↓ 34% pyramidal neurons	12 cases	Loss of pyramidal neurons (↓40%) in mood-symptom–dominant HD cases	Thu et al. (2010)

Interneurons

Region		Cases		Reference
Frontal cortex	↓ PV interneurons			Ferrer et al. (1994)
Superior frontal cortex	Relative sparing of PV and NPY interneurons	11–20 cases		Cudkowicz and Kowall (1990 a,b)
Primary motor and premotor cortex	Relative sparing of CB, CR, PV interneurons	5 cases		Macdonald and Halliday (2002)
Primary motor cortex (BA 4)	Relative sparing of CB, CR, PV interneurons	13 cases	Loss of CB interneurons (↓ 57%) in motor-symptom–dominant HD cases	Kim et al. (2014)
Occipital lobe	No change in PV interneurons			Ferrer et al. (1994)
Temporal lobe	No change in PV interneurons			Ferrer et al. (1994)
Anterior cingulate cortex (BA 24)	Loss of CR (↓ 34%) and PV (↓ 45%) interneurons	13 cases	Loss of CB (↓ 71%), CR (↓ 60%), and PV (↓ 80%) interneurons in mood-symptom–dominant HD cases	Kim et al. (2014)
Cingulate gyrus	No change in PV interneurons			Cudkowicz and Kowall (1990b)

BA, Brodmann area; CB, calbindin; CR, calretinin; HD, Huntington disease; NPY, neuropeptide Y; PV, parvalbumin.

3 and 5 (Cudkowicz & Kowall, 1990a; Nana et al., 2014). A study by Hedreen, Peyser, Folstein, and Ross (1991) showed significant neuronal loss in layers 3, 5, and 6 in the prefrontal cortex. Layer 6 was found to demonstrate the greatest loss in thickness, whereas layers 3 and 5 were also atrophied. This study showed extensive degeneration of layer 6 in early-stage HD brains. Because neurons in layer 6 have major local, subcortical, and intracortical projections, this also suggested that cortical cell loss is a disease process parallel to striatal degeneration, and not a secondary process as was originally believed.

Profound loss of specific subpopulations of large pyramidal neurons in layers 3, 5, and 6 was also demonstrated in the prefrontal cortex (Rajkowska, Selemon, & Goldman-Rakic, 1998; Selemon, Rajkowska, & Goldman-Rakic, 2004; Sotrel et al., 1991). These studies have focused mainly on the prefrontal cortex, because its role in behavior suggests that neural changes may contribute to the behavioral aspects of HD. Macdonald, Halliday, Trent, and McCusker (1997) additionally reported a significant reduction and atrophy of pyramidal cells across layers 3 and 5 in the angular gyrus of the parietal lobe. In a later study, Macdonald and Halliday (2002) showed a significant reduction of pyramidal neurons in the motor cortical regions, ie, the primary motor cortex (area 4; 42% loss) and the premotor region (area 6; 49% loss). No significant change was observed in the posterior cingulate motor region (posterior part of area 24). In agreement with this study, a detailed quantitative study using stereology showed a significant loss of pyramidal neurons (27% loss) in the primary motor cortex of 12 HD cases (Thu et al., 2010). Further studies observed a significant loss of pyramidal neurons in other cortical areas including the primary sensory cortex (27% loss), middle temporal cortex (33% loss), anterior cingulate cortex (34% loss), and association areas of the frontal, parietal, and occipital lobes (Nana et al., 2014; Thu et al., 2010). In addition, distinct dystrophic neurites in layers 3, 5, and 6 were observed in various cortical areas that differ from age-related neuritic degeneration (Jackson et al., 1995).

Whereas the degeneration of cortical pyramidal neurons is well documented, relatively few studies on cortical interneurons have been conducted in the HD cortex (see Table 8.1).

Pathological studies on the cortical interneurons show relative sparing of calretinin (CR)-, and parvalbumin (PV)-expressing interneurons in the motor cortical regions (Kim et al., 2014; Macdonald & Halliday, 2002), and PV- and neuropeptide Y–expressing interneurons in the superior frontal cortex (Cudkowicz & Kowall, 1990b). In contrast, loss of CR- and PV-expressing interneurons was observed in the anterior cingulate cortex (Kim et al., 2014). Ferrer et al. (1994) also observed a significant decrease in PV-expressing interneurons in the frontal cortex; however, no significant difference was observed in the occipital and temporal lobes. These results suggest that there is a heterogeneous topographical pattern of cortical interneuron loss in HD.

Taken together, cortical degeneration in HD has been observed and reported over many years, and the postmortem assessments indicate that cortical atrophy and loss of pyramidal neurons is a neuropathological hallmark in HD. Many studies, however, were conducted on end-stage tissue from striatal neuropathological grades 2–4, with limited understanding about cortical atrophy at earlier stages of the disease before symptomatic onset. This is an important aspect of disease progression that is highlighted in the following section.

CEREBRAL CORTEX IN HUNTINGTON DISEASE: BRAIN IMAGING FINDINGS

Modern neuroimaging studies, including structural and functional magnetic resonance imaging (MRI), single-photon emission computed tomography (SPECT), and positron emission tomography (PET), facilitate the visualization of early brain changes in vivo (see Chapter 3). These techniques are largely noninvasive, allow repeated evaluations for assessment of disease progression, and are widely accessible in clinical practice. This makes them an attractive tool for biomarkers. However, no single method has been optimal and an integrative multimodal imaging approach has been recommended (Niccolini & Politis, 2014).

The findings of generalized cortical atrophy have been supported by MRI studies detecting a significant reduction in the frontal lobe (17%) and frontal white matter (28%) volume (Aylward et al., 1998), as well as the mesial temporal lobe structures (Jernigan, Salmon, Butters, & Hesselink, 1991). Cortical thinning and volume reductions during early stages of the disease have also been observed. These changes develop progressively and topographically from the posterior to anterior regions of the cortex (Fig. 8.2), with the greatest amount of thinning in the sensorimotor region (>15%) at all stages of the disease (Rosas et al., 2008). Furthermore, multicenter, longitudinal studies of premanifest and early stage HD (Biglan et al., 2009;

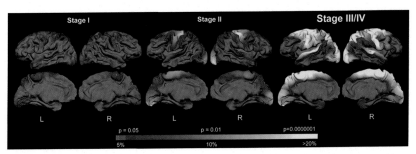

FIGURE 8.2   A model of disease progression showing regions of cortical thinning in Huntington disease (HD) subjects at different stages. The color scale represents the significance of cortical thinning compared with matched controls, from red ($p<.05$) to yellow ($p<.0000001$), as well as magnitude of thickness change, from red (5% loss) to yellow (>20% loss). *With permission from Rosas, H. D., Salat, D. H., Lee, S. Y., Zaleta, A. K., Pappu, V., Fischl, B., et al. (2008). Cerebral cortex and the clinical expression of Huntington's disease: complexity and heterogeneity.* Brain: A Journal of Neurology, 131*(Pt 4), 1057–1068.*

Tabrizi et al., 2013), have been conducted to determine and evaluate neurobiological and behavioral changes that occur in the period leading up to a diagnosis.

Besides structural changes, there is growing evidence of clinical manifestations in HD that result from changes in cortical metabolism, neuronal dysfunction, and loss of functional connectivity. Previous SPECT studies investigating neurovascular and metabolic brain changes showed widespread reduction of cerebral blood flow in 29 symptomatic (Sax et al., 1996) and 18 presymptomatic patients with HD (Hasselbalch et al., 1992). Alterations in blood flow were also observed by elevated cortical arteriolar cerebral blood volume in prodromal HD patients without obvious brain atrophy (Hua, Unschuld, Margolis, van Zijl, & Ross, 2014), indicating that changes in cerebral blood perfusion occur early in the disease process. Also, alterations of the rate of glucose uptake and its metabolism, an indicator of neuronal integrity, have been shown using ^{18}F-fluorodeoxyglucose (FDG) PET imaging (Kuwert et al., 1990). Interestingly, early decrease in cortical metabolism has been shown to be an indicator for rapid disease progression (Shin et al., 2013).

PET investigations of dopaminergic systems showed a reduction in D1 receptor binding in the temporal cortex (Ginovart et al., 1997), and D2 receptor density in the temporal and frontal areas of symptomatic and premanifest patients with HD (Pavese et al., 2010). This suggests that cortical dopaminergic abnormalities parallel the reduction of D1 and D2 receptors primarily observed in the striatum.

Several lines of study using functional MRI (fMRI) have shown alterations in brain activity in various cortical regions suggesting neuronal dysfunction, compensatory brain responses, and circuitry reorganization in the HD cortex. Data from presymptomatic HD patients have shown impaired functional connectivity between anterior cingulate and lateral prefrontal regions (Thiruvady et al., 2007). In addition, a study of 13 premanifest *HTT* gene carriers showed alterations in the activity of the anterior cingulate, sensorimotor, frontal, and temporal cortical regions (Zimbelman et al., 2007). Moreover, reduced blood oxygenation level–dependent synchrony has been observed in prodromal HD cases between the premotor cortex and caudate nucleus (Unschuld, Joel, Liu, et al., 2012), and lower functional connectivity between lateral prefrontal and parietal regions, as well as the putamen (Wolf et al., 2008). Therefore these studies suggest that prominent changes in cortical function occur early in the disease, and that there is a distinct dysfunctional network between the cortical and subcortical regions.

Consistent with this view, using diffusion tensor imaging, Rosas et al. (2006) observed white matter atrophy in early stages of the disease. These changes were detectable up to a decade before motor diagnosis (Paulsen et al., 2010). In addition, abnormal white matter connections of the sensorimotor cortex (Dumas et al., 2012) and corpus callosum (Rosas et al., 2010) have been observed, as well as a correlation between cortical gray and white matter changes with caudate atrophy (Fennema-Notestine et al., 2004), implying alterations in the corticocortical and corticostriatal connectivity.

Collectively, these neuroimaging studies provide evidence for structural and functional cortical changes that occur early in the disease process and that cortical dysfunction is a key factor underlying the pathogenesis of HD.

CEREBRAL CORTEX AND SYMPTOM HETEROGENEITY FROM HUMAN STUDIES

The neuropathological and in vivo neuroimaging studies have demonstrated regional and progressive degeneration in the HD cortex at different stages of the disease, suggesting that cortical degeneration may be related to symptom heterogeneity in HD. Despite the single-gene etiology of HD, there is remarkable variability in the types of motor, cognitive, and behavioral symptoms present in HD cases, both at clinical onset and during the course of the disease (Claes et al., 1995). Interestingly, marked differences in the symptomatic profile have been observed in monozygotic twins who inherited identical *HTT* genes (Georgiou et al., 1999).

More recently, advances in neuroimaging methods and detailed neuropathological assessments of HD brains have elucidated the cortical basis of clinical heterogeneity in HD. Importantly, a study by Rosas et al. (2008) demonstrated that patterns of regional cortical thinning are associated with varying motor disorder and cognitive deficits. For example, patients who had HD with more prominent bradykinesia and dystonia showed more significant cortical thinning in the premotor and supplementary motor areas compared with patients who had HD with chorea (Fig. 8.3). Moreover, regional cortical

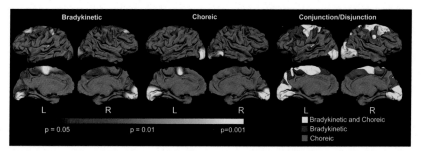

FIGURE 8.3 Relationship between differential cortical thinning and distinct motor phenotype. Huntington disease (HD) subjects with bradykinesia and chorea both showed thinning in the motor cortex and posterior regions of the brain. HD subjects with more prominent bradykinesia and dystonia additionally showed significant thinning in premotor and supplementary motor areas as indicated by the conjunction/disjunction analyses; *red* to *yellow* indicates regions of more significant correlation, from $p < .01$ to $p < .001$. *With permission from Rosas, H. D., Salat, D. H., Lee, S. Y., Zaleta, A. K., Pappu, V., Fischl, B., et al. (2008). Cerebral cortex and the clinical expression of Huntington's disease: complexity and heterogeneity.* Brain: A Journal of Neurology, 131(Pt 4), 1057–1068.

thinning correlated with functional decline as measured by the Total Functional Capacity scale.

A study by Hobbs et al. (2010) showed a correlation between higher internal capsule atrophy and a decline in motor scores. A correlation between alterations in white matter tract and cognitive performance was also observed in premanifest HD patients (Paulsen et al., 2010; Rosas et al., 2006). Using fMRI, Unschuld, Joel, Pekar, et al. (2012) have shown that Stroop-related activity of the ventromedial prefrontal cortex correlated significantly with depressive symptoms in prodromal HD patients. Also, anterior cingulate cortex atrophy has been found to correlate with emotion and depression clinical symptoms in early HD (Hobbs et al., 2011).

In line with in vivo imaging investigations, recent pathological studies (see Table 8.1) showed an association between variable cortical degeneration with specific motor and mood symptoms of HD (Kim et al., 2014; Nana et al., 2014; Thu et al., 2010). In particular, there was an association between significant pyramidal cell loss in the primary motor cortex (45% loss) in HD cases with pronounced motor symptoms, whereas significant pyramidal cell loss in the anterior cingulate cortex (40% loss) was associated with HD cases with major mood disorder (Thu et al., 2010) (Fig. 8.4).

A study after Thu et al. (2010) has shown that clinical variability also correlates with variable patterns of interneuron degeneration (Kim et al., 2014). In the motor cortex, a significant loss of calbindin (CB) interneurons (57%) was observed in HD cases dominated by motor symptoms. In contrast, the anterior cingulate cortex showed significant loss of the three interneuron populations (71% loss of CB, 60% loss of CR, and 80% loss of PV interneurons) only in HD cases with major mood disorder. Interestingly, alterations in the expression of the three calcium-binding proteins (CB, CR, and PV) have been implicated in mood-related disorders such as depression (Rajkowska, O'Dwyer, Teleki, Stockmeier, & Miguel-Hidalgo, 2007), epilepsy (DeFelipe, 1999), schizophrenia, and bipolar disorder (Benes & Berretta, 2001), suggesting that the changes in cortical γ-aminobutyric acid–transmitting interneurons contribute, in particular, to abnormalities in neuropsychiatric diseases and limbic-related cortical circuits in HD. Moreover, this study showed that interneuron cell loss was only observed where there was significant pyramidal neuronal loss (Fig. 8.5), suggesting that disruption of the interneuron–pyramidal neuron interaction may be a major contributing factor in the pathophysiology of HD.

Extending these studies, a later investigation (Nana et al., 2014) encompassing six more representative cortical regions from the same HD cases showed a widespread heterogeneous loss of neurons across the frontal, parietal, temporal, and occipital cortical lobes (Fig. 8.6). The results demonstrate that cortical cell loss is remarkably variable both within and between HD cases, and that HD cases with dominant motor symptoms relate to neuronal loss in the sensorimotor, secondary visual, and association cortices in the frontal, parietal, and temporal lobes, whereas HD cases with dominant mood symptoms relate to

Primary motor cortex (BA 4)

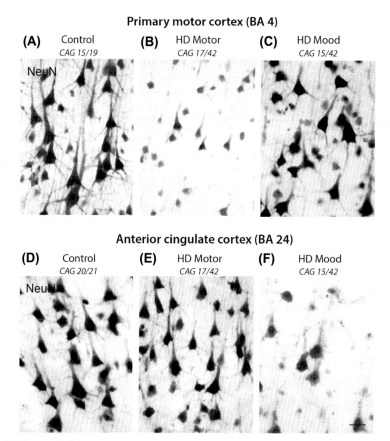

(A) Control
CAG 15/19

(B) HD Motor
CAG 17/42

(C) HD Mood
CAG 15/42

NeuN

Anterior cingulate cortex (BA 24)

(D) Control
CAG 20/21

(E) HD Motor
CAG 17/42

(F) HD Mood
CAG 15/42

NeuN

FIGURE 8.4   Cell loss in the (A–C) primary motor cortex and (D–F) anterior cingulate cortex relates to motor and mood symptoms in Huntington disease *(HD)*, respectively. (B) Marked cell loss in the motor cortex in HD motor-symptom–dominant cases compared with matched controls (A). (F) In contrast, marked cell loss in the cingulate cortex is shown in HD mood-symptom–dominant cases compared with controls (D). *BA*, Brodmann area (Scale bar = 30 μm.) *Adapted from Thu, D. C., Oorschot, D. E., Tippett, L. J., Nana, A. L., Hogg, V. M., Synek, B. J., et al. (2010). Cell loss in the motor and cingulate cortex correlates with symptomatology in Huntington's disease,* Brain: A Journal of Neurology, *133(Pt 4), 1094–1110.*

neuronal loss in the anterior cingulate and association cortices in the frontal, parietal, and temporal lobes. These studies clearly indicate the basis of cortical degeneration in different functional brain regions that underpin specific symptom profiles in HD.

Combined with evidence that the cortical changes parallel manifestation of motor, cognitive, and behavioral symptoms, these studies underscore the key role of cortical pathology and its relationship to symptom variation in HD. In addition, transgenic HD models show alterations in cortical neuronal signaling, which precede neuronal loss, suggesting dysfunction of cortical networks

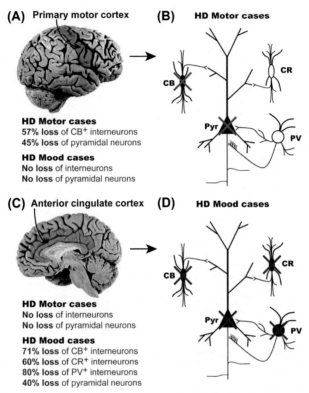

FIGURE 8.5   Interneuron and pyramidal cell loss in the primary motor cortex (A and B) and anterior cingulate cortex (C and D) relates to motor and mood symptoms in Huntington disease *(HD)*, respectively. Significant reductions of both calbindin *(CB)* interneurons (57% loss) and pyramidal neurons (45% loss) is observed in the motor cortex of HD motor cases (B), whereas significant reductions of CB (71% loss), calretinin *(CR;* 60% loss), and parvalbumin *(PV;* 80% loss) interneurons and pyramidal neurons *(Pyr;* 40%) occurred in the cingulate cortex of HD mood cases (D). *With permission from Kim, E. H., Thu, D. C., Tippett, L. J., Oorschot, D. E., Hogg, V. M., Roxburgh, R., et al. (2014). Cortical interneuron loss and symptom heterogeneity in Huntington disease, Annals of Neurology, 75(5), 717–727.*

occurs at early stages of HD. The following sections focus on the cellular dysfunctions and disease mechanisms that constitute the development of the HD phenotype.

DYSFUNCTIONAL CORTICOSTRIATAL NETWORK IN HUNTINGTON DISEASE ANIMAL MODELS

As in the human disease, cortical changes are fundamental to the onset and progression of the HD phenotype in models of HD (Laforet et al., 2001). One of the most extensively studied models of HD is the transgenic R6/2 mouse expressing expanded Htt N-terminal fragment (~150 CAG repeats). These

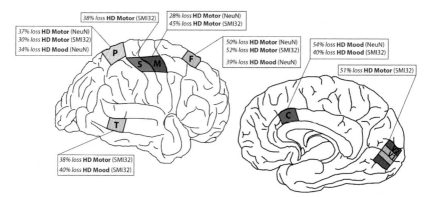

FIGURE 8.6   Cell loss across eight cortical regions in Huntington disease *(HD)*. The HD motor symptom cases show most significant cell loss in the primary motor *(M)*, sensory *(S)*, and secondary visual *(V2)* cortices, and association areas in the frontal *(F)*, parietal *(P)*, and temporal *(T)* cortices. In comparison, HD mood symptom cases show most prominent cell loss in the anterior cingulate cortex *(C)*, and association areas across frontal *(F)*, parietal *(P)*, temporal *(T)* cortices. *V1,* Primary visual cortex. *Adapted from Nana, A. L., Kim, E. H., Thu, D. C., Oorschot, D. E., Tippett, L. J., Hogg, V. M., et al. (2014). Widespread heterogeneous neuronal loss across the cerebral cortex in Huntington's disease,* Journal of Huntington's Disease, *3(1), 45–64.*

transgenic animals display rapid disease progression with overt behavioral symptoms observed as early as 4–5 weeks of age. Other widely used transgenic models of HD include mice that express the full-length human *HTT* gene, using yeast artificial chromosome (YAC) or bacterial artificial chromosome (BAC). These animals show behavioral changes around 6 months of age, and pathological changes by 12 months of age (Cepeda, Wu, Andre, Cummings, & Levine, 2007). Along with these full-length models, knock-in models represent another important class in terms of recapitulating the adult-onset HD because of its gradual disease course. An important step in understanding HD pathogenesis was the development of conditional knockout mouse models of the disease. These models allow the expression of the mutant Htt protein to be turned on or off in discrete neuronal populations using a Cre-loxP expression system; therefore the toxic effects of mutant Htt can be localized to precise cellular origins. In particular, studies in the Cre-loxP conditional knockout mouse model, where cortical and/or striatal cells selectively express mutant Htt, showed that dysfunction of cortical neurons was essential to the development of significant behavioral and motor deficits (Gu et al., 2007). Moreover, changes in ion channel function and synaptic communication between cortical neurons and striatal MSNs via the corticostriatal pathway occur early in the disease process, and have been implicated as an important factor for the development of HD phenotype (Cepeda et al., 2007).

The sequence of functional alterations has been discerned empirically by electrophysiological recordings from cortical and striatal neurons in R6/1, R6/2, and YAC mouse models. In the early phase, in vitro recordings of striatal MSNs show intrinsic alterations in cell membrane properties such as reduced cell capacitance, increased membrane input resistance, and depolarized resting membrane potentials (Klapstein et al., 2001). Comparable intrinsic membrane alterations also occur in cortical pyramidal neurons, which are more apparent at later stages of the disease (Cummings et al., 2009, 2006). This is paralleled by decreased sensitivity to glutamate N-methyl-D-aspartate receptor (NMDAR)–mediated responses in cortical pyramidal neurons (Andre, Cepeda, Venegas, Gomez, & Levine, 2006). These changes ultimately render cortical neurons hyperexcitable and alter the cortical output, which is thought to underlie motor and cognitive impairments in the R6/2 mice. Interestingly, alterations in glutamate NMDAR-mediated responses in striatal MSNs have also been observed (Zeron et al., 2002), which suggests that changes in NMDAR function may predispose striatal neurons to excitotoxic damage as a result of impaired cortical output.

Consistent with this view, increased firing rate in cortical neurons has been observed in freely behaving, symptomatic R6/2 mice in vivo (Walker, Miller, Fritsch, Barton, & Rebec, 2008). Impaired cortical pyramidal neuron activity is further supported by a reduction in correlated firing and coincident bursting between simultaneously recorded pairs of cortical neurons (Walker et al., 2008), and electrocorticograms in vivo (Stern, 2011). Also, altered correlated neuronal activity has been related to behavioral changes (Walker, Ummel, & Rebec, 2011), suggesting that deficient synchronous activity in cortical neurons underscores HD manifestations. In addition, alterations in cortical neuron spike rate and burst activity, which is important for information transmission and synaptic plasticity, has been shown in these R6/2 mice. Indeed, impaired cortical plasticity has been observed in HD (Cummings et al., 2007). Interestingly, the loss of cortical plasticity was reversed by the activation of dopamine receptors (Dallerac et al., 2011). This suggests that, along with dysregulation of glutamate release, changes in presynaptic receptors including dopamine D2, metabotropic glutamate, and endocannabinoid CB1 receptors, which have been shown to be down regulated in HD (Luthi-Carter et al., 2000), may further contribute to alterations in cortical processing.

Hyperexcitability in cortical networks is further compounded by dysfunctional cortical interneurons, which cause an imbalance between excitatory and inhibitory inputs to pyramidal neurons. A study in Cre-loxP conditional HD mice showed that the interaction between interneurons and pyramidal neurons was necessary to produce motor deficits and cortical degeneration (Gu et al., 2005). Furthermore, previous studies using transgenic mouse models of HD (BACHD, R6/2, YAC128, CAG140 knock-in) have shown pronounced alterations in the inhibitory actions of interneurons in the sensorimotor cortex (Cummings et al., 2009; Spampanato, Gu, Yang, & Mody, 2008). These studies suggest that the loss of inhibitory action of cortical interneurons can contribute significantly to early pathophysiological changes in HD.

The progressive synaptic dysfunction resulting from altered cortical excitation has been examined by observing glutamate release in the corticostriatal pathway at different stages of disease progression in R6/2 and YAC128 mice. The results demonstrated a biphasic age-dependent pattern. First, increased glutamate release and α-amino-3-hydroxy-5-methyl-4-isoxazolepropionic acid (AMPA) receptor–mediated synaptic currents evoked by cortical stimulation were observed during the early phase of the disease, before the onset of a behavioral HD phenotype (Joshi et al., 2009). This was followed by a later phase with significantly reduced glutamate release and AMPA synaptic currents after the development of a behavioral HD phenotype. The susceptibility to excitotoxic stress also progressed in a biphasic manner, so that YAC128 mice first displayed increased sensitivity to NMDAR-mediated synaptic currents in the presymptomatic phase, which was followed by reduced currents in the symptomatic mice (Graham et al., 2009).

In summary, the dysregulation of glutamate release by cortical pyramidal neurons to striatal MSNs via the corticostriatal pathway is a critical factor in the development of HD pathosis and phenotype. Compensatory mechanisms are in place, as evidenced by a biphasic release of glutamate, but these mechanisms can have deleterious effects in the disease process. These effects are the result of combined presynaptic and postsynaptic alterations, and can be further modulated by cortical interneurons that shape cortical excitability. These changes correlate well with observed changes in postmortem HD human brain studies.

HUNTINGTON DISEASE PATHOGENESIS: MECHANISMS AND PATHWAYS IN RELATION TO CORTEX

A key feature of HD pathogenesis has been ascribed to genetically determined, cell-autonomous neuronal degeneration in the striatum and cortex associated with the mutant *HTT* gene. Studies using postmortem HD tissue (Hodges et al., 2006) and mouse models of HD (Luthi-Carter et al., 2000) have shown that the expanded CAG repeat of the *HTT* gene interacts with a large number of genes. In addition, although fairly minor, somatic and germline CAG repeat instability has also been shown in various HD models and human HD tissue (Pearson, Nichol Edamura, & Cleary, 2005), which has been implicated in differential cell degeneration in HD. It is also important to note the influence of epigenetic prenatal and postnatal environmental factors on the *HTT* gene mutation (van Dellen, Blakemore, Deacon, York, & Hannan, 2000).

In terms of Htt protein, converging evidence from molecular, cell, and mouse model studies indicate that HD arises predominantly from a toxic gain-of-function from abnormal folding of mutant Htt protein (Ross & Tabrizi, 2011). HD shares a common "protein misfolding" phenomenon observed in other neurodegenerative diseases such as Alzheimer disease and Parkinson disease (Ross & Poirier, 2004). Elucidating the exact molecular mechanisms for mutant Htt cytotoxicity is an ongoing challenge. The mutant Htt shows a similar expression level and regional distribution to the wild-type Htt in the brain (Aronin et al., 1995), but a difference in Htt epitope localization has been observed, and abnormal accumulation of N-terminal fragments of mutant Htt have been found in the nucleus, cytoplasm, and dystrophic neurites in HD brains (DiFiglia et al., 1997).

The accumulation of mutant Htt was found more often in the cortex than in the striatum (Sapp et al., 1999), and abundant neuropil aggregates have been detected in the cortex before symptomatic development (Gutekunst et al., 1999). Within the cortex, the cells tend to display combinations of nuclear and cytoplasmic, as well as neuropil, aggregations (Herndon et al., 2009), with the highest levels of intranuclear inclusions found in juvenile cases with high CAG repeat length.

The important steps of the aggregate toxicity hypothesis involve proteolysis, nuclear translocation, and aggregation leading to detrimental cellular interactions. The mutant Htt possesses a higher likelihood of proteolytic cleavage than its wild-type counterpart (Goldberg et al., 1996), and the smaller, soluble truncated N-terminal fragments are suggested to be more toxic (Martindale et al., 1998) than the formation of inclusions (Arrasate, Mitra, Schweitzer, Segal, & Finkbeiner, 2004). Also, the toxicity has been associated with nuclear translocation (Saudou, Finkbeiner, Devys, & Greenberg, 1998). Furthermore, the mutant Htt protein undergoes extensive posttranslational modifications that influence abnormal conformational changes, aggregation propensity (Thakur et al., 2009), and clearance by the ubiquitin–proteasome system and autophagy (Bennett et al., 2007; Martinez-Vicente et al., 2010). The Htt protein has many interaction partners, particularly at the N-terminus, suggesting a potential role of Htt–protein interactions in the pathogenesis of HD (Li & Li, 2004). These interactions lead to a complex set of impaired cellular metabolic pathways including transcription, excitotoxicity, oxidative stress, energy metabolism, and synaptic transmission in the striatum, cerebral cortex, and other regions throughout the brain (Ross & Tabrizi, 2011).

Besides the cell-autonomous processes, another important disease mechanism entails cell–cell interactions. One of the proposed mechanisms of cell death in HD involves early changes and major alterations in the corticostriatal pathway (Cepeda et al., 2007). The striatal MSNs receive extensive excitatory glutamatergic input from the pyramidal neurons from all regions of the cerebral cortex; both of these cell types are greatly affected in HD. In addition, early dysfunction between cortical inhibitory interneurons and pyramidal neurons (Gu et al., 2005; Spampanato et al., 2008) may further exacerbate the disease process and alter the ability of pyramidal neurons to release glutamate. Excess glutamate in the striatum is also thought to make striatal MSNs particularly vulnerable to NMDAR-mediated excitotoxic damage (Zeron et al., 2002). This is further compounded by glial cell contribution to excitotoxicity (Bradford et al., 2009; Shin et al., 2005). In addition, mutant Htt has been shown to reduce the production and transport of brain-derived neurotrophic factor (BDNF), a prosurvival factor produced by cortical neurons necessary for striatal neuron survival, via the corticostriatal pathway (Zuccato & Cattaneo, 2007). The massive loss of striatal MSNs in turn influence the striatopallidal and striatonigral projections, and the subsequent relay of information to the thalamus and the cortex, affecting structures that participate in the basal–ganglia–thalamocortical circuitry.

Collectively, these studies provide accumulating mechanistic evidence that the communication between the cortex and striatum plays a major role in the initiation and development of the HD phenotype, and that dysfunction between the cortical interneurons and pyramidal neurons, and striatal MSNs via the corticostriatal pathway are critical in the pathogenesis of HD.

THERAPEUTIC ASPECTS AND FUTURE DIRECTIONS

The majority of therapeutic strategies used in HD are designed to ameliorate the primary symptomatology of the HD condition, ie, psychiatric agents to control behavioral symptoms, motor sedatives, cognitive enhancers, and neuroprotective agents (Handley, Naji, Dunnett, & Rosser, 2006). Neuronal dysfunction and cell death in HD are the result of a combination of interrelated pathological processes that operate in a complicated way. Here, some of the current HD therapeutic targets related to the neuropathology of the cerebral cortex will be discussed.

Excitotoxicity: Excitotoxicity is considered to be one of the major causes of cell death in HD. Excitotoxicity relies on increased glutamate release and NMDAR activity, ultimately resulting in impaired calcium signaling and cell death. Riluzole-mediated blockade of the excessive glutamate release from the corticostriatal terminals was one of the first attempts to counteract excitotoxicity in HD (Guyot et al., 1997). Other strategies include decreasing the activity of NMDARs using a glutamate antagonist (lamotrigine), a noncompetitive inhibitor of NMDAR (remacemide) (Ferrante et al., 2002; Schilling, Coonfield, Ross, & Borchelt, 2001), or blockade of NMDARs (memantine) (Lee et al., 2006). Most of the drugs mentioned have been shown to be neuroprotective in HD animal models and cultured cells, but unfortunately no significant beneficial results have been observed in patients with HD.

BDNF: Previous studies have suggested that reduced levels of BDNF contribute to HD phenotypes (Zuccato & Cattaneo, 2007). These findings have generated considerable excitement about establishing a BDNF therapy for HD (see Chapter 2). Some of the possible strategies to increase the levels of BDNF in HD are administration of recombinant BDNF, gene therapy, BDNF mimics, and BDNF-releasing cell grafts (Zuccato, Valenza, & Cattaneo, 2010). These possible strategies, however, are still under extensive preclinical investigations.

Autophagy of Htt inclusions: Autophagy, or cellular self-digestion, is a cellular pathway involved in degradation of proteins and organelles. Despite promising data from using antiaggregation compounds in cell-based assays, and nonmammalian HD models (ie, *Drosophila*) (Doumanis, Wada, Kino, Moore, & Nukina, 2009), few convincing results have been observed in mouse models of HD (Zuccato et al., 2010). Therefore many have shifted their focus to drugs that stimulate aggregate clearance. In fact, the list of new drugs that up-regulate autophagy and enhance the clearance of mutant Htt is growing. It is, however, crucial to assess the safety of these compounds and their ability to induce autophagy in mouse models (and larger animal models) of HD.

Targeting mutant *HTT* RNA with RNA interference: Using striatal delivery of adeno-associated virus (AAV)1–short hairpin RNA (shRNA) directed against human mutant messenger (mRNA), Harper et al. (2005) observed a reduction in the levels of mutant *HTT* mRNA and protein in the striatum of N171-82Q mice. The shRNA was designed to reduce the expression of the mutant human *HTT* gene without affecting the expression of the wild-type copy of the gene. Silencing the pathogenic gene was shown to prevent behavioral and neuropathological symptoms in these HD mice. Another study reported similar results when AAV5 was used to deliver two different human *HTT*-specific shRNAs into the striatum of R6/1 mice (Denovan-Wright, Rodriguez-Lebron, Lewin, & Mandel, 2008). Small-interference RNA (siRNA) can also be used as an alternative strategy to knock down mutant *HTT* expression, and seems to be safer and more effective than shRNAs (Snove & Rossi, 2006). However, the RNA interference (RNAi)–based strategies are only desired if they can specifically select and silence the mutant allele and avoid the potential side effects caused by a partial reduction in the expression of the normal *HTT* gene and loss of its beneficial effects in the brain (Zuccato et al., 2010).

One of the current challenges in the field of HD is to identify and target the heterozygous single nucleotide polymorphisms that are selectively associated with the disease-causing allele. Indeed, increasing numbers of disease-linked polymorphisms are now being identified, which suggests that a majority of HD patients may be treatable by individualized allele-specific RNAi that selectively targets the mutant *HTT* mRNA (Aronin, 2006). Despite the promising potential therapeutic applications of siRNA-based strategies, many technical issues remain unsolved. These include the stability of the silencing, the delivery modes, timing, and cellular targets (Aronin, 2006). Because the loss of striatal MSNs is one of the main pathological hallmarks of HD, many RNAi-based therapeutic strategies have been designed to selectively target these cells. However, recent evidence presented here suggests major pathosis of the cerebral cortex and alterations in the corticostriatal pathway in HD, indicating that a broader treatment regimen to include the cerebral cortex should be considered.

CONCLUSION

It has long been known that the cerebral cortex is not a homogeneous structure, as evidenced by the heterogeneous cellular composition identified by the Brodmann cortical classification. Furthermore, genetic studies show that neurons in different regions of the cerebral cortex have a variable genetic expression profile, which defines their particular subtype (Molyneaux, Arlotta, Menezes, & Macklis, 2007). This suggests that specific cell types across the cerebral cortex and basal ganglia may interact differently with the mutant *HTT* gene and cause variable degeneration of cortical and striatal neurons. The cellular toxic effects involve both cell-autonomous and cell–cell interaction mechanisms. These processes could be an underlying factor in the major susceptibility of the human forebrain in HD and cellular variability that lead to the heterogeneous HD symptom profile.

REFERENCES

Andre, V. M., Cepeda, C., Venegas, A., Gomez, Y., & Levine, M. S. (2006). Altered cortical glutamate receptor function in the R6/2 model of Huntington's disease. *Journal of Neurophysiology*, *95*(4), 2108–2119.

Andrew, S. E., Goldberg, Y. P., Kremer, B., Telenius, H., Theilmann, J., Adam, S., et al. (1993). The relationship between trinucleotide (CAG) repeat length and clinical features of Huntington's disease. *Nature Genetics*, *4*(4), 398–403.

Aronin, N. (2006). Target selectivity in mRNA silencing. *Gene Therapy*, *13*(6), 509–516.

Aronin, N., Chase, K., Young, C., Sapp, E., Schwarz, C., Matta, N., et al. (1995). CAG expansion affects the expression of mutant huntingtin in the Huntington's disease brain. *Neuron*, *15*(5), 1193–1201.

Arrasate, M., Mitra, S., Schweitzer, E. S., Segal, M. R., & Finkbeiner, S. (2004). Inclusion body formation reduces levels of mutant huntingtin and the risk of neuronal death. *Nature*, *431*(7010), 805–810.

Aylward, E. H., Anderson, N. B., Bylsma, F. W., Wagster, M. V., Barta, P. E., Sherr, M., et al. (1998). Frontal lobe volume in patients with Huntington's disease. *Neurology*, *50*(1), 252–258.

Benes, F. M., & Berretta, S. (2001). GABAergic interneurons: implications for understanding schizophrenia and bipolar disorder. *Neuropsychopharmacology: Official Publication of the American College of Neuropsychopharmacology*, *25*(1), 1–27.

Bennett, E. J., Shaler, T. A., Woodman, B., Ryu, K. Y., Zaitseva, T. S., Becker, C. H., et al. (2007). Global changes to the ubiquitin system in Huntington's disease. *Nature*, *448*(7154), 704–708.

Biglan, K. M., Ross, C. A., Langbehn, D. R., Aylward, E. H., Stout, J. C., Queller, S., et al. (2009). Motor abnormalities in premanifest persons with Huntington's disease: the PREDICT-HD study. *Movement Disorders: Official Journal of the Movement Disorder Society*, *24*(12), 1763–1772.

Bradford, J., Shin, J. Y., Roberts, M., Wang, C. E., Li, X. J., & Li, S. (2009). Expression of mutant huntingtin in mouse brain astrocytes causes age-dependent neurological symptoms. *Proceedings of the National Academy of Sciences USA*, *106*(52), 22480–22485.

Bruyn, G. W. (1968). Huntington's chorea: historical, clinical and laboratory synopsis. In P. J. Vinken, & G. W. Bruyn (Eds.), *Handbook of clinical neurology Vol. 6.* (pp. 298–378) (Amsterdam: North-Holland).

Cepeda, C., Wu, N., Andre, V. M., Cummings, D. M., & Levine, M. S. (2007). The corticostriatal pathway in Huntington's disease. *Progress in Neurobiology*, *81*(5–6), 253–271.

Claes, S., Van Zand, K., Legius, E., Dom, R., Malfroid, M., Baro, F., et al. (1995). Correlations between triplet repeat expansion and clinical features in Huntington's disease. *Archives of Neurology*, *52*(8), 749–753.

Cudkowicz, M., & Kowall, N. W. (1990a). Degeneration of pyramidal projection neurons in Huntington's disease cortex. *Annals of Neurology*, *27*(2), 200–204.

Cudkowicz, M., & Kowall, N. W. (1990b). Parvalbumin immunoreactive neurons are resistant to degeneration in Huntington's disease cerebral cortex. *Journal of Neuropathology and Experimental Neurology*, *49*(3), 345.

Cummings, D. M., Andre, V. M., Uzgil, B. O., Gee, S. M., Fisher, Y. E., Cepeda, C., et al. (2009). Alterations in cortical excitation and inhibition in genetic mouse models of Huntington's disease. *The Journal of Neuroscience: The Official Journal of the Society for Neuroscience, 29*(33), 10371–10386.

Cummings, D. M., Milnerwood, A. J., Dallerac, G. M., Vatsavayai, S. C., Hirst, M. C., & Murphy, K. P. (2007). Abnormal cortical synaptic plasticity in a mouse model of Huntington's disease. *Brain Research Bulletin, 72*(2–3), 103–107.

Cummings, D. M., Milnerwood, A. J., Dallerac, G. M., Waights, V., Brown, J. Y., Vatsavayai, S. C., et al. (2006). Aberrant cortical synaptic plasticity and dopaminergic dysfunction in a mouse model of Huntington's disease. *Human Molecular Genetics, 15*(19), 2856–2868.

Dallerac, G. M., Vatsavayai, S. C., Cummings, D. M., Milnerwood, A. J., Peddie, C. J., Evans, K. A., et al. (2011). Impaired long-term potentiation in the prefrontal cortex of Huntington's disease mouse models: rescue by D1 dopamine receptor activation. *Neurodegenerative Diseases, 8*(4), 230–239.

DeFelipe, J. (1999). Chandelier cells and epilepsy. *Brain: A Journal of Neurology, 122*(Pt 10), 1807–1822.

van Dellen, A., Blakemore, C., Deacon, R., York, D., & Hannan, A. J. (2000). Delaying the onset of Huntington's in mice. *Nature, 404*(6779), 721–722.

Denovan-Wright, E. M., Rodriguez-Lebron, E., Lewin, A. S., & Mandel, R. J. (2008). Unexpected off-targeting effects of anti-huntingtin ribozymes and siRNA in vivo. *Neurobiology of Disease, 29*(3), 446–455.

DiFiglia, M., Sapp, E., Chase, K. O., Davies, S. W., Bates, G. P., Vonsattel, J. P., et al. (1997). Aggregation of huntingtin in neuronal intranuclear inclusions and dystrophic neurites in brain. *Science, 277*(5334), 1990–1993.

Doumanis, J., Wada, K., Kino, Y., Moore, A. W., & Nukina, N. (2009). RNAi screening in *Drosophila* cells identifies new modifiers of mutant huntingtin aggregation. *PLoS One, 4*(9), e7275.

Duff, K., Paulsen, J. S., Beglinger, L. J., Langbehn, D. R., Stout, J. C., PREDICT HD Investigators of the Huntington Study Group, et al. (2007). Psychiatric symptoms in Huntington's disease before diagnosis: the predict-HD study. *Biological Psychiatry, 62*(12), 1341–1346.

Dumas, E. M., van den Bogaard, S. J., Ruber, M. E., Reilman, R. R., Stout, J. C., Craufurd, D., et al. (2012). Early changes in white matter pathways of the sensorimotor cortex in premanifest Huntington's disease. *Human Brain Mapping, 33*(1), 203–212.

Dunlap, C. B. (1927). Pathologic changes in Huntington's chorea. *Archives of Neurology & Psychiatry, 18*, 867–943.

Fennema-Notestine, C., Archibald, S. L., Jacobson, M. W., Corey-Bloom, J., Paulsen, J. S., Peavy, G. M., et al. (2004). In vivo evidence of cerebellar atrophy and cerebral white matter loss in Huntington disease. *Neurology, 63*(6), 989–995.

Ferrante, R. J., Andreassen, O. A., Dedeoglu, A., Ferrante, K. L., Jenkins, B. G., Hersch, S. M., et al. (2002). Therapeutic effects of coenzyme Q10 and remacemide in transgenic mouse models of Huntington's disease. *The Journal of Neuroscience: The Official Journal of the Society for Neuroscience, 22*(5), 1592–1599.

Ferrer, I., Kulisevsky, J., Gonzalez, G., Escartin, A., Chivite, A., & Casas, R. (1994). Parvalbumin immunoreactive neurons in the cerebral cortex and striatum in Huntington's disease. *Neurodegeneration, 3*(2), 169–173.

Georgiou, N., Bradshaw, J. L., Chiu, E., Tudor, A., O'Gorman, L., & Phillips, J. G. (1999). Differential clinical and motor control function in a pair of monozygotic twins with Huntington's disease. *Movement Disorders: Official Journal of the Movement Disorder Society, 14*(2), 320–325.

Ginovart, N., Lundin, A., Farde, L., Halldin, C., Backman, L., Swahn, C. G., et al. (1997). PET study of the pre- and post-synaptic dopaminergic markers for the neurodegenerative process in Huntington's disease. *Brain: A Journal of Neurology*, *120*(Pt 3), 503–514.

Goldberg, Y. P., Nicholson, D. W., Rasper, D. M., Kalchman, M. A., Koide, H. B., Graham, R. K., et al. (1996). Cleavage of huntingtin by apopain, a proapoptotic cysteine protease, is modulated by the polyglutamine tract. *Nature Genetics*, *13*(4), 442–449.

Graham, R. K., Pouladi, M. A., Joshi, P., Lu, G., Deng, Y., Wu, N. P., et al. (2009). Differential susceptibility to excitotoxic stress in YAC128 mouse models of Huntington disease between initiation and progression of disease. *The Journal of Neuroscience: The Official Journal of the Society for Neuroscience*, *29*(7), 2193–2204.

Gu, X., Andre, V. M., Cepeda, C., Li, S. H., Li, X. J., Levine, M. S., et al. (2007). Pathological cell–cell interactions are necessary for striatal pathogenesis in a conditional mouse model of Huntington's disease. *Molecular Neurodegeneration Other Titles: MN*, *2*, 8.

Gu, X., Li, C., Wei, W., Lo, V., Gong, S., Li, S. H., et al. (2005). Pathological cell–cell interactions elicited by a neuropathogenic form of mutant huntingtin contribute to cortical pathogenesis in HD mice. *Neuron*, *46*(3), 433–444.

Gutekunst, C. A., Li, S. H., Yi, H., Mulroy, J. S., Kuemmerle, S., Jones, R., et al. (1999). Nuclear and neuropil aggregates in Huntington's disease: relationship to neuropathology. *The Journal of Neuroscience: The Official Journal of the Society for Neuroscience*, *19*(7), 2522–2534.

Guyot, M. C., Palfi, S., Stutzmann, J. M., Maziere, M., Hantraye, P., & Brouillet, E. (1997). Riluzole protects from motor deficits and striatal degeneration produced by systemic 3-nitropropionic acid intoxication in rats. *Neuroscience*, *81*(1), 141–149.

Halliday, G. M., McRitchie, D. A., Macdonald, V., Double, K. L., Trent, R. J., & McCusker, E. (1998). Regional specificity of brain atrophy in Huntington's disease. *Experimental Neurology*, *154*(2), 663–672.

Handley, O. J., Naji, J. J., Dunnett, S. B., & Rosser, A. E. (2006). Pharmaceutical, cellular and genetic therapies for Huntington's disease. *Clinical Science (Lond)*, *110*(1), 73–88.

Harper, P. S. (1992). The epidemiology of Huntington's disease. *Human Genetics*, *89*(4), 365–376.

Harper, S. Q., Staber, P. D., He, X., Eliason, S. L., Martins, I. H., Mao, Q., et al. (2005). RNA interference improves motor and neuropathological abnormalities in a Huntington's disease mouse model. *Proceedings of the National Academy of Sciences USA*, *102*(16), 5820–5825.

Hasselbalch, S. G., Oberg, G., Sorensen, S. A., Andersen, A. R., Waldemar, G., Schmidt, J. F., et al. (1992). Reduced regional cerebral blood flow in Huntington's disease studied by SPECT. *Journal of Neurology, Neurosurgery & Psychiatry*, *55*(11), 1018–1023.

Hedreen, J. C., Peyser, C. E., Folstein, S. E., & Ross, C. A. (1991). Neuronal loss in layers V and VI of cerebral cortex in Huntington's disease. *Neuroscience Letters*, *133*(2), 257–261.

Herndon, E. S., Hladik, C. L., Shang, P., Burns, D. K., Raisanen, J., & White, C. L., 3rd. (2009). Neuroanatomic profile of polyglutamine immunoreactivity in Huntington disease brains. *Journal of Neuropathology and Experimental Neurology*, *68*(3), 250–261.

Hobbs, N. Z., Henley, S. M., Ridgway, G. R., Wild, E. J., Barker, R. A., Scahill, R. I., et al. (2010). The progression of regional atrophy in premanifest and early Huntington's disease: a longitudinal voxel-based morphometry study. *Journal of Neurology, Neurosurgery & Psychiatry*, *81*(7), 756–763.

Hobbs, N. Z., Pedrick, A. V., Say, M. J., Frost, C., Dar Santos, R., Coleman, A., et al. (2011). The structural involvement of the cingulate cortex in premanifest and early Huntington's disease. *Movement Disorders: Official Journal of the Movement Disorder Society*, *26*(9), 1684–1690.

Hodges, A., Strand, A. D., Aragaki, A. K., Kuhn, A., Sengstag, T., Hughes, G., et al. (2006). Regional and cellular gene expression changes in human Huntington's disease brain. *Human Molecular Genetics*, *15*(6), 965–977.

Hua, J., Unschuld, P. G., Margolis, R. L., van Zijl, P. C., & Ross, C. A. (2014). Elevated arteriolar cerebral blood volume in prodromal Huntington's disease. *Movement Disorders: Official Journal of the Movement Disorder Society, 29*(3), 396–401.

Huntington, G. (1872). On chorea. *The Medical and Surgical Reporter, 26,* 317–321.

Huntington's Disease Collaborative Research Group. (1993). A novel gene containing a trinucleotide repeat that is expanded and unstable on Huntington's disease chromosomes. *Cell, 72*(6), 971–983.

Huntington Study Group. (1996). Unified Huntington's disease rating scale: reliability and consistency. Huntington Study Group. *Movement Disorders: Official Journal of the Movement Disorder Society, 11*(2), 136–142.

Jackson, M., Gentleman, S., Lennox, G., Ward, L., Gray, T., Randall, K., et al. (1995). The cortical neuritic pathology of Huntington's disease. *Neuropathology and Applied Neurobiology, 21*(1), 18–26.

Jernigan, T. L., Salmon, D. P., Butters, N., & Hesselink, J. R. (1991). Cerebral structure on MRI. II. Specific changes in Alzheimer's and Huntington's diseases. *Biological Psychiatry, 29*(1), 68–81.

Joshi, P. R., Wu, N. P., Andre, V. M., Cummings, D. M., Cepeda, C., Joyce, J. A., et al. (2009). Age-dependent alterations of corticostriatal activity in the YAC128 mouse model of Huntington disease. *The Journal of Neuroscience: The Official Journal of the Society for Neuroscience, 29*(8), 2414–2427.

Kim, E. H., Thu, D. C., Tippett, L. J., Oorschot, D. E., Hogg, V. M., Roxburgh, R., et al. (2014). Cortical interneuron loss and symptom heterogeneity in Huntington disease. *Annals of Neurology, 75*(5), 717–727.

Klapstein, G. J., Fisher, R. S., Zanjani, H., Cepeda, C., Jokel, E. S., Chesselet, M. F., et al. (2001). Electrophysiological and morphological changes in striatal spiny neurons in R6/2 Huntington's disease transgenic mice. *Journal of Neurophysiology, 86*(6), 2667–2677.

Kuwert, T., Lange, H. W., Langen, K. J., Herzog, H., Aulich, A., & Feinendegen, L. E. (1990). Cortical and subcortical glucose consumption measured by PET in patients with Huntington's disease. *Brain: A Journal of Neurology, 113*(Pt 5), 1405–1423.

Laforet, G. A., Sapp, E., Chase, K., McIntyre, C., Boyce, F. M., Campbell, M., et al. (2001). Changes in cortical and striatal neurons predict behavioral and electrophysiological abnormalities in a transgenic murine model of Huntington's disease. *The Journal of Neuroscience: The Official Journal of the Society for Neuroscience, 21*(23), 9112–9123.

Langbehn, D. R., Hayden, M. R., Paulsen, J. S., (2010). CAG-repeat length and the age of onset in Huntington disease (HD): a review and validation study of statistical approaches. *American Journal of Medical Genetics. Part B, Neuropsychiatric Genetics: The Official Publication of the International Society of Psychiatric Genetics, 153B*(2), 397–408.

Lange, H. W. (1981). Quantitative changes of telencephalon, diencephalon, and mesencephalon in Huntington's chorea, postencephalitic, and idiopathic parkinsonism. *Verhandlungen der Anatomischen Gesellschaft, 75,* 923–925.

Lawrence, A. D., Watkins, L. H., Sahakian, B. J., Hodges, J. R., & Robbins, T. W. (2000). Visual object and visuospatial cognition in Huntington's disease: implications for information processing in corticostriatal circuits. *Brain: A Journal of Neurology, 123*(Pt 7), 1349–1364.

Lee, S. T., Chu, K., Park, J. E., Kang, L., Ko, S. Y., Jung, K. H., et al. (2006). Memantine reduces striatal cell death with decreasing calpain level in 3-nitropropionic model of Huntington's disease. *Brain Research, 1118*(1), 199–207.

Li, S. H., & Li, X. J. (2004). Huntingtin–protein interactions and the pathogenesis of Huntington's disease. *Trends in Genetics, 20*(3), 146–154.

Luthi-Carter, R., Strand, A., Peters, N. L., Solano, S. M., Hollingsworth, Z. R., Menon, A. S., et al. (2000). Decreased expression of striatal signaling genes in a mouse model of Huntington's disease. *Human Molecular Genetics, 9*(9), 1259–1271.

Macdonald, V., & Halliday, G. (2002). Pyramidal cell loss in motor cortices in Huntington's disease. *Neurobiology of Disease, 10*(3), 378–386.

Macdonald, V., Halliday, G. M., Trent, R. J., & McCusker, E. A. (1997). Significant loss of pyramidal neurons in the angular gyrus of patients with Huntington's disease. *Neuropathology and Applied Neurobiology, 23*(6), 492–495.

Mahant, N., McCusker, E. A., Byth, K., Graham, S., & Huntington Study Group (2003). Huntington's disease: clinical correlates of disability and progression. *Neurology, 61*(8), 1085–1092.

Marder, K., Zhao, H., Myers, R. H., Cudkowicz, M., Kayson, E., Kieburtz, K., et al. (2000). Rate of functional decline in Huntington's disease. Huntington Study Group. *Neurology, 54*(2), 452–458.

Martindale, D., Hackam, A., Wieczorek, A., Ellerby, L., Wellington, C., McCutcheon, K., et al. (1998). Length of huntingtin and its polyglutamine tract influences localization and frequency of intracellular aggregates. *Nature Genetics, 18*(2), 150–154.

Martinez-Vicente, M., Talloczy, Z., Wong, E., Tang, G., Koga, H., Kaushik, S., et al. (2010). Cargo recognition failure is responsible for inefficient autophagy in Huntington's disease. *Nature Neuroscience, 13*(5), 567–576.

Molyneaux, B. J., Arlotta, P., Menezes, J. R., & Macklis, J. D. (2007). Neuronal subtype specification in the cerebral cortex. *Nature Reviews. Neuroscience, 8*(6), 427–437.

de la Monte, S. M., Vonsattel, J. P., & Richardson, E. P., Jr. (1988). Morphometric demonstration of atrophic changes in the cerebral cortex, white matter, and neostriatum in Huntington's disease. *Journal of Neuropathology and Experimental Neurology, 47*(5), 516–525.

Nana, A. L., Kim, E. H., Thu, D. C., Oorschot, D. E., Tippett, L. J., Hogg, V. M., et al. (2014). Widespread heterogeneous neuronal loss across the cerebral cortex in Huntington's disease. *Journal of Huntington's Disease, 3*(1), 45–64.

Nance, M. A. (1998). Huntington disease: clinical, genetic, and social aspects. *Journal of Geriatric Psychiatry and Neurology, 11*(2), 61–70.

Niccolini, F., & Politis, M. (2014). Neuroimaging in Huntington's disease. *World Journal of Radiology, 6*(6), 301–312.

Paulsen, J. S., Nopoulos, P. C., Aylward, E., Ross, C. A., Johnson, H., Magnotta, V. A., et al. (2010). Striatal and white matter predictors of estimated diagnosis for Huntington disease. *Brain Research Bulletin, 82*(3–4), 201–207.

Pavese, N., Politis, M., Tai, Y. F., Barker, R. A., Tabrizi, S. J., Mason, S. L., et al. (2010). Cortical dopamine dysfunction in symptomatic and premanifest Huntington's disease gene carriers. *Neurobiology of Disease, 37*(2), 356–361.

Pearson, C. E., Nichol Edamura, K., & Cleary, J. D. (2005). Repeat instability: mechanisms of dynamic mutations. *Nature Reviews. Genetics, 6*(10), 729–742.

Pringsheim, T., Wiltshire, K., Day, L., Dykeman, J., Steeves, T., & Jette, N. (2012). The incidence and prevalence of Huntington's disease: a systematic review and meta-analysis. *Movement Disorders: Official Journal of the Movement Disorder Society, 27*(9), 1083–1091.

Rajkowska, G., O'Dwyer, G., Teleki, Z., Stockmeier, C. A., & Miguel-Hidalgo, J. J. (2007). GABAergic neurons immunoreactive for calcium binding proteins are reduced in the prefrontal cortex in major depression. *Neuropsychopharmacology: Official Publication of the American College of Neuropsychopharmacology, 32*(2), 471–482.

Rajkowska, G., Selemon, L. D., & Goldman-Rakic, P. S. (1998). Neuronal and glial somal size in the prefrontal cortex: a postmortem morphometric study of schizophrenia and Huntington disease. *Archives of General Psychiatry, 55*(3), 215–224.

Rosas, H. D., Lee, S. Y., Bender, A. C., Zaleta, A. K., Vangel, M., Yu, P., et al. (2010). Altered white matter microstructure in the corpus callosum in Huntington's disease: implications for cortical "disconnection. *Neuroimage*, *49*(4), 2995–3004.

Rosas, H. D., Salat, D. H., Lee, S. Y., Zaleta, A. K., Pappu, V., Fischl, B., et al. (2008). Cerebral cortex and the clinical expression of Huntington's disease: complexity and heterogeneity. *Brain: A Journal of Neurology*, *131*(Pt 4), 1057–1068.

Rosas, H. D., Tuch, D. S., Hevelone, N. D., Zaleta, A. K., Vangel, M., Hersch, S. M., et al. (2006). Diffusion tensor imaging in presymptomatic and early Huntington's disease: selective white matter pathology and its relationship to clinical measures. *Movement Disorders: Official Journal of the Movement Disorder Society*, *21*(9), 1317–1325.

Ross, C. A., & Poirier, M. A. (2004). Protein aggregation and neurodegenerative disease. *Nature Medicine* (Suppl. 10), S10–S17.

Ross, C. A., & Tabrizi, S. J. (2011). Huntington's disease: from molecular pathogenesis to clinical treatment. *Lancet Neurology*, *10*(1), 83–98.

Sapp, E., Penney, J., Young, A., Aronin, N., Vonsattel, J. P., & DiFiglia, M. (1999). Axonal transport of N-terminal huntingtin suggests early pathology of corticostriatal projections in Huntington disease. *Journal of Neuropathology and Experimental Neurology*, *58*(2), 165–173.

Saudou, F., Finkbeiner, S., Devys, D., & Greenberg, M. E. (1998). Huntingtin acts in the nucleus to induce apoptosis but death does not correlate with the formation of intranuclear inclusions. *Cell*, *95*(1), 55–66.

Sax, D. S., Powsner, R., Kim, A., Tilak, S., Bhatia, R., Cupples, L. A., et al. (1996). Evidence of cortical metabolic dysfunction in early Huntington's disease by single-photon-emission computed tomography. *Movement Disorders: Official Journal of the Movement Disorder Society*, *11*(6), 671–677.

Schilling, G., Coonfield, M. L., Ross, C. A., & Borchelt, D. R. (2001). Coenzyme Q10 and remacemide hydrochloride ameliorate motor deficits in a Huntington's disease transgenic mouse model. *Neuroscience Letters*, *315*(3), 149–153.

Selemon, L. D., Rajkowska, G., & Goldman-Rakic, P. S. (2004). Evidence for progression in frontal cortical pathology in late-stage Huntington's disease. *Journal of Comparative Neurology*, *468*(2), 190–204.

Shin, J. Y., Fang, Z. H., Yu, Z. X., Wang, C. E., Li, S. H., & Li, X. J. (2005). Expression of mutant huntingtin in glial cells contributes to neuronal excitotoxicity. *The Journal of Cell Biology*, *171*(6), 1001–1012.

Shin, H., Kim, M. H., Lee, S. J., Lee, K. H., Kim, M. J., Kim, J. S., et al. (2013). Decreased metabolism in the cerebral cortex in early-stage Huntington's disease: a possible biomarker of disease progression? *Journal of Clinical Neurology*, *9*(1), 21–25.

Snove, O., Jr., & Rossi, J. J. (2006). Toxicity in mice expressing short hairpin RNAs gives new insight into RNAi. *Genome Biol*, *7*(8), 231.

Sotrel, A., Paskevich, P. A., Kiely, D. K., Bird, E. D., Williams, R. S., & Myers, R. H. (1991). Morphometric analysis of the prefrontal cortex in Huntington's disease. *Neurology*, *41*(7), 1117–1123.

Spampanato, J., Gu, X., Yang, X. W., & Mody, I. (2008). Progressive synaptic pathology of motor cortical neurons in a BAC transgenic mouse model of Huntington's disease. *Neuroscience*, *157*(3), 606–620.

Stern, E. A. (2011). Functional changes in neocortical activity in Huntington's disease model mice: an in vivo intracellular study. *Frontiers in Systems Neuroscience*, *5*, 47.

Stout, J. C., Paulsen, J. S., Queller, S., Solomon, A. C., Whitlock, K. B., Campbell, J. C., et al. (2011). Neurocognitive signs in prodromal Huntington disease. *Neuropsychology*, *25*(1), 1–14.

Tabrizi, S. J., Scahill, R. I., Owen, G., Durr, A., Leavitt, B. R., Roos, R. A., et al. (2013). Predictors of phenotypic progression and disease onset in premanifest and early-stage Huntington's disease in the TRACK-HD study: analysis of 36-month observational data. *Lancet Neurology*, *12*(7), 637–649.

Tellez-Nagel, I., Johnson, A. B., & Terry, R. D. (1974). Studies on brain biopsies of patients with Huntington's chorea. *Journal of Neuropathology and Experimental Neurology*, *33*(2), 308–332.

Thakur, A. K., Jayaraman, M., Mishra, R., Thakur, M., Chellgren, V. M., Byeon, I. J., et al. (2009). Polyglutamine disruption of the huntingtin exon 1 N terminus triggers a complex aggregation mechanism. *Nature Structural & Molecular Biology*, *16*(4), 380–389.

Thiruvady, D. R., Georgiou-Karistianis, N., Egan, G. F., Ray, S., Sritharan, A., Farrow, M., et al. (2007). Functional connectivity of the prefrontal cortex in Huntington's disease. *Journal of Neurology, Neurosurgery & Psychiatry*, *78*(2), 127–133.

Thu, D. C., Oorschot, D. E., Tippett, L. J., Nana, A. L., Hogg, V. M., Synek, B. J., et al. (2010). Cell loss in the motor and cingulate cortex correlates with symptomatology in Huntington's disease. *Brain: A Journal of Neurology*, *133*(Pt 4), 1094–1110.

Unschuld, P. G., Joel, S. E., Liu, X., Shanahan, M., Margolis, R. L., Biglan, K. M., et al. (2012). Impaired corticostriatal functional connectivity in prodromal Huntington's disease. *Neuroscience Letters*, *514*(2), 204–209.

Unschuld, P. G., Joel, S. E., Pekar, J. J., Reading, S. A., Oishi, K., McEntee, J., et al. (2012). Depressive symptoms in prodromal Huntington's disease correlate with Stroop-interference related functional connectivity in the ventromedial prefrontal cortex. *Psychiatry Research*, *203*(2–3), 166–174.

Vonsattel, J. P., Keller, C., & Cortes Ramirez, E. P. (2011). Huntington's disease: neuropathology. *Handbook of Clinical Neurology*, *100*, 83–100.

Vonsattel, J. P., Myers, R. H., Stevens, T. J., Ferrante, R. J., Bird, E. D., & Richardson, E. P., Jr. (1985). Neuropathological classification of Huntington's disease. *Journal of Neuropathology and Experimental Neurology*, *44*(6), 559–577.

Waldvogel, H. J., Kim, E. H., Tippett, L. J., Vonsattel, J. P., & Faull, R. L. (2014). The neuropathology of Huntington's disease. *Current Topics in Behavioral Neurosciences*.

Walker, A. G., Miller, B. R., Fritsch, J. N., Barton, S. J., & Rebec, G. V. (2008). Altered information processing in the prefrontal cortex of Huntington's disease mouse models. *The Journal of Neuroscience: The Official Journal of the Society for Neuroscience*, *28*(36), 8973–8982.

Walker, A. G., Ummel, J. R., & Rebec, G. V. (2011). Reduced expression of conditioned fear in the R6/2 mouse model of Huntington's disease is related to abnormal activity in prelimbic cortex. *Neurobiology of Disease*, *43*(2), 379–387.

Wolf, R. C., Sambataro, F., Vasic, N., Schonfeldt-Lecuona, C., Ecker, D., & Landwehrmeyer, B. (2008). Aberrant connectivity of lateral prefrontal networks in presymptomatic Huntington's disease. *Experimental Neurology*, *213*(1), 137–144.

Zeron, M. M., Hansson, O., Chen, N., Wellington, C. L., Leavitt, B. R., Brundin, P., et al. (2002). Increased sensitivity to *N*-methyl-D-aspartate receptor-mediated excitotoxicity in a mouse model of Huntington's disease. *Neuron*, *33*(6), 849–860.

Zimbelman, J. L., Paulsen, J. S., Mikos, A., Reynolds, N. C., Hoffmann, R. G., & Rao, S. M. (2007). fMRI detection of early neural dysfunction in preclinical Huntington's disease. *Journal of the International Neuropsychological Society: JINS*, *13*(5), 758–769.

Zuccato, C., & Cattaneo, E. (2007). Role of brain-derived neurotrophic factor in Huntington's disease. *Progress in Neurobiology*, *81*(5–6), 294–330.

Zuccato, C., Valenza, M., & Cattaneo, E. (2010). Molecular mechanisms and potential therapeutical targets in Huntington's disease. *Physiological Reviews*, *90*(3), 905–981.

Chapter 9

Cortical Manifestations in Amyotrophic Lateral Sclerosis

A.J. Moszczynski, M.J. Strong
Western University, London, ON, Canada

BACKGROUND

Amyotrophic lateral sclerosis (ALS) is the most common adult-onset neurodegenerative disease of the motor system. Although the earliest clinical description of ALS appeared in the thesis of Aran (1850), it was Charcot J.M. and Joffroy A (1869) who coalesced the findings of progressive degeneration of both upper (descending supraspinal) and lower motor neurons into a single diagnostic entity. The net effect of this degeneration is a progressive loss of motor function, culminating in paralysis and death generally within 3–5 years of symptom onset (Strong, 2003).

Although neuropsychological changes in ALS were historically considered to be rare (Hudson A.J., 1993), the contemporary view is that 45–55% of patients with ALS will develop a neuropsychological syndrome reflective of frontotemporal dysfunction, including a frontotemporal dementia (FTD), behavioral or cognitive impairment (ALSbi and ALSci, respectively), language impairment, or deficits in social cognition (Abrahams, Newton, Niven, Foley, & Bak, 2014; Elamin et al., 2011; Montuschi et al., 2015; Oh et al., 2014; Strong et al., 2009; Strong, Grace, Orange, & Leeper, 1996). The presence of a neuropsychological syndrome in ALS is prognostically relevant because affected patients will have a significantly shorter survival than if ALS occurs in isolation (Elamin et al., 2011; Hu et al., 2013).

NEUROPSYCHOLOGICAL MANIFESTATIONS OF FRONTOTEMPORAL DYSFUNCTION IN AMYOTROPHIC LATERAL SCLEROSIS

The neuropsychological manifestations of ALS can range from impairments in cognition or behavior, deficits in social cognition or theory of mind (ToM), or as an FTD consistent with either the Neary or Hodges criteria (Hodges & Miller,

The Cerebral Cortex in Neurodegenerative and Neuropsychiatric Disorders.
http://dx.doi.org/10.1016/B978-0-12-801942-9.00009-4
223

2001; Neary et al., 1998; Strong, 2008; Strong et al., 2009). Rare presentations can include progressive nonfluent aphasia or semantic dementia, suggesting a continuum with FTD. Approximately 2–4% of patients who have ALS will develop concomitant Alzheimer disease (AD) (Consonni et al., 2013).

Impairments in language, including deficits in naming, comprehension, and spelling, occur in upwards of 35% of patients (Abrahams et al., 2014). Deficits can be further subdivided into impairment in action verbs but not cognitive verbs, with the former showing a positive association with impairments in executive functioning (York et al., 2014). These latter findings are associated with significant gray matter atrophy in the left precentral gyrus, left cingulate gyrus, and right medial frontal gyrus. As will be discussed, these observations begin to highlight the regional selectivity of the frontotemporal dysfunction in ALS.

Impairments in verbal fluency are commonly observed. In a meta-analysis of published studies, Raaphorst and colleagues observed that among those individuals with cognitive impairment, impairments in verbal fluency, visual memory, and immediate verbal recall each had a significant effect size (Raaphorst, De, Linssen, De Haan, & Schmand, 2010).

Behavioral dysfunction has been observed in upwards of 40% of patients with ALS and can include apathy, behavioral disinhibition, irritability, loss of sympathy/empathy, perseverative or stereotypic behavior, or changes in eating behavior (Abrahams et al., 2014; van der Hulst, Bak, & Abrahams, 2014; Lomen-Hoerth et al., 2003). An increased incidence of psychotic symptoms has been observed in those individuals with ALS-FTD (Lillo, Garcin, Hornberger, Bak, & Hodges, 2010). Deficits in ToM have been described in a significant proportion of patients who have ALS and are characterized as an inability to represent others' intentions and beliefs and thus the ability to predict others' behavior by attributing independent mental states to them (Adenzato, Cavallo, & Enrici, 2010). These deficits can be observed even in the absence of overt evidence of dementia (Meier, Charleston, & Tippett, 2010). Consistent with pathology of the orbitofrontal cortex, impairments range from apathy through to greater difficulty in identifying emotional expression or reductions in emotional attributions while sparing intentional attributions (and thus a reduced ability to recognize others' emotional states) (Cerami et al., 2014). ToM deficits correlate with diffuse cortical atrophy [determined by magnetic resonance imaging (MRI)] with a specific accentuation in the left superior precentral gyrus, left paracentral gyrus, and right precentral gyrus (Agosta et al., 2012).

MOLECULAR, CLINICAL, AND NEUROPATHOLOGICAL CORRELATES OF FRONTOTEMPORAL DYSFUNCTION IN AMYOTROPHIC LATERAL SCLEROSIS

Approximately 10% of ALS cases are genetic in origin (Al-Chalabi et al., 2012; Renton, Chio, & Traynor, 2014) (Table 9.1). Although the mechanism(s) by which many of these mutations induce neuronal degeneration are uncertain,

TABLE 9.1 Genes Associated With Amyotrophic Lateral Sclerosis and Their Overlap With Frontotemporal Dementia

Protein	Gene	OMIM	Functional Changes	FTD	ALS	ALS-FTD	PLS/Other	References
Superoxide dismutase 1	SOD1	147450	Oxidative stress		+		+ (SBMA, PMA)	Rosen et al. (1993)
Senataxin	SETX	608465	DNA/RNA processing		+		+	Chen et al. (2004)
Spastin	SPAST	604277	NFL, cytoskeleton, microtubule deficits		+		+	Munch, Rolfs, and Meyer, 2008; Wharton et al. (2003)
Fused in sarcoma	FUS	137070	Cell death (closely related to TDP)	+	+	+		Mackenzie, Rademakers, and Neumann, 2010; Vance et al. (2009)
Vesicle-associated membrane protein–associated proteins B and C	VAPB	605704	Altered axonal transport		+		+ (SMA)	Nishimura et al. (2004)
Angiogenin, ribonuclease, ribonuclease A family	ANG	105850	DNA/RNA processing		+	+	+ (PBP)	van Es et al. (2009)

Continued

TABLE 9.1 Genes Associated With Amyotrophic Lateral Sclerosis and Their Overlap With Frontotemporal Dementia—cont'd

Protein	Gene	OMIM	Functional Changes	FTD	ALS	ALS-FTD	PLS/Other	References
TAR DNA binding protein (TDP-43)	TARDBP	605078	DNA/RNA processing	+	+	+		Davidson et al. (2007), Sreedharan et al. (2008)
Factor-Induced gene 4 (FIG4) homolog, SAC1 lipid phosphatase domain containing (Saccharomyces cerevisiae)	FIG4	609390	Cell death/protein degradation		+		+	Chow et al. (2009)
Optineurin	OPTN	602432	Cell death/protein degradation		+		+ (PDB)	Maruyama et al. (2010)
Ataxin 2	ATXN 2	601517	Oxidative stress		+		+ (SCA2)	Elden et al. (2010)
Valosin-containing protein	VCP	601023	Protein degradation	+	+	+	+	Forman et al. (2006), Johnson et al. (2010), Weihl, Pestronk, and Kimonis (2009)
Ubiquilin 2	UBQLN2	300264	Protein degradation	+	+	+		Gellera et al. (2013), Ugwu et al. (2015)

Description	Symbol	OMIM	Function					Reference
Sigma nonopioid intracellular receptor 1	*SIGMAR1*	601978	Ion channel regulation		+	–		Al-Saif, Al-Mohanna, and Bohlega (2011), Belzil et al. (2013)
Profilin 1	*PFN1*	176610	NFL, cytoskeleton, microtubule deficits	+	+			Smith et al. (2015), van Blitterswijk et al. (2013)
Chromosome 9 open reading frame 72	*C9orf72*	614260		+	+	+		Renton et al. (2011)
Charged multivesicular body protein 2B	*CHMP2B*	609512	Vesicle trafficking	+	+			Cox et al. (2010)
Unc-13 homologue A (*Caenorhabditis elegans*)	*UNC13A*	609894	Synaptic neurotransmitter release	+	+	+		Shatunov et al. (2010)
D-amino-acid oxidase	*DAO*	124050	Oxidative stress		+			Mitchell et al. (2010)
Dynactin 1	*DCTN1*	601143	Altered axonal transport		+		+ (Perry syndrome)	Farrer et al. (2009), Munch et al. (2004)
Neurofilament, heavy polypeptide	*NEFH*	162230	NFL, cytoskeleton, microtubule deficits		+			Al-Chalabi et al. (1999)

Continued

TABLE 9.1 Genes Associated With Amyotrophic Lateral Sclerosis and Their Overlap With Frontotemporal Dementia—cont'd

Protein	Gene	OMIM [a]	Functional Changes	FTD	ALS	ALS-FTD	PLS/ Other	References
Peripherin	PRPH	170710	NFL, cytoskeleton, microtubule deficits		+			Corrado et al. (2011)
Sequestome 1	SQSTM1	601530	Protein degradation	+	+	+	+ (PDB)	Le Ber et al. (2013)
TAF15 RNA polymerase II, TATA box binding protein (TBP)–associated factor, 68 kDa	TAF15	601574	DNA/RNA processing		+			Hand et al. (2002)
Spastic paraplegia 11	SPG11	610844	DNA damage repair		+		+ (HSP)	Daoud et al. (2012)
Elongator acetyltransferase complex subunit 3	ELP3	612722	Projection neuron maturation		+			Simpson et al. (2009)

ALS, amyotrophic lateral sclerosis; FTD, frontotemporal dementia; HSP, hereditary spastic paraplegia; NFL, neurofilament; OMIM, Online Mendelian Inheritance in Man; PBP, progressive bulbar palsy; PDB, paget disease of bone; PLS, primary lateral sclerosis; PMA, progressive muscular atrophy; SBMA, spinal-bulbar muscular atrophy; SCA2, spinocerebellar ataxia type 2; SMA, spinal muscular atrophy; TAR, transactive response; TDP, TAR DNA-binding protein.

there are three general themes including the induction of oxidative stress (eg, mutations in *SOD1, ATXN2, DAO*), alterations in the cytoskeleton and/or impairments in axonal transport (eg, *VAPB, SPAST, DCTN1, NEFH, PRPH*), and alterations in RNA metabolism (eg, *TARDP, ANG, FUS,* and pathological hexanucleotide expansions of *C9orf72*). However, a group of genetic mutations cannot be readily bundled into these potential mechanisms including genes thought to directly give rise to ALS and those thought to be genetic modifiers (*CHMP2B, VCP, UBQLN2, SIGMAR1, PFN1, UNC13A, SQSTM1, TAF15, SPG11, ELP3*). Ultimately, however, there are few clinical features that are unique to any of the genes associated with ALS, suggesting that the motor degeneration and potentially the neuropsychological deficits are syndromic or, in the latter, reflective of specific neural network dysfunction that is independent of the underlying pathological mutation.

The theme of ALS being syndromic is supported by neuropathological studies. Consistent with the primary manifestation as a progressive loss of motor function, the hallmark of ALS is a loss of both spinal and bulbar motor neurons with degeneration of descending supraspinal innervation pathways. Affected motor neurons demonstrate a range of nuclear and cytoplasmic neuronal inclusions (NNIs and NCIs, respectively). In a blinded analysis of both sporadic and familial ALS motor neuron pathology, it was not possible to identify (by light microscopy) a "signature" pattern of neuronal inclusions of either cytoskeletal proteins or RNA-binding proteins that would allow differentiation amongst individual genotypes of ALS (Keller et al., 2012). The exception to this was *SOD1* mutations. The presence of frontotemporal dysfunction in ALS is typically indistinguishable from that occurring as an isolated FTD in which diffuse frontal and anterior temporal atrophy is accompanied by a vacuolar appearance consistent with superficial linear spongiosis throughout affected regions (Wilson, Grace, Munoz, He, & Strong, 2001). Somewhat in contrast to the pathology of affected motor neurons in ALS, cortical and subcortical neurons in cases with a syndrome of frontotemporal dysfunction tend to display an increase in transactive response DNA-binding protein 43 (TDP-43) cytosolic expression and a range of both NCIs and NNIs (Neumann et al., 2006).

Although an up-regulation of TDP-43 expression can also be seen as a response to neuronal injury (Moisse et al., 2009), the presence of both an increased expression of neuronal TDP-43 and TDP-43 immunoreactive NNIs and NCIs as major neuropathological features of both ALS and FTD suggests a common pathogenic process across the two diseases. TDP-43 has a range of activities that map to the regulation of gene expression, including such diverse functions as anchoring of chromatin, participation in splicing and RNA granule formation, the regulation of RNA translation, and participation in RNA degradation through the Dicer complex (Droppelmann, Campos-Melo, Ishtiaq, Volkening, & Strong, 2014).

The hypothesis of a continuum encompassing both ALS and FTD has been further reinforced by the discovery of a pathological expansion of a hexanucleotide repeat (GGGGCC) in *C9orf72* in both familial and sporadic ALS (DeJesus-Hernandez et al., 2011; Renton et al., 2011). The RNA associated with this expansion undergoes a unique type of repeat-associated non–ATG-initiated translation to give rise to dipeptide repeat proteins that can function as sinks for a range of RNA-binding proteins, effectively sequestering them from participating in RNA metabolism (Ash et al., 2013; Souza, Pinto, & Oliveira, 2015). It remains to be fully clarified as to whether the pathological RNA alone or the presence of dipeptides alone, or a combination of both, are sufficient to induce cell death (Hukema et al., 2014; Mizielinska et al., 2014). The neurodegeneration associated with pathological hexanucleotide expansions in *C9orf72* is typically more symmetrical than that observed with other variants of FTD and includes frontal and temporal cortices and the hippocampus, as well as deeper structures such as the striatum and thalamus (Mahoney et al., 2012).

No single pathological inclusion describes all variants of frontotemporal dysfunction in ALS. Indeed, there is increasing evidence to suggest the coexistence of several pathological protein inclusions within the same case, including the presence of both *C9orf72* and TDP-43 (Mackenzie et al., 2013) or *C9orf72* and the microtubule-associated protein tau in pathological inclusions (Bieniek et al., 2013). In lumbar spinal motor neurons, the coexistence within the same inclusion of the RNA-binding proteins TDP-43, fused in sarcoma/translocated in liposarcoma, and Rho guanine nucleotide exchange factor has been described (Keller et al., 2012). The critical point here is that although there is a tendency to describe the various neurodegenerative syndromes using nomenclature that reflects either the underlying genetic basis or the preponderance of a single proteinaceous inclusion, upon critical evaluation the syndromic nature of ALS and its associated frontotemporal syndromes is evident.

The clinical expression of pathological expansions of *C9orf72* is heterogeneous, ranging from a rapidly progressive variant with marked neuropsychological abnormalities to an atypically slow progression that may last decades (Chester et al., 2013; Kandiah et al., 2012; Khan et al., 2012). Such a range of survival is not only consistent with the syndromic nature of ALS, but also suggests that the phenotypic expression of a pathological expansion of *C9orf72* can be modified either by the presence of a second genetic mutation (the basis of oligogenic inheritance) or alternatively by either exogenous or environmental factors.

Perhaps the most controversial aspect of the pathogenesis of frontotemporal dysfunction in ALS is whether or not alterations in the metabolism of tau are present. However, distinct from the presence of a tauopathy among the previously hyperendemic focus of ALS in the Western Pacific, we have observed that tau immunoreactive glial and neuronal inclusions are a significant feature of ALSci (Yang, Sopper, Leystra-Lantz, & Strong, 2003; Yang &

Strong, 2012). Tau isolated from the frontal cortex of patients with ALSci is typically insoluble with (in contrast to AD tau) all six tau isoforms being expressed in the insoluble fraction and abnormally phosphorylated at threonine 175 (pThr175-tau) (Strong et al., 2006). Both the pattern of tau deposition and this phosphorylation state render the tau deposition of ALSci different from primary age-related tauopathy (Crary et al., 2014; Jellinger et al., 2015) and from normal tau deposition as a function of aging (Yang, Ang, & Strong, 2005). Moreover, pseudophosphorylated tau mimicking pThr175-tau forms pathological intracellular inclusions in vitro and leads to cell death (Gohar et al., 2009; Moszczynski et al., 2015).

These observations suggest that the phenotypic expression of both the motor neuron and cortical or subcortical neurodegeneration of ALS can be driven by a wide range of pathological processes, sometimes occurring as isolated metabolic syndromes or at times as a confluence of metabolic derangements. If this is the case, then the motor neuron phenotype would be expected to be uniform across all biological variants because there is a limited phenotypic reserve with which to manifest motor neuron dysfunction, specifically as a loss of motor function. The converse cannot be held for the neuropsychological manifestations because the phenotypic reserve upon which to draw for the clinical expression of a specific pathological process will be considerably greater. However, these latter manifestations are not limitless and, as discussed, are reflected in a discrete number of well-defined syndromes of frontotemporal dysfunction. As will become evident, our postulate is that these syndromes do in fact draw on a limited phenotypic reserve, but in this case, the reserve is defined by neural networks.

NEUROIMAGING CORRELATES OF IMPAIRED NEURAL NETWORK FUNCTION AS THE BASIS OF FRONTOTEMPORAL DYSFUNCTION IN AMYOTROPHIC LATERAL SCLEROSIS

The postulate that the frontotemporal syndromes of ALS are based on perturbations in neural networks finds support across a number of neuroimaging modalities, but most specifically resting state functional MRI (RS-fMRI) and diffusion tensor imaging (DTI) (see Chapter 3). RS-fMRI correlates brain regions that are activated concomitantly and has been used to compare functional network alterations in ALS and the behavioral variant of FTD (bvFTD) (Trojsi et al., 2015). This latter study highlighted the involvement of three major neural networks in both ALS and bvFTD: the salience network (SN), the default mode network (DMN), and the central executive network (CEN) (Fig. 9.1).

To visualize the networks more directly and, more specifically, to assess the integrity of neuronal pathways, DTI can be applied. The basis of DTI is the measurement of the diffusion of water along neuronal projections. Given the narrow diameter of neuronal tracts, water is more able to diffuse along the tract than across it, having an anisotropic motion, which when measured,

FIGURE 9.1 Three major networks affected in amyotrophic lateral sclerosis (ALS) and frontotemporal dementia (FTD). *Red nodes* have been shown to be dysfunctional in FTD. (A) Default mode network (DMN) areas affected in FTD include the medial prefrontal cortex *(mPFC)* and medial temporal (MT) lobes, whereas the posterior cingulate cortex *(PCC)*, ventral precuneus *(VP)*, and parietal cortex *(PC)* are less commonly implicated. The *dashed circle* indicates that the PC is superficial to the contained structures. (B) Salience network (SN) nodes including the anterior cingulate cortex *(ACC)*, insula *(In)*, and prefrontal cortex *(PFC)* are all implicated in FTD-related dementia processes. (C) Central executive network (CEN) areas affected include the dorsolateral prefrontal cortex *(dlPFC)*, whereas the posterior parietal cortex is less commonly implicated.

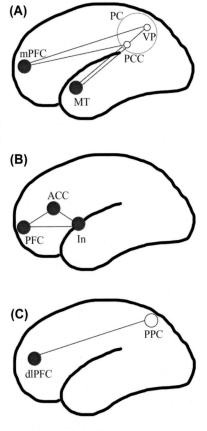

allows for an approximation of the tract direction to be generated. More myelination of tracts increases the signal because of higher water content. Therefore a reduced signal is likely to indicate reduced integrity of the connective pathways. Although not yet applied to understanding the frontotemporal dysfunction of ALS, DTI is being applied to understanding the degeneration of the corticospinal tracts as part of the neural network subserving motor function (Brettschneider, Petzold, Sussmuth, Ludolph, & Tumani, 2006; Hendrix et al., 2015; Karlsborg et al., 2004).

The concept that neural networks mediate not only the phenotypic expression of the neurodegenerative process but also can serve as "highways of disease propagation" has been supported by staging the spread of either tau protein or α-synuclein pathosis in AD and Parkinson disease (Braak & Braak, 1995; Braak et al., 2003). These observations suggest that whereas network connectivity may be affected as a whole, there are specific patterns of vulnerability within these networks. This approach to the study of neural networks has provided insight into the dysfunctional network systems in a variety of disease states in which syndrome-specific patterns of dysfunction are observed (Seeley, Crawford, Zhou, Miller, & Greicius, 2009). Extending these methodologies to evaluate the integrity of white matter tracts within the brain (structural network imaging), mathematical models in conjunction with fMRI has yielded the capacity to evaluate differences in activated brain areas comprising nodes in these networks (functional network imaging) and to ascribe differences to individual disease states (Zhou et al., 2010).

The understanding of neural networks gained through such studies can be applied to understanding the neuroanatomical origins of the frontotemporal syndromes observed in ALS. The DMN consists of regions in the medial temporal lobe (memory), medial prefrontal cortex (involved in ToM), posterior cingulate cortex, ventral precuneus, and medial, lateral, and inferior parietal cortices. The DMN is active largely during periods of wakeful rest, while the patient is not focusing on anything occurring in the outside world (ie, daydreaming) (Yan et al., 2009). Importantly, the DMN has been implicated in social cognition (Schilbach, Eickhoff, Rotarska-Jagiela, Fink, & Vogeley, 2008). The SN has been implicated in a number of psychotic disorders (Palaniyappan & Liddle, 2012). In cases of young-onset FTD, many are first diagnosed as psychotic disorders up to 5 years before FTD because of the similarity of presentation (Velakoulis, Walterfang, Mocellin, Pantelis, & McLean, 2009). It is noteworthy then that increased psychotic symptoms have been observed in ALS with FTD (Lillo et al., 2010). The SN is thought to act as a switch between the DMN and the CEN (Menon & Uddin, 2010; Sridharan, Levitin, & Menon, 2008), allowing for the focus of attention to the external world and one's inside thoughts to be prioritized and maintained. This network consists of the anterior cingulate, insula, and prefrontal cortices. The CEN is implicated in executive control (D'Esposito, 2007; Koechlin & Summerfield, 2007). The CEN (also referred to as the *frontoparietal network*) consists of the dorsolateral prefrontal cortex and posterior parietal cortex, with particular activity along the intraparietal sulcus. Importantly, the DMN and CEN have anticorrelated activations such that activation of one leads to inhibition of the other (Fox et al., 2005). Supporting dysfunction in these networks in ALS, the presence of protein inclusions in the anterior cingulate cortex paired with the signs of both ToM (van der Hulst et al., 2014) and executive control dysfunction (York et al., 2014) may indicate an SN abnormality because there are dysfunctions across all three network activities that may indicate a switching and control abnormality. Consistent with this, both ALS and FTD brains have reduced SN functioning, whereas patients with AD have an enhancement in this network and a reduction in activity of the DMN (Zhou et al., 2010).

Beyond describing the basis of the neuropsychological manifestations of ALS, the analysis of neural networks has provided insight into neural network dysfunction in ALS before the detection of executive dysfunction (Trojsi et al., 2015). When both ALS and bvFTD were compared with controls, reduced right supramarginal gyrus connectivity (reflecting CEN dysfunction) and decreased medial prefrontal cortex and insular activation (reflecting SN dysfunction) was observed in both ALS and bvFTD, although it occurred in bvFTD more than in ALS. Of note, divergence between disease states was observed, because ALS cases showed reduced posterior cingulate connectivity (reflecting DMN dysfunction), whereas bvFTD cases showed an increase in connectivity of this region along with decreased connectivity in the frontal regions of this network, indicating more widespread connectivity changes when the cognitive phenotype was present. The convergence in network dysfunction may indicate common processes at work in these separate phenotypes. Conversely, the divergence in DMN activity, along with more severe deficits in other network connectivity may be responsible for the lack of change in social cognition in some patients with ALS.

Additional network connectivity studies in patients with bvFTD have shown a reduced connectivity throughout the brain, including the anterior cingulate cortex, temporal poles, frontal gyri, and insular cortices (Agosta et al., 2013). This reduced connectivity has been determined to represent a reduction in connection efficiency and may represent a reduced ability to transfer and therefore process information (Agosta et al., 2013). Additionally, white matter integrity is compromised in the same regions as major gray matter loss, with extension to other regions with no measured gray matter atrophy (Mahoney et al., 2012). A reduction in the overall connectivity of the uncinate fasciculus has been implicated in bvFTD in distinction from other dementias, namely AD, which shares some network connectivity–change overlap with bvFTD (Mahoney et al., 2012).

Apart from the cognitive involvement, structural brain network imaging studies of patients with ALS has revealed a motor network dysfunction that correlates with the severity of disease to a larger extent than total measured atrophy (Verstraete et al., 2014). Expansion of these deficits is seen with disease progression, suggesting a spread of pathosis reminiscent of the spread of protein inclusions (reviewed in Jucker & Walker, 2013). Such a postulate would also explain a progressive diversification of symptoms, implying that this spread of dysfunctional activity along brain network paths is a key component of the disease process.

MODELS OF NEUROPSYCHOLOGICAL DYSFUNCTION IN AMYOTROPHIC LATERAL SCLEROSIS

Whereas a number of models of the motor dysfunction of ALS have been identified, there are very few that recapitulate the neuropsychological dysfunction described, and essentially none that address the integrity of neural networks. Thus although the most commonly utilized murine model for ALS harbors the G93A *SOD1* mutation seen in familial ALS, little is known regarding its impact on cognitive function in the mouse, although these mice do possess shorter dendrites in the prefrontal cortex and have reduced fear extinction (Sgobio et al., 2008).

The latter precedes the development of motor deficits. Mice harboring the G37R *SOD1* mutation have spontaneous alternation deficits on a T maze task (Filali, Lalonde, & Rivest, 2011).

Murine models of TDP-43 pathology have been developed, including the overexpression of wild-type TDP-43 (Wils et al., 2010). These mice develop spinal and cortical TDP-43 pathosis reminiscent of ALS-FTD. In a separate study, the overexpression of human wild-type TDP-43 in mice led to memory deficits in the Morris water maze as well as fear conditioning tasks (Tsai et al., 2010). The expression of mutant TDP-43 (A315T) induces both cortical and spinal motor neuron death in mice in the absence of pathological cytoplasmic TDP-43 aggregates (Wegorzewska, Bell, Cairns, Miller, & Baloh, 2009). To attempt to more precisely reflect the human disease state, Swarup and colleagues designed mouse models of human wild-type TDP-43 as well as A315T and G348C mutants that expressed TDP-43 at levels that more closely resemble that in the human CNS (Swarup et al., 2011). They found that along with motor deficits, mice developed cytoplasmic TDP-43 pathosis resembling that of ALS-FTD. Affected mice developed learning deficits on the Barnes maze test, indicative of cognitive abnormalities.

The discovery of *C9orf72* is relatively recent, and thus the development of models of cognitive dysfunction lags behind that of *SOD1* and TDP-43 models.

THERAPEUTIC STRATEGIES

Given the relatively recent increase in our understanding of both the incidence of frontotemporal dysfunction in ALS and its probable phenotypic basis in dysfunction of neural networks seemingly independent of the underlying proteinopathy, little is known regarding its treatment. Indeed, at this time, there are no studies that have specifically addressed pharmacotherapies for this aspect of the disease process.

CONCLUSIONS AND FUTURE DIRECTIONS

ALS is a clinical presentation of a group of pathologies that happen to affect the same cells through potentially different mechanisms. When patients exhibit dysexecutive syndrome, it is the result of specific network activity malfunction, such as the insula in the SN. Spread of pathosis through these networks is likely to be responsible for disease progression. Further insight into the apparent selective vulnerability of the motor and frontal cortical neurons will also be important in determining the etiology of the disease. Patient imaging with molecule-specific ligands and genotypic analysis to determine which pathologies are the most likely causes of the phenotype will be crucial for developing strategies to stop disease progression in individual patients and stratify cases based on possible mechanisms of cell death such as oxidative, RNA processing, or cytoskeletal abnormalities.

REFERENCES

Abrahams, S., Newton, J., Niven, E., Foley, J., & Bak, T. H. (2014). Screening for cognition and behaviour changes in ALS. *Amyotrophic Lateral Sclerosis & Frontotemporal Degeneration*, *15*, 9–14.

Adenzato, M., Cavallo, M., & Enrici, I. (2010). Theory of mind ability in the behavioural variant of frontotemporal dementia: an analysis of the neural, cognitive, and social levels. *Neuropsychologia*, *48*, 2–12.

Agosta, F., Canu, E., Valsasina, P., Riva, N., Prelle, A., Comi, G., et al. (2013). Divergent brain network connectivity in amyotrophic lateral sclerosis. *Neurobiology of Aging*, *34*, 419–427.

Agosta, F., Valsasina, P., Riva, N., Copetti, M., Messina, M. J., Prelle, A., et al. (2012). The cortical signature of amyotrophic lateral sclerosis. *PLoS One*, *7*, e42816.

Al-Chalabi, A., Andersen, P. M., Nilsson, P., Chioza, B., Andersson, J. L., Russ, C., et al. (1999). Deletions of the heavy neurofilament subunit tail in amyotrophic lateral sclerosis. *Human Molecular Genetics*, *8*, 157–164.

Al-Chalabi, A., Jones, A., Troakes, C., King, A., Al-Sarraj, S., & van den Berg, L. H. (2012). The genetics and neuropathology of amyotrophic lateral sclerosis. *Acta Neuropathologica*, *124*, 339–352.

Al-Saif, A., Al-Mohanna, F., & Bohlega, S. (2011). A mutation in sigma-1 receptor causes juvenile amyotrophic lateral sclerosis. *Annals of Neurology*, *70*, 913–919.

Aran, F. A. (1850). Recherches sur une maladie non encore décrite du systéme musculaire (atrophie musculaire progressive)(2e article - suite et fin). *Archives générales de medicine*, *24*, 172–214.

Ash, P. E., Bieniek, K. F., Gendron, T. F., Caulfield, T., Lin, W. L., DeJesus-Hernandez, M., et al. (2013). Unconventional translation of *C9ORF72* GGGGCC expansion generates insoluble polypeptides specific to c9FTD/ALS. *Neuron*, *77*, 639–646.

Belzil, V. V., Daoud, H., Camu, W., Strong, M. J., Dion, P. A., & Rouleau, G. A. (2013). Genetic analysis of *SIGMAR1* as a cause of familial ALS with dementia. *European Journal of Human Genetics*, *21*, 237–239.

Bieniek, K. F., Murray, M. E., Rutherford, N. J., Castanedes-Casey, M., DeJesus-Hernandez, M., Liesinger, A. M., et al. (2013). Tau pathology in frontotemporal lobar degeneration with *C9ORF72* hexanucleotide repeat expansion. *Acta Neuropathologica*, *125*, 289–302.

van Blitterswijk, M., Baker, M. C., Bieniek, K. F., Knopman, D. S., Josephs, K. A., Boeve, B., et al. (2013). Profilin-1 mutations are rare in patients with amyotrophic lateral sclerosis and frontotemporal dementia. *Amyotrophic Lateral Sclerosis and Frontotemporal Degeneration*, *14*, 463–469.

Braak, H., & Braak, E. (1995). Staging of Alzheimer's disease-related neurofibrillary changes. *Neurobiology of Aging*, *16*, 271–278.

Braak, H., Del, T. K., Rub, U., de Vos, R. A., Jansen Steur, E. N., & Braak, E. (2003). Staging of brain pathology related to sporadic Parkinson's disease. *Neurobiology of Aging*, *24*, 197–211.

Brettschneider, J., Petzold, A., Sussmuth, S. D., Ludolph, A. C., & Tumani, H. (2006). Axonal damage markers in cerebrospinal fluid are increased in ALS. *Neurology*, *66*, 852–856.

Cerami, C., Dodich, A., Canessa, N., Crespi, C., Iannaccone, S., Corbo, M., et al. (2014). Emotional empathy in amyotrophic lateral sclerosis: a behavioural and voxel-based morphometry study. *Amyotrophic Lateral Sclerosis and Frontotemporal Degeneration*, *15*, 21–29.

Charcot, J. M., & Joffroy, A. (1869). Deux cas d'atrophie musculaire progressive avec lésions de la substance grise et des faisceaux antérolatéraux de la moelle épinière. *Archives de physiologie norm et pathology*, *2*, 354–744.

Chen, Y. Z., Bennett, C. L., Huynh, H. M., Blair, I. P., Puls, I., Irobi, J., et al. (2004). DNA/RNA helicase gene mutations in a form of juvenile amyotrophic lateral sclerosis (ALS4). *The American Journal of Human Genetics*, *74*, 1128–1135.

Chester, C., de, C. M., Miltenberger, G., Pereira, S., Dillen, L., van der Zee, J., et al. (2013). Rapidly progressive frontotemporal dementia and bulbar amyotrophic lateral sclerosis in Portuguese patients with *C9orf72* mutation. *Amyotrophic Lateral Sclerosis and Frontotemporal Degeneration, 14*, 70–72.

Chow, C. Y., Landers, J. E., Bergren, S. K., Sapp, P. C., Grant, A. E., Jones, J. M., et al. (2009). Deleterious variants of *FIG4*, a phosphoinositide phosphatase, in patients with ALS. *The American Journal of Human Genetics, 84*, 85–88.

Consonni, M., Iannaccone, S., Cerami, C., Frasson, P., Lacerenza, M., Lunetta, C., et al. (2013). The cognitive and behavioural profile of amyotrophic lateral sclerosis: application of the consensus criteria. *Behavioural Neurology, 27*, 143–153.

Corrado, L., Carlomagno, Y., Falasco, L., Mellone, S., Godi, M., Cova, E., et al. (2011). A novel peripherin gene *(PRPH)* mutation identified in one sporadic amyotrophic lateral sclerosis patient. *Neurobiology of Aging, 32*, 552–556.

Cox, L. E., Ferraiuolo, L., Goodall, E. F., Heath, P. R., Higginbottom, A., Mortiboys, H., et al. (2010). Mutations in *CHMP2B* in lower motor neuron predominant amyotrophic lateral sclerosis (ALS). *PLoS One, 5*, e9872.

Crary, J. F., Trojanowski, J. Q., Schneider, J. A., Abisambra, J. F., Abner, E. L., Alafuzoff, I., et al. (2014). Primary age-related tauopathy (PART): a common pathology associated with human aging. *Acta Neuropathologica, 128*, 755–766.

D'Esposito, M. (2007). From cognitive to neural models of working memory. *Philosophical Transactions of the Royal Society of London. Series B, 362*, 761–772.

Daoud, H., Zhou, S., Noreau, A., Sabbagh, M., Belzil, V., Dionne-Laporte, A., et al. (2012). Exome sequencing reveals *SPG11* mutations causing juvenile ALS. *Neurobiology of Aging, 33*, 839.

Davidson, Y., Kelley, T., Mackenzie, I. R., Pickering-Brown, S., Du, P. D., Neary, D., et al. (2007). Ubiquitinated pathological lesions in frontotemporal lobar degeneration contain the TAR DNA-binding protein, TDP-43. *Acta Neuropathologica, 113*, 521–533.

DeJesus-Hernandez, M., Mackenzie, I. R., Boeve, B. F., Boxer, A. L., Baker, M., Rutherford, N. J., et al. (2011). Expanded GGGGCC hexanucleotide repeat in noncoding region of *C9ORF72* causes chromosome 9p-linked FTD and ALS. *Neuron, 72*, 245–256.

Droppelmann, C. A., Campos-Melo, D., Ishtiaq, M., Volkening, K., & Strong, M. J. (2014). RNA metabolism in ALS: when normal processes become pathological. *Amyotrophic Lateral Sclerosis and Frontotemporal Degeneration, 15*, 321–336.

Elamin, M., Phukan, J., Bede, P., Jordan, N., Byrne, S., Pender, N., et al. (2011). Executive dysfunction is a negative prognostic indicator in patients with ALS without dementia. *Neurology, 76*, 1263–1269.

Elden, A. C., Kim, H. J., Hart, M. P., Chen-Plotkin, A. S., Johnson, B. S., Fang, X., et al. (2010). Ataxin-2 intermediate-length polyglutamine expansions are associated with increased risk for ALS. *Nature, 466*, 1069–1075.

van Es, M. A., Diekstra, F. P., Veldink, J. H., Baas, F., Bourque, P. R., Schelhaas, H. J., et al. (2009). A case of ALS-FTD in a large FALS pedigree with a *K17I ANG* mutation. *Neurology, 72*, 287–288.

Farrer, M. J., Hulihan, M. M., Kachergus, J. M., Dachsel, J. C., Stoessl, A. J., Grantier, L. L., et al. (2009). *DCTN1* mutations in Perry syndrome. *Nature Genetics, 41*, 163–165.

Filali, M., Lalonde, R., & Rivest, S. (2011). Sensorimotor and cognitive functions in a SOD1(G37R) transgenic mouse model of amyotrophic lateral sclerosis. *Behavioural Brain Research, 225*, 215–221.

Forman, M. S., Mackenzie, I. R., Cairns, N. J., Swanson, E., Boyer, P. J., Drachman, D. A., et al. (2006). Novel ubiquitin neuropathology in frontotemporal dementia with valosin-containing protein gene mutations. *Journal of Neuropathology & Experimental Neurology, 65*, 571–581.

Fox, M. D., Snyder, A. Z., Vincent, J. L., Corbetta, M., Van Essen, D. C., & Raichle, M. E. (2005). The human brain is intrinsically organized into dynamic, anticorrelated functional networks. *Proceedings of the National Academy of Sciences USA, 102*, 9673–9678.

Gellera, C., Tiloca, C., Del, B. R., Corrado, L., Pensato, V., Agostini, J., et al. (2013). Ubiquilin 2 mutations in Italian patients with amyotrophic lateral sclerosis and frontotemporal dementia. *Journal of Neurology, Neurosurgery & Psychiatry, 84*, 183–187.

Gohar, M., Yang, W., Strong, W., Volkening, K., Leystra-Lantz, C., & Strong, M. J. (2009). Tau phosphorylation at threonine-175 leads to fibril formation and enhanced cell death: implications for amyotrophic lateral sclerosis with cognitive impairment. *Journal of Neurochemistry, 108*, 634–643.

Hand, C. K., Khoris, J., Salachas, F., Gros-Louis, F., Lopes, A. A., Mayeux-Portas, V., et al. (2002). A novel locus for familial amyotrophic lateral sclerosis, on chromosome 18q. *The American Journal of Human Genetics, 70*, 251–256.

Hendrix, P., Griessenauer, C. J., Cohen-Adad, J., Rajasekaran, S., Cauley, K. A., Shoja, M. M., et al. (2015). Spinal diffusion tensor imaging: a comprehensive review with emphasis on spinal cord anatomy and clinical applications. *Clinical Anatomy, 28*, 88–95.

Hodges, J. R., & Miller, B. (2001). The classification, genetics and neuropathology of frontotemporal dementia. Introduction to the special topic papers: Part I. *Neurocase, 7*, 31–35.

Hu, W. T., Shelnutt, M., Wilson, A., Yarab, N., Kelly, C., Grossman, M., et al. (2013). Behavior matters–cognitive predictors of survival in amyotrophic lateral sclerosis. *PLoS One, 8*, e57584.

Hudson, A. J. (1993). *Dementia and parkinsonism in amyotrophic lateral sclerosis.* B.V.: Elsevier Science Publishers, 231–240.

Hukema, R. K., Riemslagh, F. W., Melhem, S., van der Linde, H. C., Severijnen, L., Edbauer, D., et al. (2014). A new inducible transgenic mouse model for *C9orf72*-associated GGGGCC repeat expansion supports a gain-of-function mechanism in *C9orf72* associated ALS and FTD. *Acta Neuropathologica Communications, 2*, 166.

van der Hulst, E. J., Bak, T. H., & Abrahams, S. (2014). Impaired affective and cognitive theory of mind and behavioural change in amyotrophic lateral sclerosis. *Journal of Neurology, Neurosurgery & Psychiatry.*

Jellinger, K. A., Alafuzoff, I., Attems, J., Beach, T. G., Cairns, N. J., Crary, J. F., et al. (2015). Part, a distinct tauopathy, different from classical sporadic Alzheimer disease. *Acta Neuropathologica.*

Johnson, J. O., Mandrioli, J., Benatar, M., Abramzon, Y., Van Deerlin, V. M., Trojanowski, J. Q., et al. (2010). Exome sequencing reveals VCP mutations as a cause of familial ALS. *Neuron, 68*, 857–864.

Jucker, M., & Walker, L. C. (2013). Self-propagation of pathogenic protein aggregates in neurodegenerative diseases. *Nature, 501*, 45–51.

Kandiah, N., Sengdy, P., Mackenzie, I. R., Hsiung, G. Y., de Jesus-Hernandez, M., & Rademakers, R. (2012). Rapidly progressive dementia in a Chinese patient due to *C90RF72* mutation. *Canadian Journal of Neurological Sciences, 39*, 676–677.

Karlsborg, M., Rosenbaum, S., Wiegell, M., Simonsen, H., Larsson, H., Werdelin, L., et al. (2004). Corticospinal tract degeneration and possible pathogenesis in ALS evaluated by MR diffusion tensor imaging. *Amyotrophic Lateral Sclerosis and Other Motor Neuron Disorders, 5*, 136–140.

Keller, B. A., Volkening, K., Droppelmann, C. A., Ang, L. C., Rademakers, R., & Strong, M. J. (2012). Co-aggregation of RNA binding proteins in ALS spinal motor neurons: evidence of a common pathogenic mechanism. *Acta Neuropathologica, 124*, 733–747.

Khan, B. K., Yokoyama, J. S., Takada, L. T., Sha, S. J., Rutherford, N. J., Fong, J. C., et al. (2012). Atypical, slowly progressive behavioural variant frontotemporal dementia associated with *C9ORF72* hexanucleotide expansion. *Journal of Neurology, Neurosurgery & Psychiatry, 83*, 358–364.

Koechlin, E., & Summerfield, C. (2007). An information theoretical approach to prefrontal executive function. *Trends in Cognitive Sciences*, *11*, 229–235.

Le Ber, I., Camuzat, A., Guerreiro, R., Bouya-Ahmed, K., Bras, J., Nicolas, G., et al. (2013). *SQSTM1* mutations in French patients with frontotemporal dementia or frontotemporal dementia with amyotrophic lateral sclerosis. *JAMA Neurology*, *70*, 1403–1410.

Lillo, P., Garcin, B., Hornberger, M., Bak, T. H., & Hodges, J. R. (2010). Neurobehavioral features in frontotemporal dementia with amyotrophic lateral sclerosis. *Archives of Neurology*, *67*, 826–830.

Lomen-Hoerth, C., Murphy, J., Langmore, S., Kramer, J. H., Olney, R. K., & Miller, B. (2003). Are amyotrophic lateral sclerosis patients cognitively normal? *Neurology*, *60*, 1094–1097.

Mackenzie, I. R., Arzberger, T., Kremmer, E., Troost, D., Lorenzl, S., Mori, K., et al. (2013). Dipeptide repeat protein pathology in *C9ORF72* mutation cases: clinico-pathological correlations. *Acta Neuropathologica*, *126*, 859–879.

Mackenzie, I. R., Rademakers, R., & Neumann, M. (2010). TDP-43 and FUS in amyotrophic lateral sclerosis and frontotemporal dementia. *Lancet Neurology*, *9*, 995–1007.

Mahoney, C. J., Beck, J., Rohrer, J. D., Lashley, T., Mok, K., Shakespeare, T., et al. (2012). Frontotemporal dementia with the *C9ORF72* hexanucleotide repeat expansion: clinical, neuroanatomical and neuropathological features. *Brain: A Journal of Neurology*, *135*, 736–750.

Maruyama, H., Morino, H., Ito, H., Izumi, Y., Kato, H., Watanabe, Y., et al. (2010). Mutations of optineurin in amyotrophic lateral sclerosis. *Nature*, *465*, 223–226.

Meier, S. L., Charleston, A. J., & Tippett, L. J. (2010). Cognitive and behavioural deficits associated with the orbitomedial prefrontal cortex in amyotrophic lateral sclerosis. *Brain: A Journal of Neurology*, *133*, 3444–3457.

Menon, V., & Uddin, L. Q. (2010). Saliency, switching, attention and control: a network model of insula function. *Brain Structure & Function*, *214*, 655–667.

Mitchell, J., Paul, P., Chen, H. J., Morris, A., Payling, M., Falchi, M., et al. (2010). Familial amyotrophic lateral sclerosis is associated with a mutation in D-amino acid oxidase. *Proceedings of the National Academy of Sciences USA*, *107*, 7556–7561.

Mizielinska, S., Gronke, S., Niccoli, T., Ridler, C. E., Clayton, E. L., Devoy, A., et al. (2014). C9orf72 repeat expansions cause neurodegeneration in *Drosophila* through arginine-rich proteins. *Science*, *345*, 1192–1194.

Moisse, K., Mepham, J., Volkening, K., Welch, I., Hill, T., & Strong, M. J. (2009). Cytosolic TDP-43 expression following axotomy is associated with caspase 3 activation in NFL-/- mice: support for a role for TDP-43 in the physiological response to neuronal injury. *Brain Research*, *1296*, 176–186.

Montuschi, A., Iazzolino, B., Calvo, A., Moglia, C., Lopiano, L., Restagno, G., et al. (2015). Cognitive correlates in amyotrophic lateral sclerosis: a population-based study in Italy. *Journal of Neurology, Neurosurgery & Psychiatry*, *86*, 168–173.

Moszczynski, A. J., Gohar, M., Volkening, K., Leystra-Lantz, C., Strong, W., & Strong, M. J. (2015). Thr(175)-phosphorylated tau induces pathologic fibril formation via GSK3beta-mediated phosphorylation of Thr(231) in vitro. *Neurobiology of Aging*, *36*, 1590–1599.

Munch, C., Rolfs, A., & Meyer, T. (2008). Heterozygous S44L missense change of the spastin gene in amyotrophic lateral sclerosis. *Amyotrophic Lateral Sclerosis*, *9*, 251–253.

Munch, C., Sedlmeier, R., Meyer, T., Homberg, V., Sperfeld, A. D., Kurt, A., et al. (2004). Point mutations of the p150 subunit of dynactin (DCTN1) gene in ALS. *Neurology*, *63*, 724–726.

Neary, D., Snowden, J. S., Gustafson, L., Passant, U., Stuss, D., Black, S., et al. (1998). Frontotemporal lobar degeneration: a consensus on clinical diagnostic criteria. *Neurology*, *51*, 1546–1554.

Neumann, M., Sampathu, D. M., Kwong, L. K., Truax, A. C., Micsenyi, M. C., Chou, T. T., et al. (2006). Ubiquitinated TDP-43 in frontotemporal lobar degeneration and amyotrophic lateral sclerosis. *Science, 314,* 130–133.

Nishimura, A. L., Mitne-Neto, M., Silva, H. C., Richieri-Costa, A., Middleton, S., Cascio, D., et al. (2004). A mutation in the vesicle-trafficking protein VAPB causes late-onset spinal muscular atrophy and amyotrophic lateral sclerosis. *The American Journal of Human Genetics, 75,* 822–831.

Oh, S. I., Park, A., Kim, H. J., Oh, K. W., Choi, H., Kwon, M. J., et al. (2014). Spectrum of cognitive impairment in Korean ALS patients without known genetic mutations. *PLoS One, 9,* e87163.

Palaniyappan, L., & Liddle, P. F. (2012). Does the salience network play a cardinal role in psychosis? An emerging hypothesis of insular dysfunction. *Journal of Psychiatry & Neuroscience, 37,* 17–27.

Raaphorst, J., De, V. M., Linssen, W. H., De Haan, R. J., & Schmand, B. (2010). The cognitive profile of amyotrophic lateral sclerosis: a meta-analysis. *Amyotrophic Lateral Sclerosis, 11,* 27–37.

Renton, A. E., Chio, A., & Traynor, B. J. (2014). State of play in amyotrophic lateral sclerosis genetics. *Nature Neuroscience, 17,* 17–23.

Renton, A. E., Majounie, E., Waite, A., Simon-Sanchez, J., Rollinson, S., Gibbs, J. R., et al. (2011). A hexanucleotide repeat expansion in *C9ORF72* is the cause of chromosome 9p21-linked ALS-FTD. *Neuron, 72,* 257–268.

Rosen, D. R., Siddique, T., Patterson, D., Figlewicz, D. A., Sapp, P., Hentati, A., et al. (1993). Mutations in Cu/Zn superoxide dismutase gene are associated with familial amyotrophic lateral sclerosis. *Nature, 362,* 59–62.

Schilbach, L., Eickhoff, S. B., Rotarska-Jagiela, A., Fink, G. R., & Vogeley, K. (2008). Minds at rest? Social cognition as the default mode of cognizing and its putative relationship to the "default system" of the brain. *Consciousness and Cognition, 17,* 457–467.

Seeley, W. W., Crawford, R. K., Zhou, J., Miller, B. L., & Greicius, M. D. (2009). Neurodegenerative diseases target large-scale human brain networks. *Neuron, 62,* 42–52.

Sgobio, C., Trabalza, A., Spalloni, A., Zona, C., Carunchio, I., Longone, P., et al. (2008). Abnormal medial prefrontal cortex connectivity and defective fear extinction in the presymptomatic G93A *SOD1* mouse model of ALS. *Genes, Brain and Behavior, 7,* 427–434.

Shatunov, A., Mok, K., Newhouse, S., Weale, M. E., Smith, B., Vance, C., et al. (2010). Chromosome 9p21 in sporadic amyotrophic lateral sclerosis in the UK and seven other countries: a genome-wide association study. *Lancet Neurology, 9,* 986–994.

Simpson, C. L., Lemmens, R., Miskiewicz, K., Broom, W. J., Hansen, V. K., van Vught, P. W., et al. (2009). Variants of the elongator protein 3 *(ELP3)* gene associated with motor neuron degeneration. *Human Molecular Genetics, 18,* 472–481.

Smith, B. N., Vance, C., Scotter, E. L., Troakes, C., Wong, C. H., Topp, S., et al. (2015). Novel mutations support a role for profilin 1 in the pathogenesis of ALS. *Neurobiology of Aging, 36,* 1602–1627.

Souza, P. V., Pinto, W. B., & Oliveira, A. S. (2015). C9orf72-related disorders: expanding the clinical and genetic spectrum of neurodegenerative diseases. *Arquivos de Neuro-Psiquiatria, 73,* 246–256.

Sreedharan, J., Blair, I. P., Tripathi, V. B., Hu, X., Vance, C., Rogelj, B., et al. (2008). TDP-43 mutations in familial and sporadic amyotrophic lateral sclerosis. *Science, 319,* 1668–1672.

Sridharan, D., Levitin, D. J., & Menon, V. (2008). A critical role for the right fronto-insular cortex in switching between central-executive and default-mode networks. *Proceedings of the National Academy of Sciences USA, 105,* 12569–12574.

Strong, M. J. (2003). The basic aspects of therapeutics in amyotrophic lateral sclerosis. *Pharmacology & Therapeutics, 98*, 379–414.

Strong, M. J. (2008). The syndromes of frontotemporal dysfunction in amyotrophic lateral sclerosis. *Amyotrophic Lateral Sclerosis, 9*, 323–338.

Strong, M. J., Grace, G. M., Freedman, M., Lomen-Hoerth, C., Woolley, S., Goldstein, L. H., et al. (2009). Consensus criteria for the diagnosis of frontotemporal cognitive and behavioural syndromes in amyotrophic lateral sclerosis. *Amyotrophic Lateral Sclerosis, 10*, 131–146.

Strong, M. J., Grace, G. M., Orange, J. B., & Leeper, H. A. (1996). Cognition, language, and speech in amyotrophic lateral sclerosis: a review. *Journal of Clinical and Experimental Neuropsychology, 18*, 291–303.

Strong, M. J., Yang, W., Strong, W. L., Leystra-Lantz, C., Jaffe, H., & Pant, H. C. (2006). Tau protein hyperphosphorylation in sporadic ALS with cognitive impairment. *Neurology, 66*, 1770–1771.

Swarup, V., Phaneuf, D., Bareil, C., Robertson, J., Rouleau, G. A., Kriz, J., et al. (2011). Pathological hallmarks of amyotrophic lateral sclerosis/frontotemporal lobar degeneration in transgenic mice produced with TDP-43 genomic fragments. *Brain: A Journal of Neurology, 134*, 2610–2626.

Trojsi, F., Esposito, F., de, S. M., Buonanno, D., Conforti, F. L., Corbo, D., et al. (2015). Functional overlap and divergence between ALS and bvFTD. *Neurobiology of Aging, 36*, 413–423.

Tsai, K. J., Yang, C. H., Fang, Y. H., Cho, K. H., Chien, W. L., Wang, W. T., et al. (2010). Elevated expression of TDP-43 in the forebrain of mice is sufficient to cause neurological and pathological phenotypes mimicking FTLD-U. *Journal of Experimental Medicine, 207*, 1661–1673.

Ugwu, F., Rollinson, S., Harris, J., Gerhard, A., Richardson, A., Jones, M., et al. (2015). A *UBQLN2* variant of unknown significance in frontotemporal lobar degeneration. *Neurobiology of Aging, 36*, 546.

Vance, C., Rogelj, B., Hortobagyi, T., De Vos, K. J., Nishimura, A. L., Sreedharan, J., et al. (2009). Mutations in FUS, an RNA processing protein, cause familial amyotrophic lateral sclerosis type 6. *Science, 323*, 1208–1211.

Velakoulis, D., Walterfang, M., Mocellin, R., Pantelis, C., & McLean, C. (2009). Frontotemporal dementia presenting as schizophrenia-like psychosis in young people: clinicopathological series and review of cases. *The British Journal of Psychiatry, 194*, 298–305.

Verstraete, E., Polders, D. L., Mandl, R. C., Van Den Heuvel, M. P., Veldink, J. H., Luijten, P., et al. (2014). Multimodal tract-based analysis in ALS patients at 7T: a specific white matter profile? *Amyotrophic Lateral Sclerosis and Frontotemporal Degeneration, 15*, 84–92.

Wegorzewska, I., Bell, S., Cairns, N. J., Miller, T. M., & Baloh, R. H. (2009). TDP-43 mutant transgenic mice develop features of ALS and frontotemporal lobar degeneration. *Proceedings of the National Academy of Sciences USA, 106*, 18809–18814.

Weihl, C. C., Pestronk, A., & Kimonis, V. E. (2009). Valosin-containing protein disease: inclusion body myopathy with Paget's disease of the bone and fronto-temporal dementia. *Neuromuscular Disorder, 19*, 308–315.

Wharton, S. B., McDermott, C. J., Grierson, A. J., Wood, J. D., Gelsthorpe, C., Ince, P. G., et al. (2003). The cellular and molecular pathology of the motor system in hereditary spastic paraparesis due to mutation of the spastin gene. *Journal of Neuropathology & Experimental Neurology, 62*, 1166–1177.

Wils, H., Kleinberger, G., Janssens, J., Pereson, S., Joris, G., Cuijt, I., et al. (2010). TDP-43 transgenic mice develop spastic paralysis and neuronal inclusions characteristic of ALS and frontotemporal lobar degeneration. *Proceedings of the National Academy of Sciences USA, 107*, 3858–3863.

Wilson, C. M., Grace, G. M., Munoz, D. G., He, B. P., & Strong, M. J. (2001). Cognitive impairment in sporadic ALS: a pathologic continuum underlying a multisystem disorder. *Neurology, 57*, 651–657.

Yan, C., Liu, D., He, Y., Zou, Q., Zhu, C., Zuo, X., et al. (2009). Spontaneous brain activity in the default mode network is sensitive to different resting-state conditions with limited cognitive load. *PLoS One, 4*, e5743.

Yang, W., Ang, L. C., & Strong, M. J. (2005). Tau protein aggregation in the frontal and entorhinal cortices as a function of aging. *Brain Research. Developmental Brain Research, 156*, 127–138.

Yang, W., Sopper, M. M., Leystra-Lantz, C., & Strong, M. J. (2003). Microtubule-associated tau protein positive neuronal and glial inclusions in ALS. *Neurology, 61*, 1766–1773.

Yang, W., & Strong, M. J. (2012). Widespread neuronal and glial hyperphosphorylated tau deposition in ALS with cognitive impairment. *Amyotrophic Lateral Sclerosis, 13*, 178–193.

York, C., Olm, C., Boller, A., McCluskey, L., Elman, L., Haley, J., et al. (2014). Action verb comprehension in amyotrophic lateral sclerosis and Parkinson's disease. *Journal of Neurology, 261*, 1073–1079.

Zhou, J., Greicius, M. D., Gennatas, E. D., Growdon, M. E., Jang, J. Y., Rabinovici, G. D., et al. (2010). Divergent network connectivity changes in behavioural variant frontotemporal dementia and Alzheimer's disease. *Brain: A Journal of Neurology, 133*, 1352–1367.

Chapter 10

Cortical Involvement in Multiple Sclerosis

P. Bannerman
Shriners Hospital for Children, Sacramento, CA, United States

INTRODUCTION

Multiple sclerosis (MS) is a chronic neuroinflammatory disease of the brain and spinal cord causing demyelination and multiple forms of neuronal damage and, as such, should be classified as a neurodegenerative disease (Bar-Or, Rieckmann, Traboulsee, & Yong, 2011). It has been estimated that between 2.1 and 2.5 million people worldwide suffer from MS (Miller & Rhoades, 2012; Society, 2013). MS is a heterogeneous disease at two main levels. The first being that the three main subtypes of disease profile termed *relapsing-remitting MS (RRMS), secondary progressive MS (SPMS),* and *primary progressive MS (PPMS).* The second involves variations within a given subtype. RRMS reflects a profile involving an acute manifestation of clinical symptoms followed by a recovery phase (remission) that may be followed by one or multiple episodes of relapsing and remission. Heterogeneity within this most common form of MS resides not only in the number of relapsing-remitting cycles but the degree to which remission leads to total or partial clinical recovery. It begins with multiple relapsing-remitting episodes (with a gender bias of 2:1 prevalence in females versus males), which eventually culminate in a continuous progressive increase in neurological deficits, leading to SPMS. A correlation between RRMS and SPMS is that incomplete recovery from an initial MS attack is prognostic of the potential to progress to SPMS. Also, approximately 50% of patients whose RRMS symptoms have lasted for a decade will go on to develop SPMS. Heterogeneity within SPMS occurs when a subpopulation of patients selectively develop mini–B-cell follicular–like accumulations within the cerebral leptomeninges (Magliozzi et al., 2007). The third subtype of MS is PPMS and occurs in 10–15% of MS patients (with no major gender bias) and typically involves a monophasic acute attack followed by no or slight remissions before neurological disabilities steadily increase without remissions. To date, two subsets of PPMS patients have been identified, the most common of which occurs

The Cerebral Cortex in Neurodegenerative and Neuropsychiatric Disorders.
http://dx.doi.org/10.1016/B978-0-12-801942-9.00010-0

sporadically within the population and the second is familial, indicating a clear genetic disposition (Koch et al., 2008, 2010). Another difference between these subsets of PPMS patients is that those patients with familial PPMS exhibit an earlier onset of disease similar to that seen in other familial forms of neuro-degenerative disease including Alzheimer disease (see Chapter 4) and amyo-trophic lateral sclerosis (see Chapter 9).

RELEVANCE OF CORTICAL PATHOLOGY TO MULTIPLE SCLEROSIS

Why is cortical-associated pathology in patients who have MS so important to understanding clinical manifestations of the disease? The mammalian neocortex is a highly organized, complex, multilayered structure with a multitude of dif-ferent neuronal subtypes including distinct projection neurons and interspersed interneurons, which together with their elaborate dendritic/synaptic architec-ture, play a hierarchal role in cognitive functions (eg, thinking, consciousness, personality traits, decision making, memory, and language), voluntary motor control, and sensory perception. Among the various abnormal neurological defi-cits documented by neurologist Jean-Martin Charcot (1825–1893), who classi-fied MS as a distinct disease, were cognition changes, describing his patients as having a "marked enfeeblement of the memory" and "conceptions that formed slowly" alongside other motor and speech deficits. Based on accruing human, animal, and in vitro studies, we are now in a stronger position to say that cere-bral cortical pathology provides a major correlate to disability and disease pro-gression in MS patients.

CORTICAL STUDIES IN HUMAN MULTIPLE SCLEROSIS

It is true to say that our understanding of cortical [and gray matter (GM) in gen-eral] involvement in MS has only come into major focus since about the year 2000, despite the fact that neocortical lesions have been identified previously (Brownell & Hughes, 1962; Lumsden, 1970). An initial reason for this lag period was the fact that MS was primarily considered a disease of white matter (WM), involving extensive demyelination with relative axonal sparing. A landmark paradigm shift in understanding MS was the realization that subtypes of MS par-ticularly chronic/progressive forms result from disseminated axonopathy (the axonal hypothesis). Salient findings were: (1) the immunohistochemical dem-onstration of deficits in axonal transport (ie, flowopathy) and transection in MS, as detected using antibodies to amyloid precursor protein (Bitsch, Schuchardt, Bunkowski, Kuhlmann, & Bruck, 2000; Ferguson, Matyszak, Esiri, & Perry, 1997; Kuhlmann, Lingfeld, Bitsch, Schuchardt, & Bruck, 2002) and hypophos-phorylated neurofilament heavy chains (Trapp et al., 1998; Trapp, Ransohoff, & Rudick, 1999); and (2) the use of proton nuclear magnetic resonance studies that demonstrated loss of the most abundant (10 mM) neuronal-derived amino acid

N-acetyl-ʟ-aspartate (NAA) (Bjartmar, Kidd, Mork, Rudick, & Trapp, 2000; Davie et al., 1995; Leary et al., 1999; Lee et al., 2000) in patients with MS. The loss of NAA signifies compromised neuronal metabolism and/or loss of axons. Up to this point there was no reference to GM injury in the neurodegeneration equation. This omission was largely because of the fact that conventional magnetic resonance imaging (MRI) imaging techniques (eg, T2-weighted and gadolinium-enhanced T1-weighted sequences) were geared to detecting axonal demyelinating lesions in WM but were insensitive to detecting GM lesions (Geurts et al., 2005). It was also becoming increasingly evident that the detection of WM lesions in vivo, no matter how disseminated, could account for cognitive (DeLuca, Yates, Beale, & Morrow, 2015), neuropsychiatric, and motor deficit dysfunction in MS (Calabrese, Rinaldi, Poretto, & Gallo, 2011; Chiaravalloti & DeLuca, 2008; Filippi et al., 2012; Lazeron et al., 2000).

Crucial evidence supporting cortical involvement in MS deficits came from numerous histopathological studies using (1) basic histological staining procedures (eg, Luxol Fast Blue, oil red O) and (2) antibodies to myelin components such as myelin basic protein (MBP) and proteolipid protein (PLP). These studies showed clear evidence of cortical demyelination, thereby establishing a major contributor to cortical pathological changes (Albert, Antel, Bruck, & Stadelmann, 2007; Bo, 2009; Kidd et al., 1999; Kutzelnigg et al., 2005; Peterson, Bo, Mork, Chang, & Trapp, 2001). An important advantage of immunohistochemical analysis over basic histological staining methods is that the former is far more sensitive in detecting demyelination in diffuse regions of myelination, eg, cerebral cortex, compared with, for instance, Luxol Fast Blue staining. Based on the listed studies, the classification of cortical demyelinating lesions has evolved and been rationalized as follows: type I lesions, also termed *leukocortical lesions*, involve the cortex and underlying subcortical WM of the corpus callosum; type II, or intracortical lesions, are selectively and focally located within the cortical GM; type III, subpial lesions, extend from the pial surface into varying depths of the underlying cortical layers; and type IV lesions extend from the pial surface into the subcortical WM. Despite this focus on demyelination, it is also important to acknowledge that immunohistochemical studies have demonstrated evidence of varying degrees of remyelination in autopsied tissue, thereby signifying a potentially important recovery mechanism, which may also contribute to the heterogeneity of neurological deficits seen in MS patients (Albert et al., 2007; Chang et al., 2012). Other studies have provided evidence that neuronal loss from apoptosis and axonal transection can occur alongside demyelination in the MS cortex (Magliozzi et al., 2010; Peterson et al., 2001), although again, these do not represent a consistent finding in all autopsied MS tissue. A caveat of focusing on neuronal loss selectively via apoptosis is that neurons may undergo cell death by necrosis, for example, as a result of excitotoxicity caused directly by elevated glutamate levels and/or indirectly by compromised inhibitory γ-aminobutyric acid–transmitting inputs and paracrine accumulation of cytotoxic inflammatory mediators including chemokines, cytokines, and reactive oxygen species (Stadelmann, Wegner, & Bruck, 2011). For this reason it is important to quantify total neuronal numbers using a neuron specific marker, although even this approach can be problematic if its normal expression is decreased as a result of disease-induced neuronopathy (Burns et al., 2014).

Using improved (often termed *nonconventional*) MRI modalities, including magnetized transfer ratio (MTR) [or magnetized transfer imaging (MTI)], diffusion-weighted fluid-attenuated inversion recovery (FLAIR), and double inversion recovery (DIR) (see Chapter 3 and Londono & Mora, 2014; Rovira, Auger, & Alonso, 2013), which provide quantitative cortical metrics, it is now clear that the neocortex undergoes significant atrophy during the course of MS (Calabrese et al., 2011; Dalton et al., 2004; De Stefano et al., 2003; Roosendaal et al., 2011). Both conventional and nonconventional MRI have also benefited to varying degrees by the introduction of MRI scanners with higher field intensity magnets of 3, 7, and up to 9.4 T, compared with normal scanners operating at 1.5 T (Filippi, Evangelou, et al., 2014; Harrison et al., 2015; Pellicano et al., 2010; Pham, Meng, Chu, & Chan, 2012; Yao et al, 2014). The main advantage of using higher field strength is that it increases the signal-to-noise ratio of detection, providing higher resolution images.

With the aid of these improved imaging modalities, it has been shown that cortical lesions may occur before the detection of traditional WM lesions. Conventional MRI criteria are still the most widely used for predicting the likelihood of clinically definite MS developing in a patient with an initial clinically isolated episode (CIS). However, given that cortical GM lesions can predate WM lesions, a case can be made that in the future, GM MRI detection should be routinely used to provide an earlier prediction of clinically definite MS developing in a patient with a CIS. In a literature review of the use of nonconventional MRI to improve MS diagnosis (see Table 1 in Honce, 2013), DIR imaging was a prominent modality successfully used in detecting cortical lesions. This then begs the question as to whether cortical lesions detected by DIR should be standard practice as part of the MRI monitoring process for all MS patients. There were conflicting responses to this question (Calabrese & De Stefano, 2014; Chard, 2014). Whereas there is agreement as to the value of using DIR to access cortical pathosis compared with nonconventional MRI techniques, DIR preferentially detects intracortical lesions and is less sensitive to detecting subpial and leukocortical lesions. Moreover, DIR technology has already spawned the development of an improved form of itself, namely phase sensitive inversion recovery that provides both higher resolution and better discrimination at the GM–WM interface in leukocortical lesions (Sethi et al., 2012, 2013). What is abundantly clear is that the combined use of the discussed techniques has demonstrated that cortical and other deeper GM atrophy is a major correlate to cognitive and motor disability in MS patients. Given the relative thinness of cortical GM and the fact that it contains a high density of layered projection neurons along with interspersed interneurons and an extensively complex synaptic architecture, atrophy will have profound effects on hierarchal cortical function.

The ability to detect cortical GM lesions has also uncovered correlations with MS-associated fatigue, a condition experienced by 50–80% of MS patients (Bisht et al., 2015; Krupp, 2006; Lerdal, Celius, Krupp, & Dahl, 2007). MS-related fatigue is cognitive and/or physical and profoundly affects the individual's quality of life. Physical fatigue may result from loss and/or atrophy of motor neurons (Bannerman et al., 2005; Gruppe, Recks, Addicks, & Kuerten, 2012; Vogt et al., 2009), resulting in a smaller, less effective number of primary and secondary motor neurons trying to control normal skeletal muscle function. Cognitive fatigue, however, manifests as a decrease or inability to maintain mental tasks during the course of continuous information-processing–speed testing (Chiaravalloti & DeLuca, 2008; Chiaravalloti, Genova, & DeLuca, 2015; Schwid, Covington, Segal, & Goodman, 2002). It also indirectly affects physical fatigue by decreasing the "willingness" to perform a physical activity, which may be directly related to the patient suffering from depression, resulting in social withdrawal from family and friends, self-pity, self-awareness of disability, and overall pessimism. The fact that MS typically affects people between the ages of 20 and 50 years, a time frame associated with peaks in their careers, compounds feelings of depression. Physical disability and fatigue typically result in poor job performance, including a reduction in work hours. Although studies investigating cortical involvement in MS fatigue are in their infancy, several MRI studies have provided correlations between cortical atrophy within the central sulcus and precentral gyrus in fatigued versus nonfatigued patients with RRMS (Riccitelli et al., 2011). In contrast, atrophy within the corpus callosum was found to be an independent risk factor associated with fatigue (Yaldizli et al., 2011). Using higher resolution 3T MRI, another study found an association between parietal lobe cortical atrophy and MS fatigue (Mainero et al., 2009; Pellicano et al., 2010; Tallantyre et al., 2010). These findings represent another instance in which cortical GM atrophy is not a primary consequence of archetypal WM lesions.

What underlying pathology could account for cortical atrophy during the course of MS? Contending suspects include demyelination, neuronal loss, neuronopathy, dendritopathy, synaptopathy, and axonopathy. Also, what compensatory events lead to varying degrees of clinical recovery in RRMS and/or prolong survival during the course of this chronic neurodegenerative disease? The important parameters are: (1) remyelination in WM and GM, (2) reestablishment of presynaptic/postsynaptic contacts in GM, and (3) synaptic plasticity if reestablishment of contacts does not occur or is incomplete. Here we will focus on cortical GM and subcortical WM.

As described, demyelination and remyelination have been demonstrated in autopsied cortical tissue, reflecting both deleterious injury and recovery processes, respectively. The importance of encouraging remyelination in MS (see Fig. 10.1) in general cannot be overestimated because the process not only helps restore saltatory conduction but also encourages mutual paracrine-mediated trophic support between axons and oligodendrocytes and provides a protective

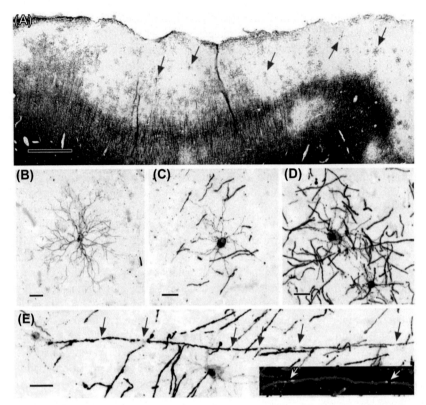

FIGURE 10.1 **Active remyelination in subpial cortical lesions.** (A) Subpial cortical lesions contain oligodendrocytes in various stages of differentiation *(arrows)* (scale bar = 1 mm). (B) Premyelinating oligodendrocytes with PLP-positive cell bodies and multiple processes are present, but actively-myelinating oligodendrocytes with proteolipid protein (PLP)–positive cell bodies and processes extending to multiple myelin internodes are more prevalent (C and D). (C and D) Myelin-internodal lengths are relatively short, which supports the interpretation that these oligodendrocytes are actively remyelinating axons. (E) Individual axons are ensheathed by multiple-short myelin internodes *(inset; arrows* indicate nodes of Ranvier). *Inset,* Remyelinated fibers also show molecular maturation as demonstrated by the appropriate distribution of the paranodal protein, Caspr *(yellow)*; *red* is PLP staining [(B–E) scale bars = 20 μm].

sheath to reduce the toxic effects of inflammatory agents on "naked" demyelinated axons (Hagemeier, Bruck, & Kuhlmann, 2012). With regards to heterogeneity in MS phenotypes, the reasons why remyelination in some MS patients and in particular those with SPMS (Patrikios et al., 2006) is unsuccessful are not known. However, one correlation exists when comparing demyelination versus remyelination in long-term progressive forms of MS, in that higher grade inflammatory lesions and demyelination have been reported in SPMS, whereas conversely in PPMS, patients exhibit less inflammation and remyelination was significantly evident (Bramow et al., 2010). These results suggest that in general, inflammatory responses in SPMS are more robust compared with PPMS.

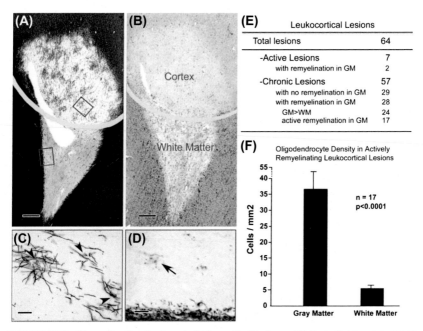

FIGURE 10.2   Remyelination in chronic leukocortical lesions. (A) Proteolipid protein (PLP) immunohistochemistry of a leukocortical lesion shows significant remyelination in the demyelinated cortex compared with the demyelinated white matter (*WM*) (*yellow line* shows the boundary between cortex and WM). (B) Major histocompatibility complex MHC class II staining identifies this lesion as chronic. (C) Magnification of the *red box* in A. The PLP-positive cells in demyelinated cortex have features of actively-remyelinating oligodendrocyte. (D) Magnification of the *blue box* in A. However, those in demyelinated WM often extend dystrophic processes with no apparent connection to myelin internodes. (E) Twenty-eight chronic leukocortical lesions (49%) show evidence of remyelination. Of these, 24 show a greater extent of remyelination in the gray matter (*GM*) compared with that in the WM, and 17 of these 24 (70%) show evidence of active remyelination. (F) The density of oligodendrocytes in the GM portion of the actively remyelinating lesions greatly exceeds the oligodendrocyte density in the WM portion ($p < .0001$). [(A and B) Scale bars = 400 μm; (C and D) scale bars = 50 μm; (F) error bars represent standard error of mean.]

Another aspect of cortical remyelination is that it is more prominent in subpial versus leukocortical lesions (compare Fig. 10.1 with Figs. 10.2 and 10.3). Fig. 10.2B also shows the presence of major histocompatibility complex (MHC) II–positive cells in the cortex and WM indicating the persistence of activated microglia and/or monocyte derived macrophages. Fig. 10.3 also demonstrates a correlation between astrogliotic scarring and relative ability to remyelinate in that "reactive" astrocytes form dense gliotic scars in WM compared with their paucity in the cortical GM, where remyelination is comparatively successful. Studies have shown that reactive astrocytes express a number of molecules that inhibit oligodendrocyte differentiation and therefore the ability to perform functional remyelination. Such inhibitory molecules include CD44 and versican, and hence their inclusion in Fig. 10.3. Such studies emphasize the fact that

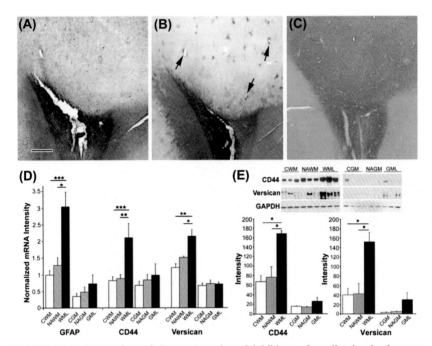

FIGURE 10.3 **Comparison of the astrocytosis and inhibitors of myelination in the gray matter (GM) and white matter (WM) portions of leukocortical lesions.** GM portions of leukocortical lesions have fewer reactive astrocytes compared with the WM portions. (A) Glial fibrillary acidic protein (*http://www.ncbi.nlm.nih.gov/pmc/articles/PMC3535551/figure/F3/ Fig. 10.3. GFAP*) immunoreactivity is much greater in the WM portion of the lesion compared with the GM portion. The same pattern is seen in sections stained for CD44 (B) and hyaluronan (C). (B) Occasional CD44-positive astrocytes are present in cortical lesions and commonly associate with blood vessels (*arrows*). (D) Messenger RNAs (mRNAs) encoding GFAP, CD44, and versican are significantly increased in WM portions of leukocortical lesions (WML) compared with normal-appearing WM (NAWM) from the same patients with multiple sclerosis (MS) and WM from controls (CWM) without neurological diseases. Levels of these mRNAs are lower in the GM portions of leukocortical lesions, normal appearing GM (NAGM), and control GM (CGM). (E) Western blot analysis confirms increased protein levels of CD44 and versican in WM portions of leukocortical lesions. *GAPDH*, Glyceraldehyde 3-phosphate dehydrogenase. [(A, B, and C) Scale bar = 500 μm; (D and E) error bars represent standard error of mean; *, $p < 0.05$; **, $p < 0.01$; ***, $p < 0.005$.]

astrocytes are considered major players in maintaining CNS innate immunity (Farina, Aloisi, & Meinl, 2007; Moreno et al., 2013).

Another emerging aspect of cortical involvement in MS is the use of biopsy and autopsy in cortical GM to perform gene expression studies in the MS disease process (Dutta, 2013). Genome-wide microanalysis using microdissected material from MS and experimental autoimmune encephalomyelitis (EAE) autopsy tissue revealed that 80% of MS-related genes were associated with microglial/monocyte-derived macrophage, T-cell inflammation, oxidative stress, DNA damage and repair, remyelination, and regenerative processes (Fischer et al.,

2013; Guerreiro-Cacais et al., 2015 for analogous studies using experimental autoimmune encephalitis models).

In RRMS, it is known that remission of disease symptoms involves, in part, remyelination of demyelinated axons. However, are other compensatory mechanisms brought into play to compensate for more serious neuronopathy, dendritopathy, and synaptopathy in the cerebral cortex? To this end, investigators have employed a number of functional testing and multiple MRI modalities to provide evidence of the role of synaptic plasticity in repairing cortical circuitry during RRMS. The use of paired associative stimulation (PAS) (Di Lazzaro et al., 2009; Ziemann et al., 2008) provides a means of detecting synaptic long-term potentiation (LTP) and synaptic plasticity in the recovery phase of RRMS. In a recent study, PAS-induced LTP was found to be in the normal range (controls) in patients showing complete clinical remission but was reduced in patients exhibiting reduced or lack of recovery (Mori et al., 2013). The use of this technology in patients with chronic/progressive subtypes of MS could help optimize potential therapeutic intervention before the disease process becomes irreversible and deficits therefore become permanent.

Whereas the focus of this chapter is to understand the role of cortical pathology and its contribution to neurological deficits in patients with MS, it needs to be emphasized that cognitive deficits in MS patients can involve neural damage to other GM structures including the hippocampus, thalamus, and other subcortical nuclei, as well as the WM tracts connecting these structures (Chiaravalloti & DeLuca, 2008; DeLuca et al., 2015).

IN VIVO MODELS OF MULTIPLE SCLEROSIS CORTICAL PATHOLOGY

Despite the major importance of histopathological studies using autopsied MS tissue, they only provided details of the final stages of disease. Also, biopsy samples are rarely acquired during the course of MS except in patients with severe relapsing disease progression. Routine MRI techniques provide the mainstay in monitoring disease evolution, progression, and remissions, particularly in WM tracts, but do not furnish cellular details including pathogenic interactions between adaptive/innate immune cells (activation and infiltration of T cells, neutrophils, monocyte-derived macrophages) and neural cells during the entire course of MS. In particular, what are the spatial and temporal roles of these cell types in mediating axonopathy, neuronopathy, dendritopathy throughout the course of RRMS and more chronic/progressive subtypes of MS? Such knowledge is necessary to tune potential therapeutic intervention before the disease process becomes irreversible and deficits therefore become permanent. Unfortunately, most of the clinically approved disease-modifying drug (DMD) treatments in MS are not effective in progressive and in particular PPMS forms of MS. Hence there is an overwhelming need for chronic models of MS to develop long-term neuroprotective strategies to prevent permanent disability.

Indeed, of 10 approved DMDs to treat RRMS only mitoxantrone is approved for the treatment of SPMS (Hartung et al., 2002), with the caveat that its chronic use is associated with cardiotoxicity (Ghalie et al., 2002).

The bulk of our knowledge regarding cellular mechanisms leading to neuroinflammation and clinical deficits in MS derives from EAE models of the disease along with in vitro studies. The first species to elicit experimentally induced encephalomyelitis was, inadvertently, a human model. This stemmed from the vaccination of patients against the rabies virus, the inoculums of which contained killed virus that became contaminated with myelin components during the isolation procedure. Some of these patients subsequently developed motor deficits (Stuart & Krikorian, 1933) analogous to early EAE models using crude CNS preparations. More recently, EAE has been induced in a wide range of species using immunogens ranging from crude CNS extracts to specific encephalogenic myelin protein peptides (eg, PLP 139–151 and myelin oligodendrocyte protein peptide [MOG 35–55], henceforth termed *PLPp-EAE* and *MOGp-EAE*, respectively), the direct adoptive transfer of myelin protein encephalogenic T cells as either a polyclonal mixed cell population from lymph nodes/spleen or as a cloned monospecific T-cell population. It was utilization of the encephalitic T-cell model in Lewis rats that directly lead to the development of the humanized monoclonal antibody natalizumab as a second tier DMD to treat patients with severe RRMS (Yednock et al., 1992). Other models of MS involve virally induced myelitic disease to mimic the potential involvement of viruses in the etiology of MS, along with the use of chemically induced (eg, cuprizone, lysolecithin) demyelination. The viral, adoptive T-cell transfer, and chemically induced models do not require initial induction of the innate and adaptive immune responses to CNS antigens. I refer the reader to comprehensive reviews of pros and cons of the various MS models (Robinson, Harp, Noronha, & Miller, 2014; Denic et al., 2011; Steinman & Zamvil, 2005; Croxford, Kurschus, & Waisman, 2011; van der Star et al., 2012; Guerreiro-Cacais et al., 2015).

EAE studies have been performed in nonhuman primates to provide a more species-relevant disease model using, in particular, the marmoset model after MOGp inoculation (Pomeroy, Jordan, Frank, Matthews, & Esiri, 2008, 2010; Pomeroy, Matthews, Frank, Jordan, & Esiri, 2005). These studies have highlighted demyelinated lesions in the neocortex alongside evidence of axonopathy, neuronopathy, synaptic loss, and gliosis. The paucity of EAE studies in nonhuman primates and the limited number of animals used in the studies is primarily the result of the prohibitive expense in terms of animal purchase and husbandry. These constraints limit their use in preclinical trials regarding the testing of DMDs in treating MS, although it should be noted that the early testing and proven efficacy of glatiramer acetate (GA) to ameliorate EAE in rhesus monkeys accelerated the future use of this first-line drug in the treatment of RRMS (Teitelbaum, Meshorer, Hirshfeld, Arnon, & Sela, 1971).

The use of murine models of EAE predominate in MS research, partly because of the low cost of mouse purchases and husbandry along with the increasing availability of constitutive or conditional knockout/knock-in mice for MS-related genes and transgenic mice with selective cell-type and even organelle reporter-gene expression. These mouse models have greatly added to our understanding of autoimmune myelitic disease. Fig. 10.4 demonstrates the use of neuronal Thy1-enhanced yellow fluorescent protein (EYFP)–expressing transgenic mice in conjunction with confocal microscopy to demonstrate apical dendritopathy in cortical neurons in MOGp-EAE (Spence et al., 2014). Murine EAE models have provided a platform for both primary preclinical testing of DMDs and as secondary (proof-of-concept) models to investigate the underlying cellular mechanisms and interactions between neural and immune cells that accompany potentially efficacious immunomodulatory/neuroprotective actions of therapeutic agents tested in other model systems (proof-of-concept testing). As a primary preclinical testing ground, murine models are not without their problems because there are instances where DMDs found to be efficacious in

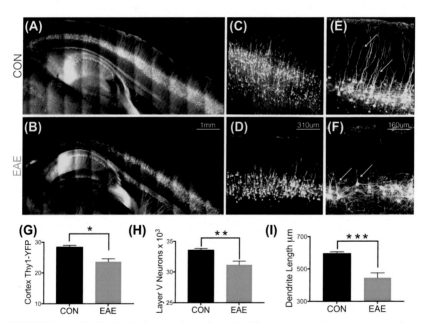

FIGURE 10.4 **Cortical pathology.** A three-dimensional image stack of Thy1-enhanced yellow fluorescent protein (EYFP)–positive neurons in the cerebral cortex and hippocampus from healthy control *(CON)* (A) and experimental autoimmune encephalomyelitis *(EAE)* mice (B). Layer 5 pyramidal neurons in healthy control (C) and EAE mice (D). Apical dendrites *(arrows)* from healthy control (E) and EAE mice (F). (G) EAE mice demonstrated a 17% decrease in Thy1-EYFP expression in the cerebral cortex compared with healthy control mice. H, EAE mice demonstrated a loss of 7% of layer 5 pyramidal neurons compared with healthy control mice. (I) EAE mice demonstrated a decrease in dendrite length of 25% compared with healthy control mice. ($n=5$; *, $p=.0038$, **, $p=.013$, ***, $p=.0001$. *T*-test analysis. Error bars indicate standard error of mean).

mice with EAE proved either ineffective or produced serious side effects when used in human clinical trials (eg, see Steinman & Zamvil, 2005). Aside from basic (ie, evolutionary differences) between the murine and human immune systems (Mestas & Hughes, 2004), two major reasons for the failure of murine-tested DMDs in humans are: (1) many preclinical studies in mice involved prophylactic administration of the DMD before development of neurological deficits, and (2) an inability to detect side effects in mice. The first issue can be rectified by ensuring mice are treated therapeutically by administering the potential DMD after the development of neurological deficits as stipulated by Animals in Research: Reporting In Vivo Experiments and other guidelines (Baker & Amor, 2012; Vesterinen et al., 2010). There is no absolute solution to potential side effects after translation from murine to human subjects other than performing studies in higher animal species and/or more rigorous clinical testing of EAE murine tissue, for example, analyzing cell counts and performing liver function tests of blood samples during the course of treatment and more comprehensive histological/immunohistochemical examination of nervous and immune system tissue.

PLPp-EAE and MOGp-EAE are the two premium murine EAE paradigms, the former being a relapsing-remitting model and the second a chronic MS model. With respect to MOGp-EAE, the choice of mouse strain is critical because MOGp inoculation in the 129/SvEv mouse strain results in an RRMS model (Zhang et al., 2006). The chronic plateau profile of neurological disability inherent to the MOGp-EAE model in C57BL/6 mice implicates a chronic yet nonprogressive involvement of neuronal damage. This profile is, however, deceptive because the stable chronic profile representation is resultant of: (1) the inherent variability of clinical symptoms ranging from no disease (score 0) to moribund (score 4.5) and death (score of 5), (2) waning acute subpial inflammation in the spinal cord over time (Bannerman & Hahn, 2007; Bannerman et al., 2005), and, most importantly, (3) progressive loss of axons in the corticospinal tract (CST) after the acute phase of neurological deficits (Gruppe et al., 2012; Liu, Li, Zhang, Elias, & Chopp, 2008; Soulika et al., 2009). Based on (3), the model, in effect, mimics progressive axonopathy in the CST as seen in chronic primary progressive forms of MS. In the Soulika et al. (2009) study, advantage was taken of the selective expression of EYFP in cortical somatosensory neurons (Bareyre, Kerschensteiner, Misgeld, & Sanes, 2005) to specifically label CST axons in the ventral aspect of the dorsal funiculus.

As for human autopsy analysis, the immunohistochemical study of EAE tissue plays a crucial role in providing spatial detail in the detection of both neural and inflammatory cells in specific locations within the CNS using an abundance of cell-type specific markers. The routine ability to label different cell types with multiple fluorochrome-labeled antibodies/ligands in conjunction with high-resolution confocal microscopy analysis has provided major insights into the interactions between neural and inflammatory cells in situ. Unbiased stereology can be reliably used to quantify numbers of specific cell types/subpopulations in selective locations (Burns et al., 2014). However, problems arise when attempting to quantify total numbers of, for example, inflammatory cells in lesions within the CNS, because the latter are typically disseminated throughout the brain and spinal cord. Moreover, because of variations in section thickness and antibody penetration from one experiment to another, immunohistochemistry is not a reliable method for quantifying different cell types based on varying levels of expression of the same marker [eg, discriminating between cluster of differentiation (CD45)- and CD11b-positive microglia and macrophages expressing high versus low levels of these cell surface antigens]. This is where fluorescence-activated cell sorting (FACS) techniques come into their own, as a result of being able to quantify isolatable, dissociated cells based on their expression of single or multiple (including intracellular) markers and, moreover, their ability to discriminate between cells based on relative expression levels of the same marker. For example, in normal mice, Iba1$^+$ (ionized calcium-binding adaptor molecule 1) CD45^{low}-expressing microglia can be sorted from Iba1$^+$ CD45^{high}-expressing monocyte-derived macrophages. Unfortunately, this phenotypic distinction is not functional in EAE mice when both activated microglia and infiltrating macrophages up-regulate their expression of CD45 and other inflammatory markers including, MHC class II markers, CD11b, and inducible nitric oxide synthetase (iNOS), the latter of which produces reactive radicals causing paracrine cellular damage (see in vitro studies below). The main downside of FACS analysis is that it typically requires the isolation of significant numbers of cells for accurate quantification, which in EAE sometimes requires the pooling of both brain and spinal cord tissue [eg, low numbers of neutrophils in early EAE lesions (Soulika et al., 2009)]. Obviously, no specific spatial discrimination of the original location of cells is possible with FACS. Not surprisingly, the combined use of immunohistochemistry and FACS analysis are used in EAE studies.

The location of the cortex immediately below the skull has allowed the use of two-photon confocal microscopy to perform live imaging of microglial cell migration in normal and early EAE-induced cortical disruptions in the blood–brain barrier. Thus after small window excisions of the skin and skull, these studies have not only visualized the active migration of microglia in the normal cortex but have also shown their active recruitment to early blood–brain barrier leakage mediated by the normal plasma constituent fibrinogen in EAE (Davalos et al., 2012; Yang, Parkhurst, Hayes, & Gan, 2013).

MRI scanners capable of imaging small animals are becoming increasingly available (often as core facilities), which provide brain imaging in EAE models both in vivo and ex vivo (Levy Barazany et al., 2014; MacKenzie-Graham et al., 2012 a,b). Importantly, these studies have demonstrated cortical atrophy in EAE mice mimicking that seen in MS patients.

Because CST axonopathy is a major feature of MOGp-EAE and chronic MS, we investigated whether or not neuronal loss/neuronopathy in upper motor neurons in cortical layer 5 occurs as a result of axonopathy in their axons in the spinal cord. For this study we used immunohistochemical neuronal markers enriched in layer 5 of the adult motor cortex including Emx1, encephalopsin, and annexin V along with the panneuronal marker NeuN (Burns et al., 2014). Some important and surprising results of this study were: (1) that NeuN immunoreactivity is not a reliable marker of neuronal numbers, potentially giving false negative results, ie, neuronal loss particularly in the acute phase of EAE; (2) the presence of recovery phases during the course of the disease with respect to cortical neuronopathy (Fig. 10.5), synaptopathy, and demyelination/remyelination (Fig. 10.6), including a chronic recovery period; and (3) that other layers aside from layer V demonstrated these phasic pertubations (see Figs. 10.5 and 10.6). We also found the same phasic changes when using markers for dendritopathy and postsynaptic protein expression (unpublished data). Whereas the observed remyelination of the motor cortex is consistent with evidence obtained from autopsy samples of patients with chronic MS, it remains to be determined whether the recovery of presynaptic and postsynaptic proteins in the cortex reflects repair of preexisting synapses and/or synaptic readjustments signifying synaptic plasticity as detected by MTR spectroscopy in patients with MS. However, it is noteworthy that in another MOGp-EAE study, where mice were immunized twice with MOGp rather than once and presumably suffered a more aggressive autoimmune

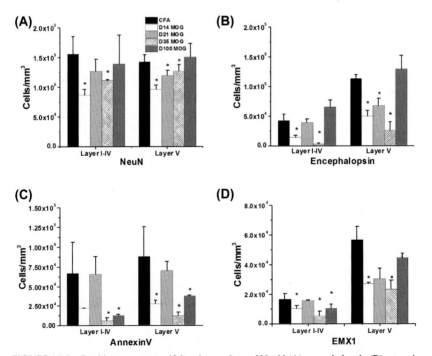

FIGURE 10.5 Bar histograms quantifying the numbers of NeuN (A), encephalopsin (B), annexin V (C), and EMX1 (D) in layer 5 and layers 1–4 in the motor strip of control and EAE mice at days 14, 21, 35, and 100 post–MOGp vaccination. Data was obtained using nonbiased stereology. (Data are mean ± standard error of mean, $n = 3$, *, $p < .05$ vs. control values).

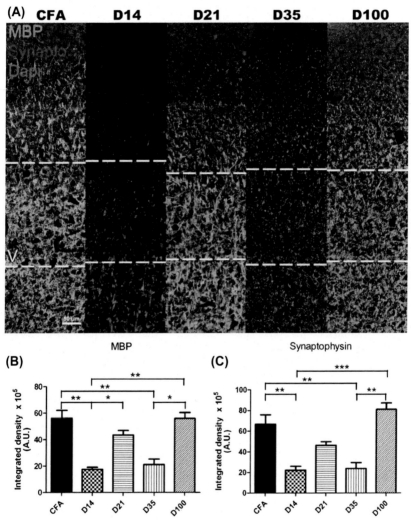

FIGURE 10.6 (A) Immunofluorescence panels showing myelin basic protein (MBP)–positive (*green*) and synaptophysin-positive (*red*) in layers 1 through 6 (layer 5 delineated by *white dashes*) in the S1HL region of the motor cortex in CFA and D14, D21, D35, and D100 MOGp-EAE mice. Nuclei are labeled with 4′,6-diamidino-2-phenylindole (DAPI) (*blue*, scale bar = 50 μm). (B and C) Relative integrated density panels in arbitrary units (a.u.) for MBP and synaptophysin immunolabelling in CFA and D14, D21, D35, and D100 MOGp-EAE mice in S1HL cortical regions depicted in (A) (Bars indicate mean values ± standard error of mean and asterisks denote levels of significance between levels, *, $p \le .05$ and **, $p \le 0.01$, ***, $p \le .001$). Note the transient decreases in immunolabelling at day D14 and D35 compared with both CFA and D100 MOGp-EAE mice.

response, the study discerned: (1) inflammatory subpial, leukocortical, and intracortical lesions that correspond to type I, II, and III lesions described; and (2) neuronal apoptosis was detected in the cortex (Fig. 10.7). Taken together, these two subtly different MOGp-EAE studies have replicated the spectrum, or more specifically, conflicting differences obtained from autopsied histopathological studies of cortical pathology as described, regarding: (1) the presence of chronic demyelination versus chronic remyelination, (2) absence/presence of neuronal apoptosis, and (3) major variations in the detection of the three subtypes of cortical lesions obtained from patients with MS.

A recurrent finding using biopsied/autopsied MS tissue is that within the cortical GM there are few adaptive immune cells, particularly inflammatory T cells. Instead, T cells are primarily localized in the underlying corpus callosum with activated microglial/monocyte-derived macrophages being the predominant immune cell type present in the cortical GM. This histopathology is also evident in MOGp-EAE (Fig. 10.8). This raises the question as to what elicits such widespread neuronopathy, demyelination, and synaptic loss throughout the layers of the cortex. Likely candidates mediating neural damage are inflammatory cytokines. Although typically associated with effects accentuating inflammatory responses via immune cells, inflammatory cytokines such as tumor necrosis factor (TNF) α and interleukin (IL) 1 can also induce direct neural damage by perturbing synaptic transmission, including causing excitotoxic neuronal damage as well as demyelination (and inhibiting remyelination) (Centonze et al., 2009, 2010; Musumeci et al., 2011; Rossi et al., 2011; see in vitro studies below). Whereas the paracrine release of these cytokines from activated immune cells may cause such diffuse pathology, this does not easily explain the cortical damage during the early acute phase of EAE (see Fig. 10.8), that is, when activated Iba1-positive cells are not evident. Unlike IL-1, TNFα can enter the CNS from the periphery via endothelial transport. By combining two-photon microscopy and neutralization of peripherally produced TNFα, it has been shown that this treatment prevented synaptic abnormalities in the layer-5 somatosensory neurons typically seen in EAE. Such findings suggest that cytokine-mediated CNS damage could occur before disruption of the blood–brain barrier.

There is evidence that persistent activation of innate immunity is correlated to poor functional recovery in both the PLP-induced model of RRMS (Rasmussen et al., 2007) and the MOGp-induced chronic model of MS (Soulika et al., 2009). Is this primarily because of the presence of activated microglia or infiltrating macrophages? Adding to the complexity of this issue was the identification of M1 versus M2 subpopulations of these cells. In murine EAE models, the most prevalent subpopulation of these activated cells is the classical proinflammatory M1-type microglia/macrophage followed by the alternatively activated "good" M2-type cells (Jiang, Jiang, & Zhang, 2014). Thus a major problem for neurobiologists studying neuroinflammatory diseases or their models is the inability to distinguish between activated forms of both microglia and monocyte-derived macrophages. However, one methodology has

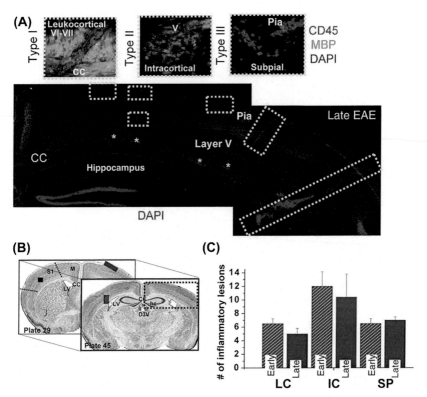

FIGURE 10.7 Forebrain pathology during chronic experimental autoimmune encephalomyelitis (EAE). (A) Representative "late EAE" (day 40 after EAE induction) coronal brain slice (a montage of three separate images from the same brain section) stained with 4′,6-diamidino-2-phenylindole (*DAPI, red*) is imaged at 4×. The total number of inflammatory lesions (*yellow dashed boxes*) per whole brain section was significantly increased at all time points compared with controls. Consecutive sections were immunostained with microglia marker: cluster of differentiation (*CD45, red*), myelin basic protein (*MBP, green*), and DAPI (*blue/red*), and 40× magnification images are shown to emphasize the different types of cortical lesions. In addition, there were also a number of purely WM-inflammatory lesions (*), specifically in the corpus callosum (*CC*). (B) Area under the *gray dashed box* imaged at 4× magnification shown in (A). Coronal brain slices stained with DAPI corresponded approximately to plates 29–48 in the atlas of Franklin and Paxinos (1997). The inflammatory lesions were found in various areas of the brain and were divided into the following three groups: type I, leukocortical (*blue*); type II, intracortical, *(black)*; and type III, subpial (*red*). (C) Quantification of the number of lesions in brain slices corresponding to plates 29–48 in the atlas of Franklin and Paxinos showed more intracortical lesions compared with leukocortical and subpial lesions. There was no significant difference in lesion numbers of early versus late EAE points. Four mice were used for quantification. *D3V*, Third ventricle; *IC*, intracortical; *hc*, hippocampus; *LC*, leukocortical; *LV*, lateral ventricle; *M*, motor cortex; *S1*, somatosensory cortex; *SP*, subpial.

come to the forefront to unambiguously discriminate between activated forms of parenchyma microglia and peripherally invading monocyte-derived macrophages in EAE. Using the established Cre-Lox genetic manipulation, transgenic mice have been generated where the Cre-recombinase activity is conditionally

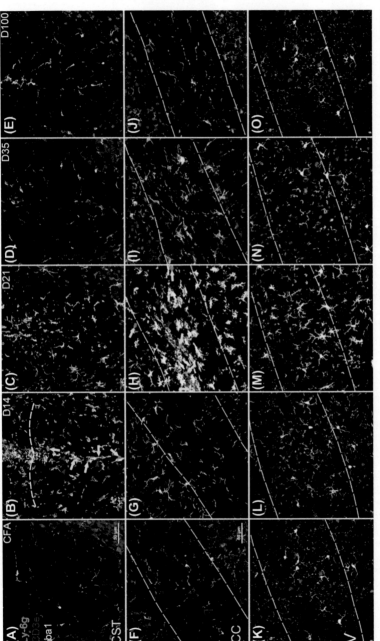

FIGURE 10.8   Triple labeled confocal micrographs showing the presence of Ly6G-positive neutrophils (*green with yellow arrows*), cluster of differentiation (CD) 3-positive T cells (*red with purple arrowheads*) and Iba1-positive microglia/macrophages (*white*) in the corticospinal tract (*CST*) (A–E), corpus callosum (CC) (F–J) and layer 5 of the motor cortex (K–O) in CFA and D14, D21, D35, and D100 MOGp-EAE mice. Within the CST (ventral aspect of the dorsal funiculus, delineated by *area below dashed line in B*), inflammatory infiltrates typically include neutrophils, T cells, and microglia/macrophages by D14. However, within both layer 5 of the cortex and the underlying CC, an overt inflammatory response was absent at D14 but evident at D21 post-MOGp, and although neutrophils and T cells were present in the CC, they were largely absent within the cortex. Also, note the difference in morphology of Iba1-positive cells in the cortex (ramified appearance) versus those in the CC (with both ameboid and ramified morphologies) (scale bar = 50 μm).

driven by cells expressing the active fractalkine receptor CX_3CR1 (CX_3CR-1^{CreER} mice) after tamoxifen administration. This allows specific manipulation of floxed gene inserts, whether they code for reporter protein expression (eg, EYFP) or knock in/out the expression of genes relevant to neuroinflammation (Goldmann et al., 2013; Parkhurst et al., 2012). This model does not require surgery or radiographic irradiation procedures (which disrupt the blood–brain barrier) and exhibits high recombination efficiency of transgene expression. Although both microglia and cells of the monocyte lineage express CX_3CR1, this paradigm takes advantage of the fact that microglia are a permanent, self-renewing population that continually activates the CX_3CR1^{CreER} promoter after tamoxifen treatment, whereas tamoxifen-induced bone marrow CX_3CR1 expressing monocyte-derived cells are rapidly turned over and are no longer present 1 month after tamoxifen treatment. The use of the transgenic CX_3CR-1^{CreER} mouse will prove invaluable in dissecting the differential roles of activated microglia versus monocyte-derived macrophages in cortical pathology.

With regard to identifying cognitive deficits in MS, a disappointing aspect of using EAE models is the relatively short time window to perform cognitive testing before the development of motor deficits. This is in stark contrast with the ability to perform such tests in patients with MS, where cognitive testing can be performed both immediately after identification of MRI lesions and during disease progression. Because it is not possible to perform long-term cognitive testing in rodents, the cortical pathologies shown in Figs. 10.5, 10.6, and 10.7 may provide an alternative in situ assay system to prevent these perturbations employing new DMDs.

IN VITRO STUDIES RELEVANT TO CORTICAL PATHOLOGY

A recent, highly important combined use of FACS and in vitro phenotyping has led to the establishment of markers discriminating between M1- and M2-activated microglia/macrophages as described in this section. In vitro studies are also widely used to test the effects of chemokines/cytokines on mixed or purified cultures of glia and/or their progenitors. Such cultures are generally prepared from late embryonic or early postnatal rodents. To obtain viable primary neuronal cultures, embryonic tissues are required, with the notable exception of cerebellar granule neurons that can be obtained from early postnatal tissue. An alternative source of neurons is to grow neuronal stem cells in media conditions that promote neuronal differentiation, eg, from neurospheres, or growing a neuronal cell, such as the NTERA-2 teratoma cells, in medium containing retinoic acid to differentiate into NT2-N neurons (Pleasure, Page, & Lee, 1992). The inherent disadvantages of studies using these culture systems is that cell lines may exhibit different properties versus primary cultured cells, and the latter are not easily obtainable from adult sources (van der Star et al., 2012). Obviously, no in vitro system can replicate the complex cell interactions between the full complement of either neural cells and inflammatory cells that are present in GM or WM lesions. Nonetheless, culture systems have provided a wealth of information regarding CNS neuroinflammation, as exemplified:

1. Given the extensive availability of murine markers for inflammatory cell types, activated M1 and M2 cells express a $CD11b^+/CD45^{hi/lo}/MHCII^+/CD80^+/CD86^+/Ly6C^{hi}/CD206^-/iNOS^+$ and $CD11b^+/CD45^{hi/lo}/iNOS^-/CD163^+/Ly6C^{low}/CD206^+/Arg1^+/Ym1^+$ phenotype in vitro, respectively (Chhor et al., 2013). This phenotyping has been extended to the identification of these cellular subtypes in situ (Jiang et al., 2014).

2. CNS neuronal cultures, when cultured with activated T cells, cause reversible axonal flowopathy, as evidenced by interruptions in microtubule immunolabeling, and hence a clear indication of T-cell–induced flowopathy (Shriver & Dittel, 2006). This study has been significantly advanced by subsequent two-photon visualization of axonopathy in vivo in MOGp-EAE and its amelioration in the presence of inflammatory oxidative scavengers (Sorbara et al., 2014). Using the NT2-N culture system, novel neuro–immune interactions have been uncovered in that IL-1 was found to stimulate neuronal expression of macrophage inflammatory proteins 1α and 1β, and that this expression is coupled to substance P and neurokinin-1 receptor expression (Guo et al., 2003; Li et al., 2003).

3. The temporal stages of oligodendrocyte development and the effect of growth factors and inflammatory cytokines on their development, growth, and differentiation have been extensively studied in vitro (Barateiro & Fernandes, 2014; Boulanger & Messier, 2014; Balabanov et al., 2007; Grinspan, 2015; Feigenson, Reid, See, Crenshaw, & Grinspan, 2009). The ability to produce purified cultures of oligodendrocyte lineage cells (OLCs) at defined stages of development is highly relevant to MS and EAE studies, because WM lesions may contain a mixture of these cells in both evolving and remyelinating foci. These cultures are typically derived from either optic nerve (Noble, Wolswijk, & Wren, 1989; Raff, Ffrench-Constant, & Miller, 1987) or corpus callosal–enriched tissue (Grinspan, Stern, Pustilnik, & Pleasure, 1990), the latter of which is associated with cortical MS pathology. Accordingly, using corpus callosal–enriched cultures of OLCs, interferon (IFN) γ has been shown to have differential effects on them, depending on the OLC's state of differentiation. Further, the MEK-ERK signaling pathway is involved in mediating IFNγ-induced cell death in oligodendroglia progenitor cells but not in immature/mature oligodendrocytes (Horiuchi, Itoh, Pleasure, & Itoh, 2006). In clinical trials, administration of IFNγ to patients with MS exacerbated clinical deficits, whereas administration with IFNβ is a proven treatment reducing the extent of severity and frequency of relapses in RRMS. The authors went on to test the effects of IFNγ and IFNβ on oligodendroglia progenitors and found that unlike IFNγ, IFNβ did not induce apoptosis in these cells and preferentially activated interferon regulatory factor (IRF) 7, whereas IFNγ induced predominantly IRF1 and IFN8 expression. Moreover, taking

advantage of the amenability of cultured cells to transfection methodology (and small interference RNA treatment) to overexpress proteins or conversely express dominant negative forms of proteins, it was found that overexpressed IRF1 elicited apoptosis, whereas expression of a dominant negative of IRF1 increased and inhibited IFNγ-mediated apoptosis, respectively (Horiuchi, Itoh, Pleasure, Ozato, & Itoh, 2011).

4. In vitro studies using mixed cell cultures have demonstrated that reactive microglia paradoxically secrete both neurotoxic and gliotoxic mediators, as well as neurotrophic factors (Rawji & Yong, 2013). Despite the extensive phenotypic marker overlap between microglia and monocyte derived-macrophages (see earlier discussion), in vitro assays have shown that these two forms of innate immune cells exhibit differing mechanisms of transcriptional control during phagocytosis (Horiuchi et al., 2012; Prinz & Priller, 2014).

5. As mentioned above, a subpopulation of patients with SPMS develop meningeal B-cell follicles. These patients exhibit extensive cortical damage and poor prognosis. It is appropriate, therefore, that in vitro studies have elucidated a major neuroinflammatory role mediated by B cells [aside from the production of autoantibodies (Benjamins, 2013)].

6. Explant/slice culture systems have been widely used in the past to study the effects of demyelinating agents and neurotoxic agents in such mixed cell systems (van der Star et al., 2012), but are now more commonly utilized to perform acute electrophysiological studies with EAE tissue. For example, cortical brain slices from MOGp-EAE have demonstrated that the ability of callosal projection axons to transmit action potentials is compromised versus control tissue (Mangiardi et al., 2011).

CORTICAL PATHOLOGY AND THERAPEUTICS

At least 10 disease modifying drugs are available for the treatment of RRMS (Carrithers, 2014; Cross & Naismith, 2014; Wingerchuk & Carter, 2014). These include the first generation injectable drugs GA and IFNβ, oral drugs (eg, fingolimod, teriflunomide, and dimethyl fumarate), and second-generation injectable humanized monoclonals (eg, natalizumab and alemtuzumab). MRI studies have established the varying ability of these DMDs to reduce WM lesion load and to reduce rates of relapses in RRMS (Filippi, Preziosa, & Rocca, 2014). Unfortunately, given the severely limited availability of MRI technology capable of measuring cortical metrics (eg, DIR, FLAIR), relatively few studies have been performed investigating the efficacy of DMDs in reducing cortical lesions in MS. However, of note were two studies combining conventional MRI with DIR and FLAIR metrics to assess cortical thinning in patients treated with IFNβ or GA versus untreated patients (Calabrese et al., 2012) and patients treated with natalizumab, GA, or IFNβ compared with control subjects (Rinaldi et al., 2012). In the former study, cortical atrophy was significantly decreased in all treated

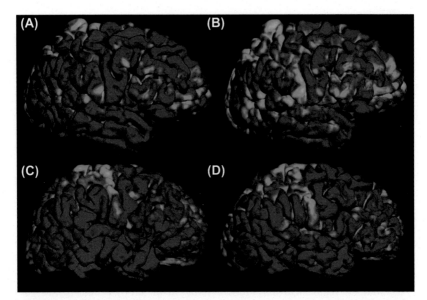

FIGURE 10.9   Three-dimensional reconstruction of the pial surface in a patient with relapsing-remitting multiple sclerosis (RRMS) treated with interferon (IFN) β1a at baseline (A) after 2 years of treatment (B) and in a patient with RRMS treated with natalizumab at baseline (C) and after 2 years (D). In *green* the cortical areas are significantly thinner than normal controls (ie, <2 standard deviations below the control's mean) are depicted. The cortical thinning is clearly faster in IFNβ-treated patient (B) than in natalizumab-treated patient (D) after 2 years of therapy.

groups compared with untreated subjects, and patients treated with subcutaneous IFNβ versus intramuscular IFNβ or GA exhibited the least amount of cortical thinning. In the second study, again all treatment groups showed less atrophy compared with untreated patients, and natalizumab outperformed both IFNβ and GA in significantly decreasing cortical lesion accumulation and cortical atrophy progression in patients with severe RRMS (Fig. 10.9).

FUTURE PERSPECTIVES

There is a paradoxical relationship between MRI imaging in patients with MS relative to EAE studies. In the former, most studies are focused on brain imaging, with relatively few studies imaging crucial spinal cord lesions (eg, chronic loss of CST axons in chronic/progressive MS). In contrast, EAE studies primarily focus on the preponderance of spinal lesions, particularly in the lumbar regions, with fewer studies focusing on brain pathology. A rapid remedy to the EAE issue would be to automatically extend these studies to include analysis of cortical pathology alongside that of the spinal cord and, importantly, analyze the entire course of the disease process (ie, preclinical, acute, and recovery/chronic phase). Also, the given models of EAE produce disseminated lesions, particularly in the spinal cord, thereby making it hard to establish causal relationships, for example, between a particular WM tract lesion and GM lesions elsewhere in the brain and spinal cord. This issue can be addressed by the development of selectively targeted EAE lesion models either directly within in the cortex/subcortical WM or indirectly in a specific spinal cord tract (Argaw et al., 2012; Kerschensteiner et al., 2004; Merkler, Ernsting, Kerschensteiner, Bruck, & Stadelmann, 2006).

The combined ability to discriminate between the roles mediated by activated microglia versus infiltrating macrophages in EAE, and to be able to distinguish between their respective M1 and M2 subtypes may be crucial in designing future therapeutic interventions. For instance, if M1 microglia are primary responsible for neural damage in MS, can drugs be targeted to prevent their activity rather than requiring systemic ablation of peripheral M1 monocyte-derived macrophages, thereby avoiding leaving the patient severely immunocompromised? Alternatively, if both M1 microglia and peripheral macrophages contribute to disease progression, can drug intervention swing the inflammatory balance from M1 to M2 microglia/macrophages, thereby ameliorating disease without causing total loss of M1 innate immune cells? Could the in vitro findings showing differences between their transcriptional control of phagocytosis be used to design DMDs to modulate these cells' activity in EAE models?

Regarding demyelination/remyelination, the in vitro findings described in this chapter may lead to therapeutic strategies to activate IFNβ and antagonize IFNγ signaling. Other culture systems have provided evidence that IFNγ and TNFα inhibit oligodendroglial progenitor differentiation to immature myelinating oligodendroglia. Again, therapeutic inventions that uncouple these negative effects of inflammatory cytokines on OLC remyelination would likely prove beneficial to the remyelinative potential in MS. However, it is unlikely that in the adult patient with me MS, OLCs will behave as per the described immature OLC, given that oligodendrocyte progenitors isolated from adult rodent CNS behave differently in vitro. It is known that NG2-positive adult oligodendrocyte progenitors are present in MS tissue, albeit in variable numbers (depending on the type of lesion, active/chronic). Can their survival, along with potentially surviving reactive mature oligodendrocytes, be promoted, and can they be persuaded to proliferate and differentiate into remyelinating cells by therapeutic intervention (Crawford, Stockley, Tripathi, Richardson, & Franklin, 2014; El Waly, Macchi, Cayre, & Durbec, 2014; McTigue & Tripathi, 2008; Staugaitis & Trapp, 2009)? Another approach would involve modulating the activity and/or reducing the negative influences of astrogliosis in WM lesions described. As well as producing inhibitory molecules such as CD44 and versican, reactive astrocytes also up-regulate their expression of cytokines such as CCL2 and CXCL10 that promote infiltration of inflammatory cells into the local CNS parenchyma, causing neural damage (Mills Ko et al., 2014; Monica Moreno et al., 2014). Decreasing the expression of these molecules would likely reduce tissue injury and promote remyelination.

I hope this chapter has emphasized the point that in vivo and in vitro studies complement each other in expanding our knowledge of the underlying mechanisms involved in MS pathology, and in particular that involving cortical involvement.

REFERENCES

Albert, M., Antel, J., Bruck, W., & Stadelmann, C. (2007). Extensive cortical remyelination in patients with chronic multiple sclerosis. *Brain Pathology, 17*(2), 129–138.

Argaw, A. T., Asp, L., Zhang, J., Navrazhina, K., Pham, T., Mariani, J. N., et al. (2012). Astrocyte-derived VEGF-A drives blood–brain barrier disruption in CNS inflammatory disease. *The Journal of Clinical Investigation, 122*(7), 2454–2468.

Baker, D., & Amor, S. (2012). Publication guidelines for refereeing and reporting on animal use in experimental autoimmune encephalomyelitis. *Journal of Neuroimmunology, 242*(1–2), 78–83.

Balabanov, R., Strand, K., Goswami, R., McMahon, E., Begolka, W., Miller, S. D., et al. (2007). Interferon-gamma-oligodendrocyte interactions in the regulation of experimental autoimmune encephalomyelitis. *The Journal of Neuroscience, 27*(8), 2013–2024.

Bannerman, P. G., & Hahn, A. (2007). Enhanced visualization of axonopathy in EAE using thy1-YFP transgenic mice. *Journal of the Neurological Sciences, 260*(1–2), 23–32.

Bannerman, P. G., Hahn, A., Ramirez, S., Morley, M., Bonnemann, C., Yu, S., et al. (2005). Motor neuron pathology in experimental autoimmune encephalomyelitis: studies in THY1-YFP transgenic mice. *Brain, 128*(Pt 8), 1877–1886.

Barateiro, A., & Fernandes, A. (2014). Temporal oligodendrocyte lineage progression: in vitro models of proliferation, differentiation and myelination. *Biochimica et Biophysica Acta, 1843*(9), 1917–1929.

Bareyre, F. M., Kerschensteiner, M., Misgeld, T., & Sanes, J. R. (2005). Transgenic labeling of the corticospinal tract for monitoring axonal responses to spinal cord injury. *Nature Medicine, 11*(12), 1355–1360.

Bar-Or, A., Rieckmann, P., Traboulsee, A., & Yong, V. W. (2011). Targeting progressive neuroaxonal injury: lessons from multiple sclerosis. *CNS Drugs, 25*(9), 783–799.

Benjamins, J. A. (2013). Direct effects of secretory products of immune cells on neurons and glia. *Journal of the Neurological Sciences, 333*(1–2), 30–36.

Bitsch, A., Schuchardt, J., Bunkowski, S., Kuhlmann, T., & Bruck, W. (2000). Acute axonal injury in multiple sclerosis: correlation with demyelination and inflammation. *Brain, 123*(Pt 6), 1174–1183.

Bisht, B., Darling, W. G., Grossmann, R. E., Shivapour, E. T., Lutgendorf, S. K., Snetselaar, L. G., et al. (2015). A multimodal intervention for patients with secondary progressive multiple sclerosis: feasibility and effect on fatigue. *Journal of Alternative and Complementary Medicine, 20*(5), 347–355.

Bjartmar, C., Kidd, G., Mork, S., Rudick, R., & Trapp, B. D. (2000). Neurological disability correlates with spinal cord axonal loss and reduced N-acetyl aspartate in chronic multiple sclerosis patients. *Annals of Neurology, 48*(6), 893–901.

Bo, L. (2009). The histopathology of grey matter demyelination in multiple sclerosis. *Acta Neurologica Scandinavica. Supplementum, 189*, 51–57.

Boulanger, J. J., & Messier, C. (2014). From precursors to myelinating oligodendrocytes: contribution of intrinsic and extrinsic factors to white matter plasticity in the adult brain. *Neuroscience, 269*, 343–366.

Bramow, S., Frischer, J. M., Lassmann, H., Koch-Henriksen, N., Lucchinetti, C. F., Sorensen, P. S., et al. (2010). Demyelination versus remyelination in progressive multiple sclerosis. *Brain, 133*(10), 2983–2998.

Brownell, B., & Hughes, J. T. (1962). The distribution of plaques in the cerebrum in multiple sclerosis. *Journal of Neurology, Neurosurgery, & Psychiatry, 25*, 315–320.

Burns, T., Miers, L., Xu, J., Man, A., Moreno, M., Pleasure, D., et al. (2014). Neuronopathy in the motor neocortex in a chronic model of multiple sclerosis. *Journal of Neuropathology and Experimental Neurology, 73*(4), 335–344.

Calabrese, M., Bernardi, V., Atzori, M., Mattisi, I., Favaretto, A., Rinaldi, F., et al. (2012). Effect of disease-modifying drugs on cortical lesions and atrophy in relapsing-remitting multiple sclerosis. *Multiple Sclerosis: Clinical and Laboratory Research, 18*(4), 418–424.

Calabrese, M., & De Stefano, N. (2014). Cortical lesion counts by double inversion recovery should be part of the MRI monitoring process for all MS patients: yes. *Multiple Sclerosis: Clinical and Laboratory Research, 20*(5), 537–538.

Calabrese, M., Rinaldi, F., Poretto, V., & Gallo, P. (2011). The puzzle of multiple sclerosis: gray matter finds its place. *Expert Review of Neurotherapeutics, 11*(11), 1565–1568.

Carrithers, M. D. (2014). Update on disease-modifying treatments for multiple sclerosis. *Clinical Therapeutics, 36*(12), 1938–1945.

Centonze, D., Muzio, L., Rossi, S., Cavasinni, F., De Chiara, V., Bergami, A., et al. (2009). Inflammation triggers synaptic alteration and degeneration in experimental autoimmune encephalomyelitis. *The Journal of Neuroscience, 29*(11), 3442–3452.

Centonze, D., Muzio, L., Rossi, S., Furlan, R., Bernardi, G., & Martino, G. (2010). The link between inflammation, synaptic transmission and neurodegeneration in multiple sclerosis. *Cell Death and Differentiation, 17*(7), 1083–1091.

Chang, A., Staugaitis, S. M., Dutta, R., Batt, C. E., Easley, K. E., Chomyk, A. M., et al. (2012). Cortical remyelination: a new target for repair therapies in multiple sclerosis. *Annals of Neurology, 72*(6), 918–926.

Chard, D. (2014). Cortical lesion counts by double inversion recovery should be part of the MRI monitoring process for all MS patients: no. *Multiple Sclerosis, 20*(5), 539–540.

Chhor, V., Le Charpentier, T., Lebon, S., Ore, M. V., Celador, I. L., Josserand, J., et al. (2013). Characterization of phenotype markers and neuronotoxic potential of polarised primary microglia in vitro. *Brain, Behavior, and Immunity, 32*, 70–85.

Chiaravalloti, N. D., & DeLuca, J. (2008). Cognitive impairment in multiple sclerosis. *Lancet Neurology, 7*(12), 1139–1151.

Chiaravalloti, N. D., Genova, H. M., & DeLuca, J. (2015). Cognitive rehabilitation in multiple sclerosis: the role of plasticity. *Frontiers in Neurology, 6*, 67.

Crawford, A. H., Stockley, J. H., Tripathi, R. B., Richardson, W. D., & Franklin, R. J. (2014). Oligodendrocyte progenitors: adult stem cells of the central nervous system? *Experimental Neurology, 260*, 50–55.

Cross, A. H., & Naismith, R. T. (2014). Established and novel disease-modifying treatments in multiple sclerosis. *Journal of Internal Medicine, 275*(4), 350–363.

Croxford, A. L., Kurschus, F. C., & Waisman, A. (2011). Mouse models for multiple sclerosis: historical facts and future implications. *Biochimica et Biophysica Acta, 1812*(2), 177–183.

Dalton, C. M., Chard, D. T., Davies, G. R., Miszkiel, K. A., Altmann, D. R., Fernando, K., et al. (2004). Early development of multiple sclerosis is associated with progressive grey matter atrophy in patients presenting with clinically isolated syndromes. *Brain, 127*(Pt 5), 1101–1107.

Davalos, D., Ryu, J. K., Merlini, M., Baeten, K. M., Le Moan, N., Petersen, M. A., et al. (2012). Fibrinogen-induced perivascular microglial clustering is required for the development of axonal damage in neuroinflammation. *Nature Communications, 3*, 1227.

Davie, C. A., Barker, G. J., Webb, S., Tofts, P. S., Thompson, A. J., Harding, A. E., et al. (1995). Persistent functional deficit in multiple sclerosis and autosomal dominant cerebellar ataxia is associated with axon loss. *Brain, 118*(Pt 6), 1583–1592.

De Stefano, N., Matthews, P. M., Filippi, M., Agosta, F., De Luca, M., Bartolozzi, M. L., et al. (2003). Evidence of early cortical atrophy in MS: relevance to white matter changes and disability. *Neurology, 60*(7), 1157–1162.

DeLuca, G. C., Yates, R. L., Beale, H., & Morrow, S. A. (2015). Cognitive impairment in multiple sclerosis: clinical, radiologic and pathologic insights. *Brain Pathology, 25*(1), 79–98.

Denic, A., Johnson, A. J., Bieber, A. J., Warrington, A. E., Rodriguez, M., & Pirko, I. (2011). The relevance of animal models in multiple sclerosis research. *Pathophysiology, 18*(1), 21–29.

Di Lazzaro, V., Dileone, M., Profice, P., Pilato, F., Oliviero, A., Mazzone, P., et al. (2009). LTD-like plasticity induced by paired associative stimulation: direct evidence in humans. *Experimental Brain Research, 194*(4), 661–664.

Dutta, R. (2013). Gene expression changes underlying cortical pathology: clues to understanding neurological disability in multiple sclerosis. *Multiple Sclerosis, 19*(10), 1249–1254.

El Waly, B., Macchi, M., Cayre, M., & Durbec, P. (2014). Oligodendrogenesis in the normal and pathological central nervous system. *Frontiers in Neuroscience, 8*, 145.

Farina, C., Aloisi, F., & Meinl, E. (2007). Astrocytes are active players in cerebral innate immunity. *Trends in Immunology, 28*(3), 138–145.

Feigenson, K., Reid, M., See, J., Crenshaw, E. B., & Grinspan, J. B. (2009). Wnt signaling is sufficient to perturb oligodendrocyte maturation. *Molecular and Cellular Neurosciences, 42*(3), 255–265.

Ferguson, B., Matyszak, M. K., Esiri, M. M., & Perry, V. H. (1997). Axonal damage in acute multiple sclerosis lesions. *Brain, 120*(Pt 3), 393–399.

Filippi, M., Evangelou, N., Kangarlu, A., Inglese, M., Mainero, C., Horsfield, M. A., et al. (2014). Ultra-high-field MR imaging in multiple sclerosis. *Journal of Neurology, Neurosurgery, & Psychiatry, 85*(1), 60–66.

Filippi, M., Preziosa, P., & Rocca, M. A. (2014). Magnetic resonance outcome measures in multiple sclerosis trials: time to rethink? *Current Opinion in Neurology, 27*(3), 290–299.

Filippi, M., Rocca, M. A., Barkhof, F., Bruck, W., Chen, J. T., Comi, G., et al. (2012). Association between pathological and MRI findings in multiple sclerosis. *Lancet Neurology, 11*(4), 349–360.

Fischer, M. T., Wimmer, I., Höftberger, R., Gerlach, S., Haider, L., Zrzavy, T., et al. (2013). Disease-specific molecular events in cortical multiple sclerosis lesions. *Brain: A Journal of Neurology, 136*(6), 1799–1815.

Franklin, K. B., & Paxinos, G. (1997). *The mouse brain in stereotaxic coordinates.* San Diego, CA: Academic Press.

Geurts, J. J., Bo, L., Pouwels, P. J., Castelijns, J. A., Polman, C. H., & Barkhof, F. (2005). Cortical lesions in multiple sclerosis: combined postmortem MR imaging and histopathology. *AJNR. American Journal of Neuroradiology, 26*(3), 572–577.

Ghalie, R. G., Edan, G., Laurent, M., Mauch, E., Eisenman, S., Hartung, H. P., et al. (2002). Cardiac adverse effects associated with mitoxantrone (Novantrone) therapy in patients with MS. *Neurology, 59*(6), 909–913.

Goldmann, T., Wieghofer, P., Muller, P. F., Wolf, Y., Varol, D., Yona, S., et al. (2013). A new type of microglia gene targeting shows *TAK1* to be pivotal in CNS autoimmune inflammation. *Nature Neuroscience, 16*(11), 1618–1626.

Grinspan, J. B. (2015). Bone morphogenetic proteins: inhibitors of myelination in development and disease. *Vitamins and Hormones, 99*, 195–222.

Grinspan, J. B., Stern, J. L., Pustilnik, S. M., & Pleasure, D. (1990). Cerebral white matter contains PDGF-responsive precursors to O2A cells. *The Journal of Neuroscience, 10*(6), 1866–1873.

Gruppe, T. L., Recks, M. S., Addicks, K., & Kuerten, S. (2012). The extent of ultrastructural spinal cord pathology reflects disease severity in experimental autoimmune encephalomyelitis. *Histology and Histopathology, 27*(9), 1163–1174.

Guerreiro-Cacais, A. O., Laaksonen, H., Flytzani, S., N'diaye, M., Olsson, T., & Jagodic, M. (2015). Translational utility of experimental autoimmune encephalomyelitis: recent developments. *Journal of Inflammation Research, 8*, 211–225.

Guo, C. J., Douglas, S. D., Lai, J. P., Pleasure, D. E., Li, Y., Williams, M., et al. (2003). Interleukin-1beta stimulates macrophage inflammatory protein-1alpha and -1beta expression in human neuronal cells (NT2-N). *Journal of Neurochemistry, 84*(5), 997–1005.

Hagemeier, K., Bruck, W., & Kuhlmann, T. (2012). Multiple sclerosis: remyelination failure as a cause of disease progression. *Histology and Histopathology, 27*(3), 277–287.

Harrison, D. M., Roy, S., Oh, J., Izbudak, I., Pham, D., Courtney, S., et al. (2015). Association of cortical lesion burden on 7-T magnetic resonance imaging with cognition and disability in multiple sclerosis. *JAMA Neurology, 72*(9), 1004–1012.

Hartung, H. P., Gonsette, R., Konig, N., Kwiecinski, H., Guseo, A., Morrissey, S. P., et al. (2002). Mitoxantrone in progressive multiple sclerosis: a placebo-controlled, double-blind, randomised, multicentre trial. *Lancet, 360*(9350), 2018–2025.

Honce, J. M. (2013). Gray matter pathology in MS: neuroimaging and clinical correlations. *Multiple Sclerosis International, 2013*, 627870.

Horiuchi, M., Itoh, A., Pleasure, D., & Itoh, T. (2006). MEK-ERK signaling is involved in interferon-gamma-induced death of oligodendroglial progenitor cells. *Journal of Biological Chemistry, 281*(29), 20095–20106.

Horiuchi, M., Itoh, A., Pleasure, D., Ozato, K., & Itoh, T. (2011). Cooperative contributions of interferon regulatory factor 1 (IRF1) and IRF8 to interferon-gamma-mediated cytotoxic effects on oligodendroglial progenitor cells. *Journal of Neuroinflammation, 8*, 8.

Horiuchi, M., Wakayama, K., Itoh, A., Kawai, K., Pleasure, D., Ozato, K., et al. (2012). Interferon regulatory factor 8/interferon consensus sequence binding protein is a critical transcription factor for the physiological phenotype of microglia. *Journal of Neuroinflammation, 9*, 227.

Jiang, Z., Jiang, J. X., & Zhang, G. X. (2014). Macrophages: a double-edged sword in experimental autoimmune encephalomyelitis. *Immunology Letters, 160*(1), 17–22.

Kerschensteiner, M., Stadelmann, C., Buddeberg, B. S., Merkler, D., Bareyre, F. M., Anthony, D. C., et al. (2004). Targeting experimental autoimmune encephalomyelitis lesions to a predetermined axonal tract system allows for refined behavioral testing in an animal model of multiple sclerosis. *The American Journal of Pathology, 164*(4), 1455–1469.

Kidd, D., Barkhof, F., McConnell, R., Algra, P. R., Allen, I. V., & Revesz, T. (1999). Cortical lesions in multiple sclerosis. *Brain, 122*(Pt 1), 17–26.

Koch, M., Uyttenboogaart, M., Heerings, M., Heersema, D., Mostert, J., & De Keyser, J. (2008). Progression in familial and nonfamilial MS. *Multiple Sclerosis, 14*(3), 300–306.

Koch, M., Zhao, Y., Yee, I., Guimond, C., Kingwell, E., Rieckmann, P., et al. (2010). Disease onset in familial and sporadic primary progressive multiple sclerosis. *Multiple Sclerosis, 16*(6), 694–700.

Krupp, L. (2006). Fatigue is intrinsic to multiple sclerosis (MS) and is the most commonly reported symptom of the disease. *Multiple Sclerosis, 12*(4), 367–368.

Kuhlmann, T., Lingfeld, G., Bitsch, A., Schuchardt, J., & Bruck, W. (2002). Acute axonal damage in multiple sclerosis is most extensive in early disease stages and decreases over time. *Brain, 125*(Pt 10), 2202–2212.

Kutzelnigg, A., Lucchinetti, C. F., Stadelmann, C., Bruck, W., Rauschka, H., Bergmann, M., et al. (2005). Cortical demyelination and diffuse white matter injury in multiple sclerosis. *Brain, 128*(Pt 11), 2705–2712.

Lazeron, R. H., Langdon, D. W., Filippi, M., van Waesberghe, J. H., Stevenson, V. L., Boringa, J. B., et al. (2000). Neuropsychological impairment in multiple sclerosis patients: the role of (juxta) cortical lesion on FLAIR. *Multiple Sclerosis, 6*(4), 280–285.

Leary, S. M., Davie, C. A., Parker, G. J., Stevenson, V. L., Wang, L., Barker, G. J., et al. (1999). 1H magnetic resonance spectroscopy of normal appearing white matter in primary progressive multiple sclerosis. *Journal of Neurology, 246*(11), 1023–1026.

Lee, M. A., Blamire, A. M., Pendlebury, S., Ho, K. H., Mills, K. R., Styles, P., et al. (2000). Axonal injury or loss in the internal capsule and motor impairment in multiple sclerosis. *Archives of Neurology, 57*(1), 65–70.

Lerdal, A., Celius, E. G., Krupp, L., & Dahl, A. A. (2007). A prospective study of patterns of fatigue in multiple sclerosis. *European Journal of Neurology, 14*(12), 1338–1343.

Levy Barazany, H., Barazany, D., Puckett, L., Blanga-Kanfi, S., Borenstein-Auerbach, N., Yang, K., et al. (2014). Brain MRI of nasal MOG therapeutic effect in relapsing-progressive EAE. *Experimental Neurology, 255*, 63–70.

Li, Y., Douglas, S. D., Pleasure, D. E., Lai, J., Guo, C., Bannerman, P., et al. (2003). Human neuronal cells (NT2-N) express functional substance P and neurokinin-1 receptor coupled to MIP-1 beta expression. *Journal of Neuroscience Research, 71*(4), 559–566.

Liu, Z., Li, Y., Zhang, J., Elias, S., & Chopp, M. (2008). Evaluation of corticospinal axon loss by fluorescent dye tracing in mice with experimental autoimmune encephalomyelitis. *Journal of Neuroscience Methods, 167*(2), 191–197.

Londono, A. C., & Mora, C. A. (2014). Nonconventional MRI biomarkers for in vivo monitoring of pathogenesis in multiple sclerosis. *Neurology: Neuroimmunology & Neuroinflammation, 1*(4), e45.

Lumsden, C. E. (1970). *The neuropathology of multiple sclerosis.* Amsterdam: North Holland.

MacKenzie-Graham, A., Rinek, G. A., Avedisian, A., Gold, S. M., Frew, A. J., Aguilar, C., et al. (2012a). Cortical atrophy in experimental autoimmune encephalomyelitis: in vivo imaging. *Neuroimage, 60*(1), 95–104.

MacKenzie-Graham, A. J., Rinek, G. A., Avedisian, A., Morales, L. B., Umeda, E., Boulat, B., et al. (2012b). Estrogen treatment prevents gray matter atrophy in experimental autoimmune encephalomyelitis. *Journal of Neuroscience Research, 90*(7), 1310–1323.

Magliozzi, R., Howell, O., Vora, A., Serafini, B., Nicholas, R., Puopolo, M., et al. (2007). Meningeal B-cell follicles in secondary progressive multiple sclerosis associate with early onset of disease and severe cortical pathology. *Brain, 130*(Pt 4), 1089–1104.

Magliozzi, R., Howell, O. W., Reeves, C., Roncaroli, F., Nicholas, R., Serafini, B., et al. (2010). A gradient of neuronal loss and meningeal inflammation in multiple sclerosis. *Annals of Neurology, 68*(4), 477–493.

Mainero, C., Benner, T., Radding, A., van der Kouwe, A., Jensen, R., Rosen, B. R., et al. (2009). In vivo imaging of cortical pathology in multiple sclerosis using ultra-high field MRI. *Neurology, 73*(12), 941–948.

Mangiardi, M., Crawford, D. K., Xia, X., Du, S., Simon-Freeman, R., Voskuhl, R. R., et al. (2011). An animal model of cortical and callosal pathology in multiple sclerosis. *Brain Pathology, 21*(3), 263–278.

McTigue, D. M., & Tripathi, R. B. (2008). The life, death, and replacement of oligodendrocytes in the adult CNS. *Journal of Neurochemistry, 107*(1), 1–19.

Merkler, D., Ernsting, T., Kerschensteiner, M., Bruck, W., & Stadelmann, C. (2006). A new focal EAE model of cortical demyelination: multiple sclerosis-like lesions with rapid resolution of inflammation and extensive remyelination. *Brain, 129*(Pt 8), 1972–1983.

Mestas, J., & Hughes, C. C. (2004). Of mice and not men: differences between mouse and human immunology. *The Journal of Immunology, 172*(5), 2731–2738.

Miller, A. E., & Rhoades, R. W. (2012). Treatment of relapsing-remitting multiple sclerosis: current approaches and unmet needs. *Current Opinion in Neurology, 25*(Suppl.), S4–S10.

Mills Ko, E., Ma, J. H., Guo, F., Miers, L., Lee, E., Bannerman, P., et al. (2014). Deletion of astroglial CXCL10 delays clinical onset but does not affect progressive axon loss in a murine autoimmune multiple sclerosis model. *Journal of Neuroinflammation, 11*, 105.

Moreno, M., Bannerman, P., Ma, J., Guo, F., Miers, L., Soulika, A., et al. (2014). Conditional ablation of astroglial CCL2 suppresses CNS accumulation of M1 macrophages and preserves axons in mice with MOG peptide EAE. *The Journal of Neuroscience, 34*(24), 8175–8185.

Moreno, M., Guo, F., Mills Ko, E., Bannerman, P., Soulika, A., & Pleasure, D. (2013). Origins and significance of astrogliosis in the multiple sclerosis model, MOG peptide EAE. *Journal of the Neurological Sciences, 333*(1–2), 55–59.

Mori, F., Kusayanagi, H., Nicoletti, C. G., Weiss, S., Marciani, M. G., & Centonze, D. (2013). Cortical plasticity predicts recovery from relapse in multiple sclerosis. *Multiple Sclerosis, 20*(4), 451–457.

Musumeci, G., Grasselli, G., Rossi, S., De Chiara, V., Musella, A., Motta, C., et al. (2011). Transient receptor potential vanilloid 1 channels modulate the synaptic effects of TNF-alpha and of IL-1beta in experimental autoimmune encephalomyelitis. *Neurobiology of Disease, 43*(3), 669–677.

Noble, M., Wolswijk, G., & Wren, D. (1989). The complex relationship between cell division and the control of differentiation in oligodendrocyte-type-2 astrocyte progenitor cells isolated from perinatal and adult rat optic nerves. *Progress in Growth Factor Research, 1*(3), 179–194.

Parkhurst, C. N., Yang, G., Ninan, I., Savas, J. N., Yates, J. R., 3rd, Lafaille, J. J., et al. (2012). Microglia promote learning-dependent synapse formation through brain-derived neurotrophic factor. *Cell, 155*(7), 1596–1609.

Patrikios, P., Stadelmann, C., Kutzelnigg, A., Rauschka, H., Schmidbauer, M., Laursen, H., et al. (2006). Remyelination is extensive in a subset of multiple sclerosis patients. *Brain, 129*(Pt 12), 3165–3172.

Pellicano, C., Gallo, A., Li, X., Ikonomidou, V. N., Evangelou, I. E., Ohayon, J. M., et al. (2010). Relationship of cortical atrophy to fatigue in patients with multiple sclerosis. *Archives of Neurology, 67*(4), 447–453.

Peterson, J. W., Bo, L., Mork, S., Chang, A., & Trapp, B. D. (2001). Transected neurites, apoptotic neurons, and reduced inflammation in cortical multiple sclerosis lesions. *Annals of Neurology, 50*(3), 389–400.

Pham, A. H., Meng, S., Chu, Q. N., & Chan, D. C. (2012). Loss of *Mfn2* results in progressive, retrograde degeneration of dopaminergic neurons in the nigrostriatal circuit. *Human Molecular Genetics, 21*(22), 4817–4826.

Pleasure, S. J., Page, C., & Lee, V. M. (1992). Pure, postmitotic, polarized human neurons derived from NTERA 2 cells provide a system for expressing exogenous proteins in terminally differentiated neurons. *The Journal of Neuroscience, 12*(5), 1802–1815.

Pomeroy, I. M., Jordan, E. K., Frank, J. A., Matthews, P. M., & Esiri, M. M. (2008). Diffuse cortical atrophy in a marmoset model of multiple sclerosis. *Neuroscience Letters, 437*(2), 121–124.

Pomeroy, I. M., Jordan, E. K., Frank, J. A., Matthews, P. M., & Esiri, M. M. (2010). Focal and diffuse cortical degenerative changes in a marmoset model of multiple sclerosis. *Multiple Sclerosis, 16*(5), 537–548.

Pomeroy, I. M., Matthews, P. M., Frank, J. A., Jordan, E. K., & Esiri, M. M. (2005). Demyelinated neocortical lesions in marmoset autoimmune encephalomyelitis mimic those in multiple sclerosis. *Brain, 128*(Pt 11), 2713–2721.

Prinz, M., & Priller, J. (2014). Microglia and brain macrophages in the molecular age: from origin to neuropsychiatric disease. *Nature Reviews. Neuroscience, 15*(5), 300–312.

Raff, M. C., Ffrench-Constant, C., & Miller, R. H. (1987). Glial cells in the rat optic nerve and some thoughts on remyelination in the mammalian CNS. *The Journal of Experimental Biology, 132*, 35–41.

Rasmussen, S., Wang, Y., Kivisakk, P., Bronson, R. T., Meyer, M., Imitola, J., et al. (2007). Persistent activation of microglia is associated with neuronal dysfunction of callosal projecting pathways and multiple sclerosis-like lesions in relapsing-remitting experimental autoimmune encephalomyelitis. *Brain, 130*(Pt 11), 2816–2829.

Rawji, K. S., & Yong, V. W. (2013). The benefits and detriments of macrophages/microglia in models of multiple sclerosis. *Clinical & Developmental Immunology, 2013*, 948976.

Riccitelli, G., Rocca, M. A., Forn, C., Colombo, B., Comi, G., & Filippi, M. (2011). Voxelwise assessment of the regional distribution of damage in the brains of patients with multiple sclerosis and fatigue. *AJNR. American Journal of Neuroradiology, 32*(5), 874–879.

Rinaldi, F., Calabrese, M., Seppi, D., Puthenparampil, M., Perini, P., & Gallo, P. (2012). Natalizumab strongly suppresses cortical pathology in relapsing-remitting multiple sclerosis. *Multiple Sclerosis, 18*(12), 1760–1767.

Robinson, A. P., Harp, C. T., Noronha, A., & Miller, S. D. (2014). The experimental autoimmune encephalomyelitis (EAE) model of MS: utility for understanding disease pathophysiology and treatment. *Handbook of Clinical Neurology, 122*, 173–189.

Roosendaal, S. D., Bendfeldt, K., Vrenken, H., Polman, C. H., Borgwardt, S., Radue, E. W., et al. (2011). Grey matter volume in a large cohort of MS patients: relation to MRI parameters and disability. *Multiple Sclerosis, 17*(9), 1098–1106.

Rossi, S., De Chiara, V., Furlan, R., Musella, A., Cavasinni, F., Muzio, L., et al. (2011). Abnormal activity of the Na/Ca exchanger enhances glutamate transmission in experimental autoimmune encephalomyelitis. *Brain, Behavior, and Immunity, 24*(8), 1379–1385.

Rovira, A., Auger, C., & Alonso, J. (2013). Magnetic resonance monitoring of lesion evolution in multiple sclerosis. *Therapeutic Advances in Neurological Disorders, 6*(5), 298–310.

Schwid, S. R., Covington, M., Segal, B. M., & Goodman, A. D. (2002). Fatigue in multiple sclerosis: current understanding and future directions. *Journal of Rehabilitation Research and Development, 39*(2), 211–224.

Sethi, V., Muhlert, N., Ron, M., Golay, X., Wheeler-Kingshott, C. A., Miller, D. H., et al. (2013). MS cortical lesions on DIR: not quite what they seem? *PLoS One, 8*(11), e78879.

Sethi, V., Yousry, T. A., Muhlert, N., Ron, M., Golay, X., Wheeler-Kingshott, C., et al. (2012). Improved detection of cortical MS lesions with phase-sensitive inversion recovery MRI. *Journal of Neurology, Neurosurgery, & Psychiatry, 83*(9), 877–882.

Shriver, L. P., & Dittel, B. N. (2006). T-cell–mediated disruption of the neuronal microtubule network: correlation with early reversible axonal dysfunction in acute experimental autoimmune encephalomyelitis. *The American Journal of Pathology, 169*(3), 999–1011.

Society, N. M. S.. (2013). What we know about MS. http://www.nationalmssocietyorg/about-multiple-sclerosis/what-we-know-about-ms/faqs-about-ms/indexaspx.

Sorbara, C. D., Wagner, N. E., Ladwig, A., Nikic, I., Merkler, D., Kleele, T., et al. (2014). Pervasive axonal transport deficits in multiple sclerosis models. *Neuron, 84*(6), 1183–1190.

Soulika, A. M., Lee, E., McCauley, E., Miers, L., Bannerman, P., & Pleasure, D. (2009). Initiation and progression of axonopathy in experimental autoimmune encephalomyelitis. *The Journal of Neuroscience, 29*(47), 14965–14979.

Spence, R. D., Kurth, F., Itoh, N., Mongerson, C. R., Wailes, S. H., Peng, M. S., et al. (2014). Bringing CLARITY to gray matter atrophy. *Neuroimage, 101*, 625–632.

Stadelmann, C., Wegner, C., & Bruck, W. (2011). Inflammation, demyelination, and degeneration: recent insights from MS pathology. *Biochimica et Biophysica Acta, 1812*(2), 275–282.

van der Star, B. J., Vogel, D. Y., Kipp, M., Puentes, F., Baker, D., & Amor, S. (2012). In vitro and in vivo models of multiple sclerosis. *CNS & Neurological Disorders Drug Targets, 11*(5), 570–588.

Staugaitis, S. M., & Trapp, B. D. (2009). NG2-positive glia in the human central nervous system. *Neuron Glia Biology, 5*(3–4), 35–44.

Steinman, L., & Zamvil, S. S. (2005). Virtues and pitfalls of EAE for the development of therapies for multiple sclerosis. *Trends in Immunology, 26*(11), 565–571.

Stuart, G., & Krikorian, K. S. (1933). Neuroparalytic accidents complicating antirabic treatment. *British Medical Journal, 1*(3768), 501–504.

Tallantyre, E. C., Morgan, P. S., Dixon, J. E., Al-Radaideh, A., Brookes, M. J., Morris, P. G., et al. (2010). 3 Tesla and 7 Tesla MRI of multiple sclerosis cortical lesions. *Journal of Magnetic Resonance Imaging, 32*(4), 971–977.

Teitelbaum, D., Meshorer, A., Hirshfeld, T., Arnon, R., & Sela, M. (1971). Suppression of experimental allergic encephalomyelitis by a synthetic polypeptide. *European Journal of Immunology, 1*(4), 242–248.

Trapp, B. D., Peterson, J., Ransahoff, R. M., Rudick, R., Sverre, M., & Bo, L. (1998). Axonal transection in the lesions of multiple sclerosis. *New England Journal of Medicine, 338*, 278–285.

Trapp, B. D., Ransohoff, R., & Rudick, R. (1999). Axonal pathology in multiple sclerosis: relationship to neurologic disability. *Current Opinion in Neurology, 12*(3), 295–302.

Vesterinen, H. M., Sena, E. S., ffrench-Constant, C., Williams, A., Chandran, S., & Macleod, M. R. (2010). Improving the translational hit of experimental treatments in multiple sclerosis. *Multiple Sclerosis, 16*(9), 1044–1055.

Vogt, J., Paul, F., Aktas, O., Muller-Wielsch, K., Dorr, J., Dorr, S., et al. (2009). Lower motor neuron loss in multiple sclerosis and experimental autoimmune encephalomyelitis. *Annals of Neurology, 66*(3), 310–322.

Wingerchuk, D. M., & Carter, J. L. (2014). Multiple sclerosis: current and emerging disease-modifying therapies and treatment strategies. *Mayo Clinic Proceedings, 89*(2), 225–240.

Yaldizli, O., Glassl, S., Sturm, D., Papadopoulou, A., Gass, A., Tettenborn, B., et al. (2011). Fatigue and progression of corpus callosum atrophy in multiple sclerosis. *Journal of Neurology, 258*(12), 2199–2205.

Yang, G., Parkhurst, C. N., Hayes, S., & Gan, W. B. (2013). Peripheral elevation of TNF-alpha leads to early synaptic abnormalities in the mouse somatosensory cortex in experimental autoimmune encephalomyelitis. *Proceedings of the National Academy of Sciences of the United States of America, 110*(25), 10306–10311.

Yao, B., Hametner, S., van Gelderen, P., Merkle, H., Chen, C., Lassmann, H., et al. (2014). 7 Tesla magnetic resonance imaging to detect cortical pathology in multiple sclerosis. *PLoS One, 9*(10), e108863.

Yednock, T. A., Cannon, C., Fritz, L. C., Sanchez-Madrid, F., Steinman, L., & Karin, N. (1992). Prevention of experimental autoimmune encephalomyelitis by antibodies against alpha 4 beta 1 integrin. *Nature, 356*(6364), 63–66.

Zhang, Y., Wells, J., Buist, R., Peeling, J., Yong, V. W., & Mitchell, J. R. (2006). A novel MRI texture analysis of demyelination and inflammation in relapsing-remitting experimental allergic encephalomyelitis. *Medical Image Computing and Computer-Assisted Intervention, 9*(Pt 1), 760–767.

Ziemann, U., Paulus, W., Nitsche, M. A., Pascual-Leone, A., Byblow, W. D., Berardelli, A., et al. (2008). Consensus: motor cortex plasticity protocols. *Brain Stimulation, 1*(3), 164–182.

Part III

The Cerebral Cortex in Neuropsychiatric Disorders

Chapter 11

Prefrontal Cortical Abnormalities in Cognitive Deficits of Schizophrenia

N. Rajakumar
University of Western Ontario, London, ON, Canada

INTRODUCTION

Cognitive deficits are present in all patients with schizophrenia and are the most important predictor of the quality of life, ability to maintain social relationships, likelihood of being employed, and long-term disability in these patients. Available pharmacological strategies are not effective against the associated cognitive symptoms. Nevertheless, advancements in schizophrenia research are extremely promising and point to the prefrontal cortex (PFC) as an important nodal point underlying cognitive deficits. Abnormalities in intrinsic, corticocortical, and cortico–subcortical circuitries appear to contribute to the manifestation of cognitive deficits of schizophrenia. This chapter is focused on the role intrinsic abnormalities of the PFC play in mediating cognitive deficits of schizophrenia.

COGNITIVE DEFICITS REPRESENT CORE SYMPTOMS OF SCHIZOPHRENIA

Schizophrenia is a heterogeneous and chronic mental disorder that affects approximately 0.7% of the population worldwide. Schizophrenia is characterized by highly heritable and complex polygenic traits. Monozygotic twins have about 50 times greater chance of manifesting the disease, and first-degree family members have a 10 times greater chance compared with the general population. Genetic studies have concluded that multiple common genetic variants with small effects, and rare but highly penetrable de novo mutations and copy number variations with relatively larger effects contribute to the susceptibility of schizophrenia (Schizophrenia Working Group of the Psychiatric Genomics Consortium, 2014). A large number of the candidate genes described to date are involved in the development, maturation, and function of synapses. In addition to genetic predisposition, epidemiological studies have indicated that prenatal viral infections, obstetrical and

The Cerebral Cortex in Neurodegenerative and Neuropsychiatric Disorders.
http://dx.doi.org/10.1016/B978-0-12-801942-9.00011-2

277

neonatal complications, urban upbringing, and adolescent use of marijuana may increase the risk of schizophrenia. Based on these findings in combination with postmortem results indicating abnormal neuronal migration and aberrant pruning of synapses, and common occurrence of facial, cranial, and dermatoglyph abnormalities in patients, schizophrenia is considered a neurodevelopmental disorder (Pilowsky, Kerwin, & Murray, 1993).

The onset of schizophrenia is defined by the manifestations of clusters of positive or psychotic, negative, and cognitive symptoms that usually occur in the late teens or early twenties, with men developing the illness slightly earlier than women. The majority of patients also have a history of mild neuropsychological abnormalities, including disorganized thought processes, poor attention, distractibility, misperception, and subdelusional features, and mild motor abnormalities during their childhood—findings that indicate that brain abnormalities may predate the clinical diagnosis of schizophrenia. Once a diagnosis is made, patients are prescribed combinations of antipsychotic drugs that they take for their entire lives. Despite the chronic use of multiple antipsychotic drugs, the therapeutic efficacy of these drugs is limited to controlling the positive and certain negative symptoms, but they do not show any significant beneficial effects on the cognitive deficits of schizophrenia (Lieberman et al., 2005).

Cognitive deficits of schizophrenia are independent manifestations, not secondary to positive or negative symptoms. Considerable impairment of cognitive function is seen in high-risk groups before the clinical manifestation of schizophrenia (Yung & McGorry, 1996). Moreover, a significant cognitive impairment is a common feature at the time of diagnosis in the majority of cases. Consequently, cognitive deficit in schizophrenia is considered an original and core abnormality of the disease. The degree of cognitive impairment is also an important predictor of likelihood of employment, quality of life, and long-term outcome in these patients. Schizophrenia patients show deficits in a wide range of domains of cognition, including executive functioning, speed of processing, working memory, anticipation of reward and pleasure, vigilance, attention, language usage, and social cognition. These deficits are typically one to two standard deviations below the means of a control population (Keefe & Eesley, 2012).

THE PREFRONTAL CORTEX: A NODAL POINT MEDIATING COGNITIVE DEFICITS

Functional magnetic resonance imaging studies have identified activity in the PFC, posterior cingulate cortex, medial temporal lobe, inferior parietal areas, and precuneus when subjects are at rest, and the circuitry connecting these areas is referred to as the *default mode network* (Greicius, Krasnow, Reiss, & Menon, 2003). Successful performance in cognitive tasks is associated with a corresponding suppression in the default mode network activity, and this suppression is associated with increased γ-aminobutyric acid (GABA) neurotransmission (Northoff et al., 2007). Increased prefrontal cortical dopamine activity and increased nicotinic stimulation of the brain in healthy adults are correlated to increased efficiency of suppression of the default mode network, as well as better cognitive performance. Interestingly, a number of studies have described that schizophrenia patients show a profound inability to deactivate the default mode network during performance of cognitive tasks (Broyd et al., 2009). This suggests that these brain areas might be involved in the cognitive deficits of schizophrenia, and that altered neurotransmission of GABA, dopamine, and/or acetylcholine may contribute to the cognitive abnormalities.

Studies investigating individual cognitive domains in first-episode drug-naïve schizophrenia patients have identified several brain areas potentially contributing to cognitive deficits of schizophrenia. A recent meta-analysis has concluded that engaging in executive function tasks is associated with decreased activity in circuitry connecting the dorsolateral and medial parts of the PFC, anterior cingulate cortex, posterior parietal areas, and the thalamus in schizophrenia patients compared with a control population (Minzenberg et al., 2009). Similarly, patients showed decreased activity in the dorsolateral PFC, anterior cingulate cortex, and inferior parietal cortex during working memory tasks (Wolf et al., 2015). Patients also showed decreased activity in circuitry involving the dorsolateral PFC, inferior parietal cortex, and the caudate nucleus in tasks requiring sustained attention (Diwadkar et al., 2014). Despite differences in the paradigms used and heterogeneity of the patient populations studied, evidence points to abnormalities in the PFC, especially the dorsolateral PFC, and associated circuitries as contributing to cognitive deficits of schizophrenia.

Prefrontal cortical volume loss is one of the most consistent finding of in vivo imaging studies of schizophrenia patients. The volume loss has been described in first-episode drug-naïve patients and in high-risk groups, whereas those who convert to clinical schizophrenia showed an even greater volume loss in the PFC (McIntosh et al., 2011). Decreased volumes have been demonstrated in both gray and white matter, and the gray matter loss in the dorsolateral PFC corresponds to the degree of cognitive impairment in patients. Consensus is that the prefrontal cortical volume loss is a primary pathosis associated with the development of schizophrenia, and not secondary to antipsychotic medication, drug abuse, chronic course of the illness, or comorbid conditions. Postmortem studies have failed to demonstrate evidence of reactive gliosis or glial cell proliferation in schizophrenia brains, suggesting that the volume loss is not mediated by classical neurodegenerative process. Interestingly, prefrontal cortical volume continues to decrease during the first 5 years of the diagnosis and usually stops progressing further.

ABNORMALITIES INVOLVE BOTH PYRAMIDAL AND NONPYRAMIDAL NEURONS

Postmortem studies have demonstrated abnormalities in pyramidal (glutamatergic) and nonpyramidal [GABA-transmitting (GABAergic)] neurons of the dorsolateral PFC. These changes are likely associated with the primary disease process and compensatory efforts of the brain. Several well-constructed studies in primates suggest that these abnormalities are unlikely caused by chronic antipsychotic therapy or drug abuse.

In normal human PFC, pyramidal neurons are distributed in layers 2 and 3, and in layers 5 and 6, and constitute about 80% of the total neurons. Pyramidal neurons of layers 2 and 3 receive the majority of intrinsic, cortical, and thalamic afferents. Layer-2 and layer-3 pyramidal neurons project to other cortical areas, whereas those in layers 5 and 6 project to subcortical areas. Interestingly, abnormalities are consistently described in layer-2 and layer-3 pyramidal neurons of the dorsolateral PFC, whereas those in layers 5 and 6 often appear normal. Layer-3 pyramidal neurons of the dorsolateral PFC show small cell bodies and decreased dendritic arbor, and they express abnormal levels of messenger (mRNA) and protein of molecules that are important for normal synaptic transmission.

The nonpyramidal, GABA-containing neurons, on the other hand, constitute about 20% of total neurons and synapses of the dorsolateral PFC. The PFC contains several different types of GABA neurons that differ in their morphology, laminar distribution, coexpression of calcium-binding proteins and neuropeptides, firing properties, and preferential synaptic targets. The calcium-binding protein parvalbumin–containing GABA neurons and somatostatin-containing GABA neurons are particularly abnormal in the PFC of patients who have schizophrenia. These abnormalities include decreased levels of mRNA and proteins integral to proper GABAergic neurotransmission. The parvalbumin–containing neurons are fast-spiking interneurons and are of two main types: basket cells and chandelier cells. Basket cells constitute about 50% of the total GABA-containing neurons of the PFC, and because their axons preferentially form synapses onto cell bodies of pyramidal neurons, they are considered to be the main source of inhibitory control on pyramidal neuronal function. Chandelier cells, on the other hand, are a small population and each axon branches profusely and innervates exclusively the initial segments of axons of several pyramidal neurons. Thereby they are in a position to control firing of a group of pyramidal neurons. Somatostatin-containing GABA neurons form about 25% of the total interneurons of the PFC, are slow-spiking, and preferentially target apical dendrites of pyramidal neurons. In addition, basket-cell terminals synapse mainly onto α1 subunit-containing GABA-A receptors, whereas chandelier-cell terminals synapse onto α2 subunit-containing GABA-A receptors, and somatostatin-containing neuronal terminals synapse onto α5 subunit-containing GABA-A receptors.

PYRAMIDAL NEURONAL ABNORMALITIES MAY LOWER THEIR EXCITABILITY

Fewer numbers of dendritic spines, particularly on the basal dendrites of layer-3 pyramidal neurons, and a corresponding decrease in proteins specific to dendritic spines such as spinophilin are consistent findings in the dorsolateral PFC of schizophrenia brains. In addition to the loss of dendritic spines, dendrites of layer-3 pyramidal neurons are also shorter in length. Each dendritic spine of a pyramidal neuron typically forms synapses with at least one glutamatergic excitatory terminal. Consequently, the loss of dendritic spines results in decreased glutamatergic (excitatory) synapses onto layer-3 pyramidal neurons of the dorsolateral PFC in schizophrenia.

The loss of dendritic spines might be a primary pathological state in schizophrenia because a number of candidate genes of schizophrenia affect the development and function of dendritic spines. For example, the protein disrupted in schizophrenia 1 (DISC1) binds to postsynaptic density protein-95 and modulates its interaction with N-methyl-D-aspartate (NMDA) receptors, and hence it is integral to activity-dependent structural plasticity of dendritic spines (see Chapter 2). DISC1 has been identified as a candidate gene in schizophrenia. In a preclinical model, DISC1 mutant mice show small dendritic spines in pyramidal neurons of the PFC (Lee et al., 2011).

In addition to abnormalities of postsynaptic elements, postmortem studies have identified a decreased density of synaptophysin-immunoreactive puncta representing presynaptic axon terminals in the PFC of schizophrenia patients. Axon terminals in the PFC may come from collateral branches of pyramidal neuronal axons, GABA interneurons, and afferents from cortical and subcortical areas. Decreased density of afferent axon terminals from the mediodorsal thalamus and terminals containing dopamine from the ventral tegmental area have also been described in the dorsolateral PFC in schizophrenia brains. Studies have also identified reduced density of glutamate- or GABA-containing axon terminals, presumably corticocortical and intrinsic in origin. Collectively, these findings indicate reduced synaptic connections in the schizophrenia PFC. Although the precise neurochemical identity and source of terminals lost in schizophrenia PFC are not yet clearly demonstrated, considering about 80% of the synapses are excitatory in the PFC, the aforementioned changes may collectively point to a decreased excitatory tone in the PFC of schizophrenia; this concept is overwhelmingly supported by observations of NMDA-receptor antagonists, causing a schizophrenia-like phenotype in humans and animal models.

The extent of dendritic branching and axonal arbor of neurons generally correspond to their somal size and, as expected, layer-3 pyramidal neurons are smaller in the dorsolateral PFC of schizophrenia patients compared with matched controls. Despite the reduced size, the total number of neurons remains unchanged in the schizophrenia PFC. Consequently the decreased axonal and dendritic elements (collectively called *neuropil*) and smaller size neurons without change in total neuronal number are believed to be responsible for the gray matter volume loss described in the PFCs of patients who have schizophrenia (Selemon & Goldman-Rakic, 1999).

γ-AMINOBUTYRIC ACID NEURONAL CHANGES REDUCE INHIBITORY TONE IN THE PFC

GABA synthesis is regulated by two separate enzymes, 65 and 67 kDa isoforms of glutamic acid decarboxylase (GAD). They are products of two separate genes, *GAD65* and *GAD67*. Although both GAD isoforms are widely expressed in the PFC, only *GAD67* transcription is activity-dependent. Decreased levels of GAD67 mRNA and protein in upper layers of the dorsolateral PFC are common findings in schizophrenia brains, whereas GAD65 levels remain unchanged. The most marked decrease of GAD67 is seen in parvalbumin-containing GABA neurons of layers 2 and 3. GAD67 immunoreactivity is almost below detection levels in about 50% of parvalbumin-containing neurons, indicating that certain subpopulations are preferentially affected. Parvalbumin mRNA and protein levels are also decreased in layer-2 and layer-3 GABA neurons. Parvalbumin, with its very high affinity for calcium, is critical for the fast-firing capacity of these neurons, and consequently, decreased parvalbumin may impair their fast-spiking ability. Despite the reduction in GAD67 as well as parvalbumin mRNA and protein levels, the total number of parvalbumin-containing neurons of the dorsolateral PFC remains unchanged in schizophrenia. Because the number of axon terminals immunoreactive for parvalbumin and GAD67 are markedly decreased in layer 3 of the dorsolateral PFC in schizophrenia brains, it is likely that there is a decreased density of basket-cell terminals on layer 3 neurons. The aforementioned abnormalities may disrupt GABA neurotransmission and the spiking activity of basket cells, ultimately leading to reduced inhibitory tone on pyramidal neurons.

The density of mediodorsal thalamic afferent fibers and dopaminergic afferent fibers are decreased in the PFCs of patients with schizophrenia. In addition to providing direct synaptic connections on dendrites of pyramidal neurons, mediodorsal thalamic and dopaminergic afferent fibers target parvalbumin-containing basket-cell dendrites of the PFC. It appears that thalamic and dopaminergic afferents exert their main effects on pyramidal neurons via basket cells. A study employing optogenetic techniques in mice has confirmed that mediodorsal thalamic fibers form direct synaptic contacts with basket cells (Delevich, Tucciarone, Huang, & Li, 2015). These authors also found that stimulation of thalamic afferents resulted in more pronounced excitation of parvalbumin-containing basket cells in comparison with layer-3 pyramidal neurons (Delevich et al., 2015). Similarly, stimulation of ventral tegmental area resulted in suppressed pyramidal cell activity in the PFC, which is dependent on increased prefrontal cortical GABA activity (Tseng & O'Donnell, 2004). Basket cells are therefore in a position to convert excitatory influence of both thalamic and dopaminergic afferents to feedforward inhibitory control on layer-3 pyramidal neurons. Decreased density of dopaminergic and mediodorsal thalamic afferent fibers described in the schizophrenia PFC, along with abnormal basket cell function, may substantially reduce the inhibitory tone on pyramidal neurons and drive them to be hyperactive (Homayoun & Moghaddam, 2007).

Cognitive demand in normal humans is associated with a proportional increase in gamma frequency (30–80 Hz) oscillations in the PFC. Reduced gamma-band oscillation is a common feature both in patients experiencing a first episode and those with chronic schizophrenia performing cognitive tasks (Cho, Konecky, & Carter, 2006). Electrophysiological studies in animals have demonstrated that gamma-band oscillation during cognitive demand is associated with synchronized inhibition of PFC pyramidal neurons by increased activity of fast-spiking GABA interneurons. Optogenetically evoked inhibition of parvalbumin-containing GABA neurons in the PFC of mice resulted in an immediate suppression of 30–80 Hz oscillations, whereas increasing parvalbumin-containing neuronal inhibition on pyramidal neurons enhanced gamma oscillation (Sohal et al., 2009). Collectively, these results indicate that temporally synchronized inputs from parvalbumin-containing basket cells to pyramidal neurons are critical for both gamma-band oscillations and cognitive function. Basket cell abnormalities of schizophrenia outlined above may disrupt gamma-band oscillation and contribute to cognitive deficits. It is important to note that impaired gamma-band power and cognitive deficits show excellent correlation.

In addition to basket cells, somatostatin-containing neurons and chandelier neurons also show several abnormalities in schizophrenia brains. Somatostatin-containing neurons show reduced expression of GAD67 mRNA and somatostatin mRNA and protein in the dorsolateral PFC of schizophrenia brains. Interestingly, changes are severe in layers 2 and 3. In addition, the $\alpha5$ subunit of GABA-A receptors is considerably decreased in upper layers of the dorsolateral PFC, indicating reduced GABAergic inhibition by somatostatin-containing neurons in schizophrenia brains. In contrast, immunoreactivity for GABA transporter 1 (GAT1) is markedly decreased in chandelier axonal terminals contacting axonal initial segments of layer-2 and layer-3 pyramidal neurons, suggesting an effort to increase GABA levels at these synapses. Consistent with this observation, the $\alpha2$ subunit of GABA-A receptors is increased on axonal initial segments in schizophrenia PFC, potentially augmenting GABA effects on layer-2 and layer-3 pyramidal neurons. Interestingly, these changes are limited to layers 2 and 3, and not seen in layers 5 and 6. Although an overall decrease in GAD67 levels has been described in parvalbumin-containing neurons in layers 2 and 3 of the PFC in schizophrenia brains, GAD67 changes specific to chandelier neurons are not yet reported. If GABA levels are reduced in chandelier neurons, the changes in GAT1 and GABA-A receptor might be a form of compensation to offset decreased GABA synthesis.

Interestingly, GABA transmission at chandelier axonal terminal–pyramidal axon initial segment synapses has either been depolarizing or hyperpolarizing (Glickfeld, Roberts, Somogyi, & Scanziani, 2009; Szabadics et al., 2006). The same terminals might depolarize or hyperpolarize the axonal initial segment based on axoplasmic chloride ion concentration and the prevailing membrane potential of pyramidal neurons (Woodruff et al., 2011). In neuronal membranes, the chloride transporters KCC2 (potassium chloride cotransporter 2) and NKCC1 (sodium potassium chloride cotransporter 1) mediate chloride ion extrusion and intake, respectively. Reduced levels of two kinases affecting the phosphorylation status and hence function of these transporters have been described in pyramidal neurons of the dorsolateral PFC in schizophrenia brains (Lewis, Curley, Glausier, & Volk, 2012).

It has been proposed that the presumed abnormal kinase activity would allow elevated chloride concentration within the axoplasm (Lewis et al., 2012), and therefore GABA transmission at the chandelier neuronal terminal–pyramidal axon initial segment synapse may be depolarizing. If so, augmenting GABA neurotransmission as predicted from chandelier neuronal abnormalities of schizophrenia PFC would counteract reduced excitatory drive of layer-3 pyramidal neurons. A similar effect was been proposed earlier in this chapter for basket cell abnormalities. It is interesting to note that irrespective of the excitatory or inhibitory effect of chandelier terminals on the initial segment of pyramidal neurons, decreased chandelier neuronal input to pyramidal neurons may favor a schizophrenia-like phenotype because the postmitotic cortical interneuron-specific knockdown of *ErbB4*, a candidate gene of schizophrenia, resulted in a selective loss of chandelier neuronal synapses onto pyramidal neurons (Fazzari et al., 2010).

PRECLINICAL ANIMAL MODELS OF SCHIZOPHRENIA WITH PREFRONTAL CORTEX ABNORMALITIES

A large number of preclinical animal models have been reported as showing multitude of behavioral features reminiscent of schizophrenia symptoms. However, these animal models show only a few structural abnormalities identified in postmortem brains. For example, one of the most-studied animal models of schizophrenia, produced by excitotoxic lesions of the developing ventral hippocampi bilaterally at postnatal day 7 in rats, results in decreased dendritic length and reduced number of dendritic spines in layer-3 and layer-5 pyramidal neurons in the PFC (Flores, Morales-Medina, & Diaz, 2016). Daily administration of phencyclidine in adult rats for 7 days with a drug-free period of 7 days resulted in a decreased number of dendritic spines in the PFC (Hajszan, Leranth, & Roth, 2006), whereas a 30-day daily administration with a 30-day drug-free period resulted in increased spine density in PFC neurons (Flores, Wen, Labelle-Dumais, & Kolb, 2007). Nevertheless, both treatment protocols produced multiple behavioral abnormalities relevant to schizophrenia. In a separate model, rats reared in social isolation during postweaning and adolescent periods showed a decreased dendritic spine density in the PFC (Flores et al., 2016). It is important to emphasize that modeling structural abnormalities of schizophrenia is mostly unsuccessful, and a correlation of neuropathology to symptoms remains speculative.

Recently, our laboratory has identified that partial ablation of the subplate layer in the developing PFC results in misrouted mediodorsal thalamic fibers into the PFC, and these animals showed adult-onset behavioral abnormalities reminiscent of schizophrenia symptoms (Lazar, Rajakumar, & Cain, 2008; Rajakumar et al., 2004). These animals also showed reduced prefrontal cortical volume without any reduction in total neuronal number. However, synaptophysin immunoreactive puncta were decreased, indicating loss of synapses in the PFC. A corresponding decrease was also seen in spinophilin labeling, suggesting a loss of dendritic spines. In addition, the laminar organization of parvalbumin immunoreactive neurons and terminals were abnormal in layers 2 and 3, suggesting possible abnormality in basket cell function. These animals also showed decreased density of GAT1 immunoreactive terminals in upper layers of the PFC, indicating altered chandelier neuronal function.

CONCLUSIONS

Evidence overwhelmingly points to dorsolateral prefrontal cortical abnormalities contributing to cognitive deficits of schizophrenia. Pathological changes of PFC pyramidal neurons and synapses indicate that excitability of pyramidal neurons might be compromised. Abnormalities in parvalbumin-containing GABA neurons indicate that GABA neurotransmission at basket-cell terminals on PFC pyramidal neurons is suppressed, whereas GABA transmission at chandelier neuronal terminals on PFC pyramidal neurons is augmented. It is not clear whether the abnormalities identified in basket cells and chandelier cells in schizophrenia brains are compensatory mechanisms to counteract the reduced excitatory tone in the PFC, as proposed recently (Lewis et al., 2012). This is a compelling hypothesis, considering most schizophrenia candidate genes impact glutamatergic neurotransmission (eg, *DISC1*, dysbindin, *GluR1*), and in animal studies, chronic blockade of NMDA receptors recapitulates abnormalities of GABA neurons. In normal PFC, parvalbumin-containing basket cells play a critical role in transforming thalamocortical and dopaminergic excitation into inhibitory control on pyramidal neurons, and abnormalities seen in basket cells in schizophrenia brains render this mechanism ineffective and produce a state of "disconnection" of the PFC from the thalamus and mesolimbic dopamine neurons. Such disconnection may contribute to certain symptoms of schizophrenia, including some cognitive deficits. A number of these abnormalities are seen in animals with partial ablation of prefrontal cortical subplate, and this animal model may further our understanding of mechanisms underlying cognitive abnormalities of schizophrenia.

REFERENCES

Broyd, S. J., Demanuele, C., Debener, S., et al. (2009). Default-mode brain dysfunction in mental disorders: a systematic review. *Neuroscience and Biobehavioral Reviews, 33,* 279–296.

Cho, R. Y., Konecky, R. O., & Carter, C. S. (2006). Impairments in frontal cortical gamma synchrony and cognitive control in schizophrenia. *Proceedings of the National Academy of Sciences of the United States of America, 103,* 19878–19883.

Delevich, K., Tucciarone, J., Huang, Z. J., & Li, B. (2015). The mediodorsal thalamus drives feedforward inhibition in the anterior cingulate cortex via parvalbumin interneurons. *The Journal of Neuroscience, 35,* 5743–5753.

Diwadkar, V. A., Bakshi, N., Gupta, G., et al. (2014). Dysfunction and dysconnection in cortical-striatal networks during sustained attention: genetic risk for schizophrenia or bipolar disorder and its impact on brain network function. *Frontiers in Psychiatry, 5,* 50. http://dx.doi.org/10.3389/fpsyt.2014.00050.

Fazzari, P., Paternain, A. V., Valiente, M., et al. (2010). Control of cortical GABA circuitry development by Nrg1 and ErbB4 signalling. *Nature, 464,* 1376–1380.

Flores, G., Morales-Medina, J. C., & Diaz, A. (2016). Neuronal and brain morphological changes in animal models of schizophrenia. *Behavioural Brain Research, 301,* 190–203.

Flores, C., Wen, X., Labelle-Dumais, C., & Kolb, B. (2007). Chronic phencyclidine treatment increases dendritic spine density in prefrontal cortex and nucleus accumbens neurons. *Synapse, 61,* 978–984.

Glickfeld, L. L., Roberts, J. D., Somogyi, P., & Scanziani, M. (2009). Interneurons hyperpolarize pyramidal cells along their entire somatodendritic axis. *Nature Neuroscience, 12,* 21–23.

Greicius, M. D., Krasnow, B., Reiss, A. L., & Menon, V. (2003). Functional connectivity in the resting brain: a network analysis of the default mode hypothesis. *Proceedings of the National Academy of Sciences of the United States of America, 100,* 253–258.

Hajszan, T., Leranth, C., & Roth, R. H. (2006). Subchronic phencyclidine treatment decreases the number of dendritic spine synapses in the rat prefrontal cortex. *Biological Psychiatry, 60,* 639–644.

Homayoun, H., & Moghaddam, B. (2007). NMDA receptor hypofunction produces opposite effects on prefrontal cortex interneurons and pyramidal neurons. *The Journal of Neuroscience, 27,* 11496–11500.

Keefe, R. S. E., & Eesley, C. E. (2012). Neurocognitive impairments. In J. A. Lieberman, T. S. Stroup, & D. O. Perkins (Eds.), *Essentials of schizophrenia* (pp. 73–92). American Psychiatric Publishing.

Lazar, N. L., Rajakumar, N., & Cain, D. P. (2008). Injections of NGF into neonatal frontal cortex decrease social interaction as adults: a rat model of schizophrenia. *Schizophrenia Bulletin, 34,* 127–136.

Lee, F. H., Fadel, M. P., Preston-Maher, K., et al. (2011). *Disc1* point mutations in mice affect development of the cerebral cortex. *The Journal of Neuroscience, 31,* 3197–3206.

Lewis, D. A., Curley, A. A., Glausier, J. R., & Volk, D. W. (2012). Cortical parvalbumin interneurons and cognitive dysfunction in schizophrenia. *Trends in Neuroscience, 35,* 57–67.

Lieberman, J. A., Stroup, T. S., McEvoy, J. P., et al. (2005). Effectiveness of antipsychotic drugs in patients with chronic schizophrenia. *The New England Journal of Medicine, 353,* 1209–1223.

McIntosh, A. M., Owens, D. C., Moorhead, W. J., et al. (2011). Longitudinal volume reductions in people at high genetic risk of schizophrenia as they develop psychosis. *Biological Psychiatry, 69,* 953–958.

Minzenberg, M. J., Laird, A. R., Thelen, S., et al. (2009). Meta-analysis of 41 functional neuroimaging studies of executive function in schizophrenia. *Archives of General Psychiatry, 66,* 811–822.

Northoff, G., Walter, M., Schulte, R. F., et al. (2007). GABA concentrations in the human anterior cingulate cortex predict negative BOLD responses in fMRI. *Nature Neuroscience, 10,* 1515–1517.

Pilowsky, L. S., Kerwin, R. W., & Murray, R. M. (1993). Schizophrenia: a neurodevelopmental perspective. *Neuropsychopharmacology: Official Publication of the American College of Neuropsychopharmacology, 9,* 83–91.

Rajakumar, N., Leung, L. S., Ma, J., et al. (2004). Altered neurotrophin receptor function in the developing prefrontal cortex leads to adult-onset dopaminergic hyperresponsivity and impaired prepulse inhibition of acoustic startle. *Biological Psychiatry, 55,* 797–803.

Schizophrenia Working Group of the Psychiatric Genomics Consortium. (2014). Biological insights from 108 schizophrenia-associated genetic loci. *Nature, 511,* 421–427.

Selemon, L. D., & Goldman-Rakic, P. S. (1999). The reduced neuropil hypothesis: a circuit based model of schizophrenia. *Biological Psychiatry, 45*, 17–25.

Sohal, V. S., Zhang, F., Yizhar, O., et al. (2009). Parvalbumin neurons and gamma rhythms enhance cortical circuit performance. *Nature, 459*, 698–702.

Szabadics, J., Varga, C., Molnar, G., et al. (2006). Excitatory effect of GABAergic axo-axonic cells in cortical microcircuits. *Science, 311*, 233–235.

Tseng, K. Y., & O'Donnell, P. (2004). Dopamine-glutamate interactions controlling prefrontal cortical pyramidal cell excitability involve multiple signaling mechanisms. *The Journal of Neuroscience, 24*, 5131–5139.

Wolf, D. H., Satterthwaite, T. D., Calkins, M. E., et al. (2015). Functional neuroimaging abnormalities in youth with psychosis spectrum symptoms. *JAMA Psychiatry, 72*, 456–465.

Woodruff, A. R., McGarry, L. M., Vogels, T. P., et al. (2011). State-dependent function of neocortical chandelier cells. *The Journal of Neuroscience, 31*, 17872–17886.

Yung, A. R., & McGorry, P. D. (1996). The prodromal phase of first episode psychosis: past and current conceptualizations. *Schizophrenia Bulletin, 22*, 353–370.

Chapter 12

Role of the Prefrontal Cortex in Addictive Disorders

J. Renard, L. Rosen, W.J. Rushlow, S.R. Laviolette
University of Western Ontario, London, ON, Canada

INTRODUCTION

The mammalian prefrontal cortex (PFC) serves as a critical functional interface between several subcortical neural regions involved in the processing of motivationally salient, reward-related information. Evidence from both clinical and animal models of drug addiction has revealed varied roles for the PFC and its anatomical subregions in the processing of addiction-related learning, memory, and drug-seeking behaviors. Whereas addictive behaviors represent a highly heterogeneous array of underlying neurobiological and psychological processes, the process of addiction generally consists of a repeating cycle, beginning with initial exposure to highly rewarding, appetitive drug stimuli (Fig. 12.1). After chronic and ongoing use, neural motivational pathways become altered and sensitized to the appetitive effects of the drug of abuse, leading to compulsive drug-seeking behaviors. Many drugs of abuse, in particular opiate-class drugs such as morphine and heroin, have a significant physiological and psychological withdrawal syndrome that occurs when the user no longer has access to the drug or voluntarily attempts to quit. However, the drug craving and associated effects that occur during withdrawal most often lead to relapse, particularly upon exposure to environmental cues that trigger powerful associative memories linked to the rewarding properties of the drug. These memories may be linked either to the initial high that the user experienced during early exposure, or to the withdrawal alleviating effects that the drug may acquire following long-term cycles of withdrawal and relapse. Importantly, regardless of drug class or severity of dependence and withdrawal, addiction-related phenomena are invariably linked to a loss of control over behavior. This lack of inhibition of craving and drug seeking is particularly acute when the drug user is exposed to memory cues triggering relapse.

Although decades of basic neuroscience research have revealed the importance of specific neurotransmitter systems and associated neuroanatomical regions underlying the appetitive motivational properties of drugs of abuse, recent

The Cerebral Cortex in Neurodegenerative and Neuropsychiatric Disorders.
http://dx.doi.org/10.1016/B978-0-12-801942-9.00012-4

289

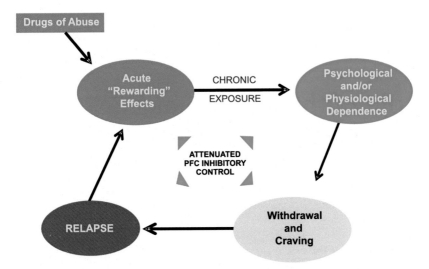

FIGURE 12.1 The cycle of addiction. Most drugs of abuse initially produce appetitive, rewarding effects that activate subcortical neural motivational systems such as the mesolimbic dopamine pathway. After chronic exposure, psychological and/or physiological dependence occurs, leading to withdrawal and drug craving when the substance is no longer available. Drug-dependent individuals are thus particularly vulnerable to relapse during states of withdrawal and craving, leading to recurring repetition of the addiction cycle. A loss of prefrontal cortex (PFC)–mediated inhibitory control over drug-related associative memories and/or impulse regulation may impact any stage of the addiction cycle.

theoretical models of addiction have emphasized the importance of both learning and memory-related abnormalities underlying the addiction cycle. Thus considerable evidence now suggests that the persistence of addictive behaviors may be related to the intractable nature of memories linked to the drug-taking experience. More importantly, this emphasis on learning and memory-related phenomena as underlying factors in addiction leads to consideration of neural mechanisms required for learning and memory-related plasticity (see Chapter 2). In addition, executive control and response inhibition phenomena are increasingly recognized as important psychological variables associated with the loss of behavioral control and emotional regulation characteristic of addiction-related compulsions. In this chapter, we will review anatomical, molecular, and behavioral evidence outlining the important role of the PFC and its associated connections with limbic brain regions involved in processing drug-related reward and withdrawal-related information. We will focus on a growing body of both clinical and basic neuroscience evidence suggesting that fundamental alterations in the PFC at the neuronal and molecular levels may lead to dysregulation of subcortical neural motivational pathways controlling reward-related learning and memory plasticity. In addition, the potential role of PFC dysfunction as an important factor underlying the loss of impulse control and executive cognitive function during the addiction process will be considered.

CLINICAL EVIDENCE FOR PREFRONTAL CORTICAL PATHOLOGY IN ADDICTION

Considerable evidence from both functional magnetic resonance imaging (fMRI) and positron emission tomography (PET) scanning studies in humans has implicated the PFC as a critical brain region for drug-related memory formation, both withdrawal and craving phenomena. Given that the primary rewarding/appetitive effects of drugs of abuse are believed to depend upon subcortical neural motivational pathways, most specifically the mesolimbic dopamine (DA) system, most clinical research into the role of the human PFC in addiction-related phenomena has focused upon the well-established role of the PFC as an integrative center for executive control, impulse regulation, and cognitive processing of emotionally relevant information arising from extrinsic inputs to the PFC. Given the anatomical complexity of the human PFC region, various brain imaging techniques including PET and fMRI have reported addiction-related effects including the anterior cingulate cortex (ACC), orbitofrontal cortex (OFC), and dorsolateral PFC (DLPFC). Such studies have examined both the effects of acute drug exposure on general PFC activity patterns, as well as cue-induced measurements of PFC activation, such as showing human subjects visual cues linked to the drug-taking experience (eg, pictures of cocaine or injection-related paraphernalia for heroin users). Such studies have revealed an important role for PFC subregions both in mediating the primary, acute effects of drug-related alterations in cognition as well as longer-term deficits in executive cognitive control, decision making, attentional processing, and addiction-related craving.

EFFECTS OF ACUTE DRUG EXPOSURE AND DRUG-RELATED CUE EXPOSURE ON HUMAN PREFRONTAL CORTEX ACTIVITY PATTERNS

Numerous studies have found acute metabolic effects in anatomically specific regions of the human PFC during exposure to various drugs of abuse (Goldstein & Volkow, 2011). For example, the severity of neuropsychological impairments observed in both alcohol- and cocaine-dependent subjects was found to correlate with specific metabolic abnormalities observed in the PFC (Goldstein et al., 2004). Furthermore, acute cocaine administration activates a variety of PFC subregions, including the anterior PFC of Brodmann area 10, the ACC and the OFC, based on fMRI analyses (Kufahl et al., 2005, 2008). Interestingly, these cocaine–PFC effects are strongly modulated by expectation state. Thus whereas PFC regions show intense activation while subjects are *expecting* to receive cocaine, activation of subcortical neural regions involved in the primary reinforcing effects of cocaine [including the nucleus accumbens (NAc), ventral tegmental area (VTA), thalamus, and amygdala] preferentially respond to *unexpected* cocaine delivery (Kufahl et al., 2008). Examining PFC activation patterns during short-term abstinence in human heroin abusers, Li et al. (2012) reported that exposure to heroin-related visual cues induced self-reported feelings of drug craving, and these effects were correlated with increased activation of DLPFC and OFC subregions. Event-related fMRI measurements in heroin-dependent subjects undergoing methadone maintenance therapy revealed that PFC responses in the OFC and ACC regions were stronger when exposed to heroin-related visual cues before receiving methadone maintenance administration, versus. posttreatment responses (Langleben et al., 2008). These effects, similar to those found with cocaine, suggest an important role for the PFC during drug-related anticipation phenomena, and may also implicate PFC activation as in important substrate for drug-related craving.

Functional connectivity between the PFC and subcortical limbic regions is also disturbed during the addiction process. For example, using fMRI, Ma et al. (2010) reported increased accumbens–ACC–OFC and amygdala–OFC connectivity, but reduced PFC–OFC connectivity during resting-state measurements of heroin-dependent subjects undergoing methadone treatment. In alcohol-dependent subjects, Claus, Ewing, Filbey, Sabbineni, and Hutchison (2011), using MRI and functional connectivity analyses during exposure to alcohol-containing beverage samples, reported increased activation in both the OFC and ACC, along with subcortical regions such as the dorsal striatum, insula, and VTA. Interestingly, these studies are largely consistent with basic addiction modeling studies in rodents, which similarly report altered connectivity and functionality between the PFC and subcortical regions during the processing of addiction-related learning and memory (Bishop, Lauzon, Bechard, Gholizadeh, & Laviolette, 2011; Gholizadeh et al., 2013; Sun & Laviolette, 2012). Human imaging studies are generally limited in terms of identifying the precise cellular and/or molecular mechanisms underlying functional connectivity alterations induced within and across the PFC during the addiction process. However, such studies reveal that chronic exposure to a variety of drugs of abuse may fundamentally alter both how specific cortical subregions may communicate with each other during drug-related cognitive processing, and also how aberrant connectivity between higher cortical regions and subcortical limbic motivational centers may represent an important phenotype associated with addiction vulnerability and persistence.

The PFC is well established as being a critical brain center for the regulation and control of attentional processes. Such cognitive processes are critical during the addiction cycle because increasing exposure to drugs of abuse invariably leads to amplification of salience attribution to drug-related cues and subsequent relapse events. For example, using fMRI analyses in dependent smokers, Janes et al. (2010) reported that attentional biases during exposure to smoking-related words during an emotional Stroop task procedure were related to abnormal activation patterns in the PFC. Specifically, cue-induced activation in the dorsal ACC correlated with attentional biases to smoking-related words. Interestingly, smokers also presented attenuated fMRI functional connectivity between an insula-containing neural network and PFC regions critical for cognitive attentional control, including the ACC and DLPFC. Given the importance of attentional biases for drug-related cues, specifically during relapse phenomena, such findings point to the importance of the PFC in signaling drug-related cue salience and distortions in underlying attentional biases.

In addition to reported immediate effects of drug exposure on PFC activity patterns and attentional processing, long-term drug abuse and withdrawal also influences PFC-dependent cognitive and executive function. For example, Rapeli et al. (2006) reported that opiate-dependent subjects undergoing early withdrawal experience profound deficits in various measures of PFC-dependent processing, including complex working memory (digit span test), executive function (Stroop and Ruff Figural Fluency tests), and tests of fluid intelligence. Interestingly, such effects were correlated with time of withdrawal and appeared worse during early versus later phases of withdrawal, suggesting some plasticity in PFC cognitive function after recovery from chronic opiate abuse.

HUMAN PREFRONTAL CORTEX REGULATION OF INHIBITORY CONTROL MECHANISMS: RELEVANCE TO ADDICTION

A critical psychological variable related to addiction vulnerability and persistence involves the ability of an individual to self-regulate behavioral impulses, particularly in instances when such behaviors lead to adverse consequences, such as the effects of chronic addiction. Indeed, impairments in the ability to control compulsive drug seeking are a critical underlying factor leading to criminality, harm to others, and/or self-harm observed in many drug-abusing subjects. Given the critical role of the PFC in executive cognitive control and impulse regulation, not surprisingly, deficits in these domains of PFC function have been linked to addiction-related phenomena.

One common test of behavioral response inhibition that recruits higher-order PFC function is the Go-No/Go Association Task. This test is designed to measure a subject's ability to either perform a cue-related task or inhibit that response under other stimulus settings, thereby measuring response-inhibition capacity. Interestingly, in a sample of chronically dependent heroin users, Fu et al. (2008) reported that cortical regions including the ACC, PFC, and inferior frontal lobe were involved importantly in response inhibition and competition. However, heroin-dependent subjects demonstrated impaired response inhibition capacity that was present even after months of abstinence, demonstrating that the effects of chronic heroin on PFC-mediated inhibitory control were persistent even in long-term withdrawal states. Psychological measures of impulsivity in heroin-dependent subjects has also been correlated with a loss in PFC gray matter volume, suggesting that structural abnormalities induced by chronic heroin exposure may similarly lead to impulse control deficits (Qiu et al., 2013).

In a sample of polysubstance-abusing subjects, Moreno-Lopez et al. (2012) performed an extensive array of neuropsychological performance tests focusing on both "hot" executive control tests (ie, self-regulation, decision making, and emotion perception) and "cold" executive control tests (ie, cognitive updating, response inhibition, and cognitive flexibility) and analyzed PET-derived regions of interest or voxel uptake measures. Not surprisingly, substance-abusing subjects displayed poor performance in terms of executive function and emotional processing measures, relative to control subjects. Interestingly, however, performance deficits in drug-dependent subjects were correlated with abnormal regional metabolism in the DLPFC, midsuperior frontal gyrus, superior and inferior temporal gyri, and inferior parietal cortex specifically while performing "cold" task measures. In contrast, deficits observed in the performance of "hot" executive functions were associated with the DLPFC, midsuperior frontal gyrus, anterior and midposterior cingulate cortices, and temporal and fusiform gyri. These findings add to the complex nature of PFC-related deficits in the context of addiction disorders and, importantly, suggest that separate PFC regions may differentially control specific aspects of cognitive/emotional valence regulation during the processing of executive cognitive functions disturbed in addiction.

THE PREFRONTAL CORTEX IN ADDICTION-RELATED NEURAL CIRCUITS

Historically, studies of the mammalian PFC in the context of addiction-related behaviors have relied upon human imaging (PET and fMRI), nonhuman primates (especially neuronal electrophysiological studies), and rodent models of addiction-related learning and memory. Given that the overwhelming bulk of our understanding of how the PFC controls reward and addiction-related behaviors comes from rodent-based basic neuroscience research approaches, a critical question concerns whether the rodent PFC can actually serve as an effective analog for the complexity of the primate PFC (see Chapter 1). Despite profound differences in subcompartmental complexity, most comparative anatomical evidence points to the rodent medial PFC (mPFC) as an analog to the primate dorsolateral prefrontal and anterior cingulate cortices (Fig. 12.2; Seamans, Lapish, & Durstewitz, 2008). Furthermore, as will be reviewed, considerable evidence from neuroanatomical, neuropharmacological, imaging, and behavioral studies most certainly demonstrates that the rodent PFC shares many important functional similarities with the primate PFC, particularly in the context of reward- and addiction-related phenomena. Finally, as will be described presently, the rodent PFC, similar to human and nonhuman primate PFC regions, has been demonstrated to strongly modulate subcortical neurochemical pathways involved in reward-related neural signaling.

The mammalian brain contains specialized regions that are involved critically in the mediation of reward-related information (Fig. 12.3). However, the mesolimbic pathway, comprising the A10 dopaminergic (DAergic) neurons of the midbrain VTA of Tsai and its associated DAergic projection fibers to the forebrain NAc is perhaps the best characterized and most widely studied of these systems. In addition, the mesocortical pathway comprises DAergic

HUMAN   RAT

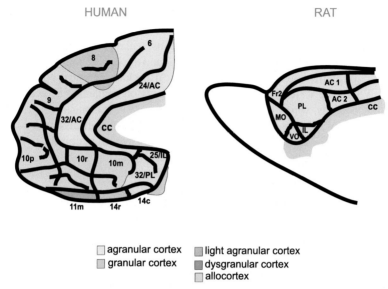

☐ agranular cortex   ▨ light agranular cortex
▨ granular cortex   ■ dysgranular cortex
                        ☐ allocortex

FIGURE 12.2   Comparative complexity of the human versus rat prefrontal cortex (PFC). Despite profound differences in compartmental complexity across species, the rat PFC serves as a useful analog of the human PFC, both in terms of its functional connectivity with various subcortical neural reward pathways and its neurochemical substrates. Numbered zones in the human cortex represent respective Brodmann areas. *AC*, Anterior cingulate; *CC*, corpus callosum; *Fr2*, frontal cortical area 2; *IL*, infralimbic; *MO*, medial orbital; *PL*, prelimbic; *VO*, ventral orbital.

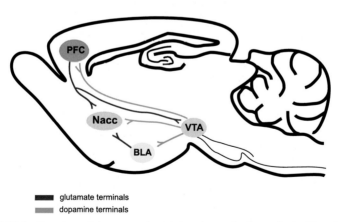

■ glutamate terminals
▨ dopamine terminals

FIGURE 12.3   Overview of drug reward-related pathways in the rat brain. Neural regions implicated in drug reward-related processing include the prefrontal cortex (PFC), ventral tegmental area (VTA), nucleus accumbens (NAc), and basolateral nucleus of the amygdala (BLA). These regions all share functional, bidirectional interconnections. Importantly, projections from the PFC region are capable of modulating neural activity patterns in all three subcortical regions, thereby serving a modulatory role in the regulation of drug-related motivational signaling.

projections originating from the A10 DAergic neurons of the VTA, sending ascending DAergic fibers to widespread areas of the PFC. Importantly, communications across these areas are in both directions, with the NAc sending projections (primarily GABAergic) back to the VTA, and the PFC sending descending outputs [primarily glutamatergic (GLUTergic)] back to neuronal populations in the VTA. The VTA itself is a heterogeneous region containing both DA and non-DA neurons, which are primarily GABAergic. The canonical understanding of how reward-related information controls DAergic transmission from the VTA involves the ability of drugs of abuse (eg, opiates) to inhibit feedforward inhibitory inputs to the VTA DA neurons, thereby releasing inhibition on DAergic output projections to reward projection areas, including the NAc, PFC, and also the basolateral nucleus of the amygdala (BLA). It is important to note that although activation of the VTA DAergic efferents are important for signaling reward-related information, there is considerable evidence that the VTA processes DA-independent reward signals via activation of the non-DAergic, GABAergic neuronal populations within the VTA (Laviolette, Gallegos, Henriksen, & van der Kooy, 2004; Laviolette & van der Kooy, 2001).

In the context of PFC–VTA interconnections, anatomical evidence suggests a complex functional relationship between VTA DAergic activity and PFC-mediated control of VTA neuronal activity. For example, excitatory projections from the PFC to the VTA synapse on dendrites of both DA and non-DA neurons in the VTA (Carr & Sesack, 2000). However, these PFC inputs to the VTA appear to differentially control VTA outputs from these different neuronal populations. Thus neurons in the PFC provide selective inputs to VTA GABAergic neurons, which then project predominantly to the NAc (ie, mesoaccumbens projections). In contrast, PFC inputs target VTA DAergic neurons that selectively project back to the PFC (ie, mesocortical projections), demonstrating a complex and bidirectional role for the PFC in controlling the output signals from the VTA (Sesack & Carr, 2002; Sesack, Deutsch, Roth, & Bunney, 1989).

Other drugs of abuse potently regulate mesolimbic and mesocortical DAergic pathways, but via different mechanisms of action. For example, nicotine can directly activate VTA DAergic neurons (Tan, Bishop, Lauzon, Sun, & Laviolette, 2009). Drugs such as amphetamine (AMPH) or cocaine can increase synaptic release of DA via actions on reuptake mechanisms within the synaptic cleft. However, regardless of the underlying mechanism, virtually all drugs of abuse share the ability to increase DAergic activity within the VTA, and hence increase levels of DA in target outputs of the VTA, including the PFC (Wise, 2004).

MODULATION OF PREFRONTAL CORTICAL NEUROTRANSMITTER RELEASE BY DRUGS OF ABUSE: EVIDENCE FROM ANIMAL MODELS

Given the anatomical locus of the PFC within the mesocorticolimbic system and its associated connections with other limbic regions critical for reward-related processing, including the VTA, BLA, and NAc (Fig. 12.3), considerable research has examined how drugs of abuse may regulate the release of neurotransmitters within the PFC. Studies in rodents using in vivo methods such as microdialysis, which measures dialysate levels of specific neurotransmitters including DA and glutamate (GLUT), have reported that exposure to a variety of drugs of abuse can potently increase the release of DA and GLUT within the PFC. For example, cocaine strongly increases the release of intra-PFC DA (Williams & Steketee, 2005a, 2005b) and GLUT (Steketee, 2005; Williams & Steketee, 2004). In terms of functional significance, the ability of psychostimulant drugs such as cocaine to modulate release and receptor expression levels of both intra-PFC DA and GLUTergic signaling substrates is critically linked to the phenomena of drug-related sensitization.

Sensitization refers to the ability of repeated exposure to a drug of abuse to sensitize neural motivational pathways (eg, the mesolimbic and mesocortical systems) to subsequent "challenge" exposures. Psychotropic drugs known to induce sensitized behaviors include psychostimulants such as nicotine, AMPH, and cocaine, or narcotics such as morphine or heroin. Animal models of drug-related sensitization phenomena generally involve measurements of psychomotor activity (eg, measures of horizontal distance traveled or rearing behaviors) during different phases of drug exposure. For example, a rat may receive five consecutive injections of cocaine, then experience a wash-out period in the home-cage environment for a specific period of time wherein no drug administration is performed. After the period of sensitization, the rat then receives an acute challenge dose of cocaine, and motor activity is measured again. In a sensitized animal, locomotor activity will be strongly enhanced (ie, hyperlocomotor activity), which is believed to indicate a sensitization of the mesolimbic/mesocortical neural motivational pathways to the effects of the drug. In general, neural reward sensitization phenomena, particularly in the mesolimbic pathway, have been linked to the pathological amplification of reward salience associated with drugs of abuse during the addiction process (Robinson & Berridge, 2000, 2001) and, as such, have been hypothesized to be an important underlying mechanism related to compulsive drug seeking and craving in both human addicts and animal models of addiction (Vanderschuren & Pierce, 2010). Simply put, sensitization is believed to underlie the ability of repeated drug exposure to pathologically heighten the motivational salience of drug-related cues. In the case of intra-PFC DA transmission, previous reports have demonstrated that PFC DAergic release dynamics are tightly regulated by the specific phase of drug exposure. For example, Williams and Steketee (2005a) reported that when measured during early stages of cocaine sensitization (eg, 1–7 days), PFC DA release was decreased. However, later stages of sensitization (eg, >30 days) were associated with strongly elevated PFC DA release after cocaine challenge.

Similar time-dependent PFC alterations during drug exposure and sensitization phenomena are found with GLUTergic transmission. GLUTergic terminals and receptors are abundant within the PFC, and excitatory GLUTergic projections from the PFC can strongly modulate subcortical neural reward regions including the NAc and VTA (Kalivas, 2004; Steketee, 2005; Wolf, 1998).

Accordingly, GLUTergic outputs from the PFC are positioned to modulate subcortical neural motivational processing, particularly in the context of drug-related reward and sensitization phenomena. For example, similar to the effects observed with DA release, repeated exposure to cocaine leads to sensitized increases in GLUT release measured in the PFC (Williams & Steketee, 2004). However, in contrast to the effects observed with DA release, time-dependent cocaine-induced sensitization in GLUT release measured in the PFC appears to occur in early (versus later) phases of drug-sensitization. Intra-PFC GLUT release is also observed during exposure to conditioned associative cues linked to the rewarding properties of cocaine (Hotsenpiller & Wolf, 2002) and GLU-Tergic projections from the PFC to the NAc are critical for cocaine cue-induced relapse to cocaine-seeking behaviors (McFarland, Lapish, & Kalivas, 2003).

ROLE OF THE PREFRONTAL CORTEX IN ADDICTION-RELATED BEHAVIORAL PHENOMENA: EVIDENCE FROM ANIMAL BEHAVIORAL PHARMACOLOGY RESEARCH

A large body of basic neuroscience research has examined how various drugs of abuse modulate neuronal activity within the PFC both in terms of acute responses to drug-related stimuli and how specific neuronal subpopulations within the PFC may be involved in the behavioral processing of addiction-related behaviors and memories. Most animal models measuring the rewarding properties of drugs of abuse rely upon either Pavlovian or operant forms of behavioral conditioning (Fig. 12.4). The most commonly used Pavlovian procedure is called *conditioned place preference* (*CPP*). This involves pairing a specific drug with a specific contextual environment. In contrast, the same subject receives a vehicle administration in an alternate environmental context. After several cycles of environmental pairings, the experimental animal is given the choice to spend time either in an environment previously paired with a drug reward stimulus (eg, morphine, AMPH, or cocaine) or the environment where the vehicle control (eg, physiological saline) exposure occurred. The amount of time the animal chooses to spend in the previously drug-paired environment is taken as a measure of the rewarding effects of the drug. Essentially, because animals are tested in the absence of the conditioning drug, the CPP test measures the extent to which the animal is willing to seek drug-associated cues based entirely on the strength of the previously formed associative memory.

In contrast, operant conditioning procedures measuring drug reward behaviors typically involve the use of intravenous self-administration (IVSA) of selected drugs via a surgically implanted indwelling catheter. In IVSA, the animal is trained to press a lever in order to obtain a discrete infusion of drug directly into the bloodstream. Lever-pressing responses may be paired with specific associative cues, such as a light or sound, delivered to the operant test chamber. The IVSA procedure is advantageous in that the drug administration is voluntary and thus more closely resembles voluntary self-administration in

OPERANT CONDITIONING:
INTRA-VENOUS DRUG
SELF-ADMINISTRATION

PAVLOVIAN CONDITIONING:
CONDITIONED PLACE PREFERENCE

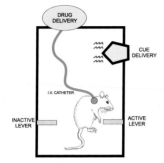

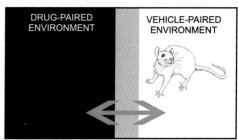

FIGURE 12.4 Common behavioral animal models of drug addiction. Operant forms of drug reward modeling involve the use of intravenous self-administration (IVSA) of drugs via voluntary lever-pressing behaviors produced by the experimental animal. Lever pressing and the subsequent delivery of the drug reward can be paired with specific associative cues such as auditory or visual stimuli. In contrast, Pavlovian forms of learning include conditioned place preference (CPP), wherein the experimental animal receives an experimenter-administered drug injection (either systemically or intracranially) and is then placed into a specific conditioning environment. After this, the animal receives a nonpsychoactive control injection (eg, saline vehicle) and is placed in the alternate environment. In this manner, the animal learns to associate the motivational effects of the drug with specific environmental cues. *IV*, Intravenous

human drug users. However, behavioral outputs can be confounded by motoric or other physiological artifacts that may be induced by the presence of the drug itself during the actual experiment. CPP is advantageous in that it can measure not only reward, but also aversive conditioning effects as well. In addition, CPP demands the recall of powerful, associative memories linked to the drug-taking experience. Its primary drawback is that because the drug exposure is administered by the experimenter (ie, nonvoluntary), CPP is perhaps a less robust analog of human drug-taking behaviors.

In terms of the general functional involvement of the PFC in the processing of drug-related addiction memories, excitotoxic lesions of the rat PFC have been shown to disrupt the encoding of cocaine-related associative reward memories. Using a CPP procedure in rats, anatomically selective lesions targeting the prelimbic region of the PFC were found to selectively impair the acquisition of cocaine reward memories, but had no effect on the formation of reward memories using AMPH or morphine (Tzschentke & Schmidt, 1998). Similarly, prelimbic PFC lesions were demonstrated to selectively block only cocaine-induced psychomotor sensitization, but not morphine or AMPH-dependent effects in rats (Tzschentke & Schmidt, 2000). Importantly, lesion studies are limited in their ability to identify discrete functional roles for complex neural regions in drug reward behaviors because they generally will indiscriminately destroy all neuronal populations (eg, both interneuron and pyramidal neurons) along with fibers of passage. Accordingly, more specific experimental approaches, including behavioral pharmacological techniques, molecular analyses, and neuronal electrophysiological recordings, have yielded a wealth of additional information pertaining to how the PFC process.

Using chronically implanted neuronal microwire recording arrays, Sun et al. (2011) demonstrated that subpopulations of neurons within the rat prelimbic cortex were capable of encoding opiate-related reward memories (Fig. 12.5). For example, during the acquisition of associative morphine-reward memories measured in a standard CPP procedure, it was found that subpopulations of PFC neurons selectively increased their firing frequency during morphine-environment conditioning sessions. In addition, PFC neurons showed specific firing patterns depending on the phase of the reward memory processing (eg, acquisition, recall, or extinction of these drug-related memories). Closer analysis of PFC neuronal activity patterns revealed important differences in terms of tonic firing rates versus neuronal firing occurring as "bursting" events (eg, action potential spikes occurring in regular tonic patterns versus bursts of irregular spike trains). Interestingly, mPFC neurons showed highly divergent patterns of burst activity during memory acquisition versus recall phases of newly acquired opiate memories, versus the extinction (ie, forgetting) of these memories. Thus whereas bursting activity did not change during recall of recent opiate memories, they found that PFC neuronal bursting strongly increased during the extinction phase of the memory.

In terms of PFC neuronal involvement in the temporal consolidation of opiate-related reward memories, inputs from the BLA are critical. For example, Gholizadeh et al. (2013) demonstrated that the acute consolidation phase of an associative morphine-reward memory (measured in a CPP procedure in rats) was dependent upon memory consolidation substrates within the BLA. However, during later phase consolidation of these drug reward memories, PFC-dependent memory consolidation substrates were recruited. Interestingly, this transfer of memory-consolidation dependence along the BLA–PFC pathway was dependent upon postlearning temporal dynamics. Thus BLA-dependent memory consolidation was only required during the first 6 hours postconditioning and was mediated through an extracellular-signal–related kinase (ERK) molecular substrate. In contrast, during later phases of memory consolidation, a PFC-dependent, calcium-calmodulin kinase α, ERK-independent memory substrate was activated within the PFC from 6 to 12 hours postlearning. These findings suggested that during later phases of addiction-related memory formation, PFC memory substrates are specifically brought online after a period of first-order memory consolidation in subcortical limbic regions such as the BLA. Indeed, inactivation of the BLA during opiate-related reward learning has been shown to increase the spontaneous firing and bursting activity of rat PFC neurons and alter the long-term memory processing associated with opiate-related conditioning effects. For example, Sun and Laviolette (2012) demonstrated that pharmacologically inactivating the rat BLA during the acquisition phase of opiate reward CPP conditioning causes a later acceleration in the extinction of previously learned opiate reward

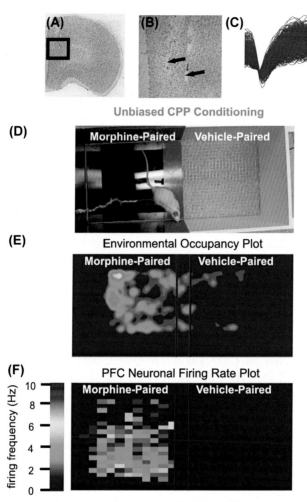

FIGURE 12.5   Prefrontal cortex (PFC) neurons encode opiate-related reward memories. (A and B) Microphotograph showing a typical intra-PFC microwire location (*black arrows*). Using microwire recordings with implanted electrode arrays directly in the rat PFC, PFC neurons can be recorded and analyzed during addiction-related reward processing. (C) A typical PFC neuronal waveform. (D) Using an unbiased conditioned place preference (CPP) procedure, neurons in the rat PFC show associative increases in firing frequency rates when the rat is reexposed to an environment where the rewarding effects of morphine were previously experienced. (E) Rats spend increased time in the morphine-paired environment, revealed with a videotaped occupancy plot recording during CPP testing. (F) Recordings of PFC activity show increased neuronal firing rates specifically when the rat experiences the morphine-paired environment.

memories reflected in associative PFC neuronal activity changes during conditioning. Furthermore, BLA inactivation switched rewarding opiate conditioning effects into behavioral aversions. Together, these findings demonstrate that specific subpopulations of neurons in the mammalian PFC are capable of differentially encoding specific phases of addiction-related memories and are governed by relatively precise temporal phases of drug reward exposure. Furthermore, such evidence implicates an important functional role for PFC neurons not only in the initial acquisition of addiction-related associative memories, but also in the later consolidation and recall of these memories.

Using neuronal labeling techniques and pharmacogenetic inactivation procedures in rats, Bossert et al. (2011) demonstrated that specific ensembles of ventral medial neurons within the rat PFC (ie, the infralimbic cortex) are activated during exposure to heroin-associated relapse-triggering cues. More importantly, directly inactivating these same neuronal ensembles revealed that context-dependent relapse to heroin self-administration could be blocked. These findings further demonstrate the specificity of PFC neuronal encoding of addiction-related memories and suggest that specific neuronal ensembles within PFC circuits are responsible for the encoding of reward-related associative memories. Thus considerable evidence now demonstrates that specific neuronal populations within the mammalian PFC are capable of encoding associative memories linked to drug-associated reward and memory formation during various phases of drug-related memory processing. As will be described in a later section, this role for the PFC in mediating cue-related memories associated with the addictive properties of drugs of abuse finds considerable support in brain imaging experiments with human drug abusers.

NEUROCHEMICAL CONTROL OF DRUG-RELATED REWARD PROCESSING IN THE PREFRONTAL CORTEX: ROLE OF DOPAMINE–GLUTAMATE INTERACTIONS IN ANIMAL MODELS

Considerable evidence has revealed how specific neurotransmitter substrates within the PFC may modulate the processing of drug-related reward information and associated memories. As noted previously, drugs of abuse powerfully modulate the release of GLUT and DA within the PFC; thus, not surprisingly, modulation of either of these receptor substrates has been shown to powerfully modulate drug-related processing and behaviors in the PFC. For example, using a CPP behavioral procedure to examine the role of GLUTergic NMDA receptor transmission in the rat PFC, Bishop et al. (2011) demonstrated that blockade of NMDA transmission via direct microinfusions of a selective NMDA receptor antagonist, or a blocker of the NMDA receptor subunit NR2B, was able to potently increase the reward salience of normally nonrewarding conditioning doses of systemic or intra-VTA morphine administration. Interestingly the ability of PFC NMDA receptor hypofunction to increase opiate reward salience was dependent upon intra-PFC DA receptor transmission, suggesting that blockade of intra-PFC NMDA transmission was able to amplify opiate reward signals via activating downstream DAergic outputs from the VTA to the PFC. The effects of intra-PFC NMDA receptor blockade were also dependent upon functional inputs from the BLA, suggesting that a state of PFC

NMDA receptor hypofunction may represent an opiate-addiction vulnerability phenotype by amplifying convergent VTA and BLA DAergic or GLUTergic inputs into the PFC.

Whereas such an effect seems paradoxical given that many drugs of abuse induce strong release of intra-PFC GLUT, considerable evidence indicates that hypofunction of NMDA receptor transmission within the PFC actually increases mesolimbic release of DA via PFC projections to the mesolimbic system. Indeed, the NMDA receptor is highly expressed in the PFC (Goebel & Poosch, 1999), and various studies have demonstrated that pharmacological modulation of the NMDA receptor can regulate subcortical DA transmission. For example, in vivo microdialysis studies performed in rats demonstrate that NMDA receptor agonists actually decrease intra-PFC levels of DA release but increase extracellular concentrations of γ-aminobutyric acid (GABA) (Del Arco & Mora, 1999, 2002, 2008). Conversely, administration of NMDA antagonists such as ketamine or phencyclidine have been shown to strongly increase the release of GLUT and DA within the rat PFC (Lorrain, Baccei, Bristow, Anderson, & Varney, 2003; Moghaddam, Adams, Verma, & Daly, 1997). These effects are most likely the result of GLUT receptor modulation of inhibitory versus excitatory influences that impinge upon either GABA transmitting (GABAergic), GLUTergic, or DAergic terminals within the PFC (Homayoun & Moghaddam, 2007; Jackson, Homayoun, & Moghaddam, 2004). Importantly, in vivo neuronal electrophysiological studies have demonstrated that pharmacological blockade of NMDA transmission can decrease inhibitory feedforward drive to PFC pyramidal output neurons through inhibition of PFC GABAergic interneurons (Homayoun & Moghaddam, 2007), providing a mechanism by which NMDA antagonists may amplify prefrontal cortical activity and subsequent downstream regulation of excitatory PFC outputs to the mesolimbic system. This PFC-mediated control of subcortical DAergic motivational signaling was further demonstrated by Tan, Rosen, Ng, Rushlow, and Laviolette (2014), where it was reported that blockade of NMDA receptor function in the rat PFC acutely activated DA neuron activity in the VTA and switched on a DA-dependent opiate reward system. Furthermore, because the rewarding effects of opiate-class drugs are normally mediated through non-DAergic VTA reward mechanisms in the drug-naïve state and only become dependent upon DA signaling once the organism is chronically exposed to opiates and in a state of withdrawal (Laviolette et al., 2004; Nader & van der Kooy, 1997), the authors further tested whether VTA DA neuron activation induced by intra-PFC NMDA receptor hypofunction may switch the processing of opiate reward into a DA-dependent mechanism. Remarkably, it was found that blockade of NMDA transmission within the PFC was capable of switching on a DA-dependent reward system, regardless of the animal's prior opiate exposure history. Interestingly, similar effects on downstream DA activity and opiate reward salience are observed with direct pharmacological blockade of α-amino-3-hydroxy-5-methyl-4-isoxazolepropionic acid (AMPA) receptors in the rat PFC (De Jaeger et al., 2013).

Given the evidence for PFC neuronal populations as critical neural substrates for the encoding and storage of drug-related associative memories, it is not surprising that the PFC is implicated also in drug relapse phenomena. GLUTergic transmission within the PFC is implicated in the processing of drug-related relapse phenomena. For example, methamphetamine self-administration in rats was shown to decrease GLUT levels measured with microdialysis in the PFC during acute exposure, but caused increased GLUTergic release during relapse to methamphetamine self-administration behaviors (Parsegian & See, 2014). In a study using cocaine IVSA in rats, analysis of expression levels of the metabotropic GLUT-1 receptor (mGLUR1) subtype in the ventral-medial PFC revealed that cocaine-associated cue exposure caused dysregulation of mGLUR1 signaling, an effect that was associated with resistance to extinction of cocaine-related associative cue memories (Ben-Shahar et al., 2013). DAergic transmission within the rat PFC is also involved in the recall of opiate-related reward memories. For example, overstimulation of the DA D1 receptor subtype in the PFC was shown to transiently suppress the recall of morphine CPP memories. Interestingly, this DA-dependent addiction memory suppression was only transient, and the memories were able to be recalled in the absence of D1 receptor activation (Lauzon, Bechard, Ahmad, & Laviolette, 2013). Together, these findings point to the importance of GLUTergic/DAergic signaling mechanisms within the mammalian PFC that can strongly modulate drug reward sensitivity and addiction vulnerability. Indeed, the functional role of the PFC in modulating mesolimbic DAergic motivational signaling suggests that disturbances in PFC function may underlie the pathological amplification in motivational salience attributed to drug of abuse and their associated cues. As will be described, evidence from human drug users suggests that such disturbances in PFC regulation of drug-associated salience attribution may be a critical underlying cause of addiction-related loss of inhibitory control over compulsive drug seeking and relapse.

CANNABINOID MODULATION OF DRUG-RELATED REWARD PROCESSING IN THE ANIMAL PREFRONTAL CORTEX–MESOLIMBIC CIRCUITRY

In addition to psychostimulants and opiate-class drugs, cannabinoid-based drugs such as marijuana (MJ) have been shown to strongly modulate PFC neuronal activity and more specifically, PFC-mediated control of subcortical reward pathways through actions on the naturally occurring cannabinoid (CB1) receptor (CB1R) subtype (Ahmad, Lauzon, de Jaeger, & Laviolette, 2013; Draycott et al., 2014; Pistis, Porcu, Melis, Diana, & Gessa, 2001). For example, systemic treatment with Δ9-tetrahydrocannabinol (THC), the psychoactive component of MJ, or with WIN 55,212-2, a synthetic CB1R agonist, increases excitability of VTA DA neurons projecting to the rat PFC (French, Dillon, & Wu, 1997) and can indirectly increase the excitability of DA neuron via an inhibition of

GABAergic neurons within the VTA (Szabo, Siemes, & Wallmichrath, 2002). Similarly, using in vivo microdialysis analysis, it has been observed that acute THC treatment increases the levels of both DA and GLUT while reducing the inhibitory GABA levels in the PFC (Pistis et al., 2002). More interestingly, it has been recently reported that direct intra-mPFC CB1 activation with a synthetic agonist, WIN55,212-2, biphasically and dose-dependently modulates spontaneous DA neuron activity in the VTA. Lower doses of WIN 55,212-2 significantly increase spontaneous firing and bursting rates of VTA DA neurons and, conversely, higher doses strongly inhibited spontaneous VTA DA neuron activity (Draycott et al., 2014). Moreover, acute THC treatment increases DA turnover (DOPAC/DA) in the rat PFC, but not in the NAc or striatum (Jentsch, Andrusiak, Tran, Bowers, & Roth, 1997). Conversely, chronic treatment with either THC or WIN 55,212-2 causes a selective and persistent (up to 14 days) reduction of DA turnover in the rat PFC, but not in the striatum (Jentsch, Verrico, Le, & Roth, 1998; Verrico, Jentsch, & Roth, 2003). Thus acute or chronic cannabinoid exposure is associated with reduced DA transmission in the mPFC, and these MJ-induced alterations in PFC function may in turn modulate subcortical neural reward pathways associated with drug addiction vulnerability and plasticity.

SUMMARY

As described in the preceding sections, considerable evidence from both clinical and animal models of addiction identifies the mammalian PFC as a critical neural region for executive control over subcortical limbic regions. Importantly, addiction represents a loss of control over primordial emotional processing centers, specifically in limbic regions, that regulate motivational and hedonic salience attribution. To the extent that the addiction process can be considered a hijacking of the brain's subcortical reward pathways by drugs of abuse, resistance to the powerful, dependence-producing effects of these stimuli must ultimately depend upon the brain's ability to control these subcortical processes through cortical control mechanisms. In this sense, a healthy PFC, capable of modulating subcortical brain reward pathways and regulating the salience of powerful, drug-related associative memories, is undoubtedly a crucial variable controlling why only certain individuals may be vulnerable to addiction-related psychological and neurophysiological alterations. Evidence from both animal models and human imaging studies described in this chapter demonstrates that cortical control of motivational neural pathways linked to the addiction process are disturbed as a result of chronic exposure to drugs of abuse. Despite a growing body of evidence in support of such a role for PFC function (and dysfunction) in the pathogenesis of addiction-related compulsive behaviors, a greater understanding of how PFC interactions with subcortical emotional processing centers is essential. Importantly, we still lack a reliable neural marker for addiction vulnerability. Given the known metabolic abnormalities and PFC-related psychological disturbances present in drug dependence, analysis of PFC function (either via prognostic imaging and/or psychological testing of PFC-related cognitive and impulse/executive control parameters) may ultimately serve as a reliable tool for addiction vulnerability screening in at-risk patient populations.

REFERENCES

Ahmad, T., Lauzon, N. M., de Jaeger, X., & Laviolette, S. R. (2013). Cannabinoid transmission in the prelimbic cortex bidirectionally controls opiate reward and aversion signaling through dissociable kappa versus μ-opiate receptor dependent mechanisms. *The Journal of Neuroscience*, *33*, 15642–15651.

Ben-Shahar, O., Sacramento, A. D., Miller, B. W., Webb, S. M., Wroten, M. G., Silva, H. E., et al. (2013). Deficits in ventromedial prefrontal cortex group 1 metabotropic glutamate receptor function mediate resistance to extinction during protracted withdrawal from an extensive history of cocaine self-administration. *The Journal of Neuroscience*, *33*, 495–506.

Bishop, S. F., Lauzon, N. M., Bechard, M. A., Gholizadeh, S., & Laviolette, S. R. (2011). NMDA receptor hypofunction in the prelimbic cortex increases sensitivity to the rewarding properties of opiates via dopaminergic and amygdalar substrates. *Cerebral Cortex*, *21*, 68–80.

Bossert, J. M., Stern, A. L., Theberge, F. R., Cifani, C., Koya, E., Hope, B. T., et al. (2011). Ventral medial prefrontal cortex neuronal ensembles mediate context-induced relapse to heroin. *Nature Neuroscience*, *14*, 420–422.

Carr, D. B., & Sesack, S. R. (2000). Projections from the rat prefrontal cortex to the ventral tegmental area: target specificity in the synaptic associations with mesoaccumbens and mesocortical neurons. *The Journal of Neuroscience*, *20*, 3864–3873.

Claus, E. D., Ewing, S. W., Filbey, F. M., Sabbineni, A., & Hutchison, K. E. (2011). Identifying neurobiological phenotypes associated with alcohol use disorder severity. *Neuropsychopharmacology*, *36*, 2086–2096.

De Jaeger, X., Bishop, S. F., Ahmad, T., Lyons, D., Ng, G. A., & Laviolette, S. R. (2013). The effects of AMPA receptor blockade in the prelimbic cortex on systemic and ventral tegmental area opiate reward sensitivity. *Psychopharmacology*, *225*, 687–695.

Del Arco, A., & Mora, F. (1999). Effects of endogenous glutamate on extracellular concentrations of GABA, dopamine, and dopamine metabolites in the prefrontal cortex of the freely moving rat: involvement of NMDA and AMPA/KA receptors. *Neurochemical Research*, *24*, 1027–1035.

Del Arco, A., & Mora, F. (2002). NMDA and AMPA/kainate glutamatergic agonists increase the extracellular concentrations of GABA in the prefrontal cortex of the freely moving rat: modulation by endogenous dopamine. *Brain Research Bulletin*, *57*, 623–630.

Del Arco, A., & Mora, F. (2008). Prefrontal cortex–nucleus accumbens interaction: in vivo modulation by dopamine and glutamate in the prefrontal cortex. *Pharmacology, Biochemistry, and Behavior*, *90*, 226–235.

Draycott, B., Loureiro, M., Ahmad, T., Tan, H., Zunder, J., & Laviolette, S. R. (2014). Cannabinoid transmission in the prefrontal cortex bi-phasically controls emotional memory formation via functional interactions with the ventral tegmental area. *The Journal of Neuroscience*, *34*, 13096–13109.

French, E. D., Dillon, K., & Wu, X. (1997). Cannabinoids excite dopamine neurons in the ventral tegmentum and substantia nigra. *Neuroreport*, *8*, 649–652.

Fu, L. P., Bi, G. H., Zou, Z. T., Wang, Y., Ye, E. M., Ma, L., et al. (2008). Impaired response inhibition function in abstinent heroin dependents: an fMRI study. *Neuroscience Letters*, *438*, 322–326.

Gholizadeh, S., Sun, N., De Jaeger, X., Bechard, M. A., Coolen, L., & Laviolette, S. R. (2013). Early versus late-phase consolidation of opiate reward memories requires distinct molecular and temporal mechanisms in the amygdala-prefrontal cortical pathway. *PLoS One, 8,* e63612.

Goebel, D. J., & Poosch, M. S. (1999). NMDA receptor subunit gene expression in the rat brain: a quantitative analysis of endogenous mRNA levels of NR1Com, NR2A, NR2B, NR2C, NR2D and NR3A. *Brain Research. Molecular Brain Research, 69,* 164–170.

Goldstein, R. Z., Leskovjan, A. C., Hoff, A. L., Hitzemann, R., Bashan, F., Khalsa, S. S., et al. (2004). Severity of neuropsychological impairment in cocaine and alcohol addiction: association with metabolism in the prefrontal cortex. *Neuropsychologia, 42,* 1447–1558.

Goldstein, R. Z., & Volkow, N. D. (2011). Dysfunction of the prefrontal cortex in addiction: neuroimaging findings and clinical implications. *Nature Reviews. Neuroscience, 12,* 652–669.

Homayoun, H., & Moghaddam, B. (2007). NMDA receptor hypofunction produces opposite effects on prefrontal cortex interneurons and pyramidal neurons. *The Journal of Neuroscience, 27,* 11496–11500.

Hotsenpiller, G., & Wolf, M. E. (2002). Extracellular glutamate levels in prefrontal cortex during the expression of associative responses to cocaine related stimuli. *Neuropharmacology, 43,* 1218–1229.

Jackson, M. E., Homayoun, H., & Moghaddam, B. (2004). NMDA receptor hypofunction produces concomitant firing rate potentiation and burst activity reduction in the prefrontal cortex. *Proceedings of the National Academy of Sciences, 101,* 8467–8472.

Janes, A. C., Pizzagalli, D. A., Richardt, S., Frederick, B., Chuzi, S., Pachas, G., et al. (2010). Brain reactivity to smoking cues prior to smoking cessation predicts ability to maintain tobacco abstinence. *Biological Psychiatry, 67,* 722–729.

Jentsch, J. D., Andrusiak, E., Tran, A., Bowers, M. B., Jr., & Roth, R. H. (1997). Delta9-Tetrahydrocannabinol increases prefrontal cortical catecholaminergic utilization and impairs spatial working memory in the rat: blockade of dopaminergic effects with HA966. *Neuropsychopharmacology, 16,* 426–432.

Jentsch, J. D., Verrico, C. D., Le, D., & Roth, R. H. (1998). Repeated exposure to delta 9-tetrahydrocannabinol reduces prefrontal cortical dopamine metabolism in the rat. *Neuroscience Letters, 246,* 169–172.

Kalivas, P. W. (2004). Glutamate systems in cocaine addiction. *Current Opinion in Pharmacology, 4,* 23–55.

Kufahl, P., Li, Z., Risinger, R., Rainey, C., Piacentine, L., Wu, G., et al. (2008). Expectation modulates human brain responses to acute cocaine: a functional magnetic resonance imaging study. *Biological Psychiatry, 63,* 222–230.

Kufahl, P. R., Li, Z., Risinger, R. C., Rainey, C. J., Wu, G., Bloom, A. S., et al. (2005). Neural responses to acute cocaine administration in the human brain detected by fMRI. *Neuroimage, 28,* 904–914.

Langleben, D. D., Ruparel, K., Elman, I., Busch-Winokur, S., Pratiwadi, R., Loughead, J., et al. (2008). Acute effect of methadone maintenance dose on brain fMRI response to heroin-related cues. *The American Journal of Psychiatry, 165,* 390–394.

Lauzon, N. M., Bechard, M., Ahmad, T., & Laviolette, S. R. (2013). Supra-normal stimulation of dopamine D1 receptors in the prelimbic cortex blocks behavioral expression of both aversive and rewarding associative memories through a cyclic-AMP-dependent signaling pathway. *Neuropharmacology, 67,* 104–114.

Laviolette, S. R., Gallegos, R. A., Henriksen, S. J., & van der Kooy, D. (2004). Opiate state controls bi-directional reward signaling via GABA$_A$ receptors in the ventral tegmental area. *Nature Neuroscience, 7,* 160–169.

Laviolette, S. R., & van der Kooy, D. (2001). GABA$_A$ receptors in the ventral tegmental area control bidirectional reward signalling between dopaminergic and non-dopaminergic neural motivational systems. *The European Journal of Neuroscience, 13,* 1009–10115.

Li, Q., Wang, Y., Zhang, Y., Li, W., Yang, W., Zhu, J., et al. (2012). Craving correlates with mesolimbic responses to heroin-related cues in short-term abstinence from heroin: an event-related fMRI study. *Brain Research, 1469,* 63–72.

Lorrain, D. S., Baccei, C. S., Bristow, L. J., Anderson, J. J., & Varney, M. A. (2003). Effects of ketamine and N-methyl-D-aspartate on glutamate and dopamine release in the rat prefrontal cortex: modulation by a group II selective metabotropic glutamate receptor agonist LY379268. *Neuroscience, 117,* 697–706.

Ma, N., Liu, Y., Li, N., Wang, C. X., Zhang, H., Jiangm, X. F., et al. (2010). Addiction related alteration in resting-state brain connectivity. *Neuroimage, 49,* 738–744.

McFarland, K., Lapish, C. C., & Kalivas, P. W. (2003). Prefrontal glutamate release into the core of the nucleus accumbens mediates cocaine-induced reinstatement of drug-seeking behavior. *The Journal of Neuroscience, 23,* 3531–3537.

Moghaddam, B., Adams, B., Verma, A., & Daly, D. (1997). Activation of glutamatergic neurotransmission by ketamine: a novel step in the pathway from NMDA receptor blockade to dopaminergic and cognitive disruptions associated with the prefrontal cortex. *The Journal of Neuroscience, 17,* 2921–2927.

Moreno-López, L., Stamatakis, E. A., Fernández-Serrano, M. J., Gómez-Río, M., Rodríguez-Fernández, A., Pérez-García, M., et al. (2012). Neural correlates of hot and cold executive functions in polysubstance addiction: association between neuropsychological performance and resting brain metabolism as measured by positron emission tomography. *Psychiatry Research, 203,* 214–221.

Nader, K., & van der Kooy, D. (1997). Deprivation state switches the neurobiological substrates mediating opiate reward in the ventral tegmental area. *The Journal of Neuroscience, 17,* 383–390.

Parsegian, A., & See, R. E. (2014). Dysregulation of dopamine and glutamate release in the prefrontal cortex and nucleus accumbens following methamphetamine self-administration and during reinstatement in rats. *Neuropsychopharmacology, 39,* 811–822.

Pistis, M., Ferraro, L., Pira, L., Flore, G., Tanganelli, S., Gessa, G. L., et al. (2002). Delta(9)-tetrahydrocannabinol decreases extracellular GABA and increases extracellular glutamate and dopamine levels in the rat prefrontal cortex: an in vivo microdialysis study. *Brain Research, 948,* 155–158.

Pistis, M., Porcu, G., Melis, M., Diana, M., & Gessa, G. L. (2001). Effects of cannabinoids on prefrontal neuronal responses to ventral tegmental area stimulation. *The European Journal of Neuroscience, 14,* 96–102.

Qiu, Y. W., Jiang, G. H., Su, H. H., Lu, X. F., Tian, J. Z., Li, L. M., et al. (2013). The impulsivity behavior is correlated with prefrontal cortex gray matter volume reduction in heroin-dependent individuals. *Neuroscience Letters, 538,* 43–48.

Rapeli, P., Kivisaari, R., Autti, T., Kähkönen, S., Puuskari, V., Jokela, O., et al. (2006). Cognitive function during early abstinence from opioid dependence: a comparison to age, gender, and verbal intelligence matched controls. *BMC Psychiatry, 6,* 9.

Robinson, T. E., & Berridge, K. C. (2000). The psychology and neurobiology of addiction: an incentive-sensitization view. *Addiction, 95*(Suppl. 2), S91–S117.

Robinson, T. E., & Berridge, K. C. (2001). Incentive-sensitization and addiction. *Addiction, 96,* 103–114.

Seamans, J. K., Lapish, C. C., & Durstewitz, D. (2008). Comparing the prefrontal cortex of rats and primates: insights from electrophysiology. *Neurotoxicity Research, 14,* 249–262.

Sesack, S. R., & Carr, D. B. (2002). Selective prefrontal cortex inputs to dopamine cells: implications for schizophrenia. *Physiology & Behavior, 77*, 513–517.

Sesack, S. R., Deutsch, A. Y., Roth, R. H., & Bunney, B. S. (1989). Topographical organization of the efferent projections of the medial prefrontal cortex in the rat: an anterograde tract-tracing study with *Phaseolus vulgaris* leukoagglutinin. *Journal of Comparative Neurology, 290*, 213–242.

Steketee, J. D. (2005). Cortical mechanisms of cocaine sensitization. *Critical Reviews in Neurobiology, 17*, 69–86.

Sun, N., Chi, N., Lauzon, N., Bishop, S., Tan, H., & Laviolette, S. R. (2011). Acquisition, extinction, and recall of opiate reward memory are signaled by dynamic neuronal activity patterns in the prefrontal cortex. *Cerebral Cortex, 21*, 2665–2680.

Sun, N., & Laviolette, S. R. (2012). Inactivation of the basolateral amygdala during opiate reward learning disinhibits prelimbic cortical neurons and modulates associative memory extinction. *Psychopharmacology, 222*, 645–661.

Szabo, B., Siemes, S., & Wallmichrath, I. (2002). Inhibition of GABAergic neurotransmission in the ventral tegmental area by cannabinoids. *The European Journal of Neuroscience, 15*, 2057–2061.

Tan, H., Bishop, S. F., Lauzon, N. M., Sun, N., & Laviolette, S. R. (2009). Chronic nicotine exposure switches the functional role of mesolimbic dopamine transmission in the processing of nicotine's rewarding and aversive effects. *Neuropharmacology, 56*, 741–751.

Tan, H., Rosen, L. G., Ng, G. A., Rushlow, W. J., & Laviolette, S. R. (2014). NMDA receptor blockade in the prelimbic cortex activates the mesolimbic system and dopamine-dependent opiate reward signaling. *Psychopharmacology, 231*, 4669–4679.

Tzschentke, T. M., & Schmidt, W. J. (1998). Discrete quinolinic acid lesions of the rat prelimbic medial prefrontal cortex affect cocaine- and MK-801-, but not morphine- and amphetamine-induced reward and psychomotor activation as measured with the place preference conditioning paradigm. *Behavioural Brain Research, 97*, 115–127.

Tzschentke, T. M., & Schmidt, W. J. (2000). Differential effects of discrete subarea-specific lesions of the rat medial prefrontal cortex on amphetamine- and cocaine-induced behavioural sensitization. *Cerebral Cortex, 10*, 488–498.

Vanderschuren, L. J., & Pierce, R. C. (2010). Sensitization processes in drug addiction. *Current Topics in Behavioral Neurosciences, 3*, 179–195.

Verrico, C. D., Jentsch, J. D., & Roth, R. H. (2003). Persistent and anatomically selective reduction in prefrontal cortical dopamine metabolism after repeated, intermittent cannabinoid administration to rats. *Synapse, 49*, 61–66.

Williams, J. M., & Steketee, J. D. (2004). Cocaine increases medial prefrontal cortical glutamate overflow in cocaine-sensitized rats: a time course study. *The European Journal of Neuroscience, 20*, 1639–1646.

Williams, J. M., & Steketee, J. D. (2005a). Time dependent effects of repeated cocaine administration on dopamine transmission in the medial prefrontal cortex. *Neuropharmacology, 48*, 51–61.

Williams, J. M., & Steketee, J. D. (2005b). Effects of repeated cocaine on the release and clearance of dopamine within the rat medial prefrontal cortex. *Synapse, 55*, 98–109.

Wise, R. A. (2004). Dopamine, learning and motivation. *Nature Reviews. Neuroscience, 5*, 483–494.

Wolf, M. E. (1998). The role of excitatory amino acids in behavioral sensitization to psychomotor stimulants. *Progress in Neurobiology, 54*, 679–720.

List of Acronyms and Abbreviations

6-OHDA 6-hydroxydopamine.
ACC Anterior cingulate cortex.
AChE Acetylcholinesterase.
AD Alzheimer's Disease.
ADB AD with Balint's syndrome.
ADNI Alzheimer's Disease Research Initiative.
ALS Amyotrophic lateral sclerosis.
ALSbi Amyotrophic lateral sclerosis with behavioral impairment.
ALSci Amyotrophic lateral sclerosis with cognitive impairment.
AMPA α-amino-3-hydroxy-5-methyl-4-isoxazolepropionic acid receptor for glutamate.
AMPH Amphetamine.
ApoE4 Apolipoprotein E4.
APP Amyloid precursor protein.
AβO β-Amyloid oligomer.
BA Broca area.
BBB Blood brain barrier.
BCAO Bilateral carotid artery occlusion.
BCAS Bilateral carotid artery stenosis.
BDNF Brain-derived neurotrophic factor.
BLA Basolateral nucleus of the amygdala.
BOLD-fMRI Blood oxygen level–dependent functional magnetic resonance imaging.
BTA-1 2-(4-Methylaminophenyl)benzothiazole.
bvFTD Behavioral variant of frontotemporal dementia.
CA *Cornu Ammonis* region of the hippocampus.
CAA Cerebral amyloid angiopathy.
CADASIL Cerebral autosomal-dominant arteriopathy with subcortical infarcts and leukoen-cephalopathy.
CB+ Calbindin-positive.
CB1R Cannabinoid receptor 1.
CBS Corticobasal syndrome.
CCA Common carotid artery.
CCK Cholecystokinin.
CDR Clinical dementia rating.
CEN Central executive network.
CFA Complete Freund's adjuvant.
CIS Clinically isolated episode.
CNS Central nervous system.
CPP Conditioned place preference.
CR+ Calretinin-positive.
CSF Cerebrospinal fluid.
CSPG Chondroitin-sulfate-proteoglycan.
CST Corticospinal tract.

CT Computed tomography.
DA Dopamine.
DAT Dopamine active transporter.
DIR -MRI Double inversion recovery-magnetic resonance imaging.
DLPFC Dorsolateral prefrontal cortex.
DMD Disease-modifying drug.
DMN Default-mode network.
DPR Dipeptide repeat.
DTI Diffusion tensor imaging.
EAE Experimental autoimmune encephalitis.
EC Entorhinal cortex.
EMG Electromyography.
ERK Extracellular-signal–related kinase.
EYFP Enhanced yellow fluorescent protein.
FACS Fluorescence-activated cell sorting.
FAD Familial Alzheimer's disease.
FDG ^{18}F-fluorodeoxyglucose.
FDG PET ^{18}F-fluorodeoxyglucose positron emission tomography.
FLAIR Fluid-attenuated inversion recovery.
FTD Frontotemporal dementia.
FTLD Frontotemporal lobar degeneration.
FUS Fused in sarcoma.
GA Glatiramer acetate.
GABA γ-Aminobutyric acid.
GAD Glutamic acid decarboxylase.
GAT-1 γ-Aminobutyric acid transporter 1.
GFP Green fluorescent protein.
GLUT Glutamate.
GM Gray matter.
GRN Progranulin gene.
GSK Glycogen synthase kinase.
GWAS Genome-wide association study.
HD Huntington disease.
HTT Huntingtin gene.
IFN Interferon.
IL Interleukin.
iPSC Induced pluripotent stem cell.
IRF Interferon regulatory factor.
IVSA Intravenous self-administration.
LOAD Late onset Alzheimer's disease.
LTD Long-term depression.
LTP Long-term potentiation.
MAP Microtubule-associated protein.
MAPT Microtubule-associated protein tau gene.
MBP Myelin basic protein.
MCI Mild cognitive impairment.
MEC Medial entorhinal cortex.
mGLUR Metabotropic glutamate receptor.
MHC II Major histocompatibility complex II.
mI Myoinositol.
MJ Marijuana.
MMSE Mini Mental State Exam.

MOG   Myelin oligodendrocyte glycoprotein.
mPFC   Medial prefrontal cortex.
MPTP   1-methyl-4-phenyl-1,2,3,6-tetrahydropyridine.
MRI   Magnetic resonance imaging.
MRS   Magnetic resonance spectroscopy.
MS   Multiple sclerosis.
MSN   Medium spiny neuron.
MT/V   Mediotemporal/visual areas.
NAA   N-Acetylaspartate.
Nac   Nucleus accumbens.
NCI   Nuclear cytoplasmic inclusion.
nfPPA   Nonfluent/agrammatic primary progressive aphasia.
NFT   Neurofibrillary tangle.
NINDS   National Institute of Neurological Disorders and Stroke.
NMDA N-methyl-D-aspartate.
NMDAR N-methyl-D-aspartate receptor for glutamate.
NMR   Nuclear magnetic resonance.
NNI   Nuclear neuronal inclusion.
NO   Nitric oxide.
NPY   Neuropeptide Y.
NT-3   Neurotrophin-3.
OFC   Orbitofrontal cortex.
OLC   Oligodendrocyte lineage cell.
PAG   Peri-aqueductal gray.
PAS   Paired associative stimulation.
PBB   Phenyl/pyridinylbutadienyl-benzothiazoles/benzothiazolium.
PCP   Phencyclidine.
PD   Parkinson's disease.
PET   Positron emission tomography.
PFC   Prefrontal cortex.
PHF   Paired helical filament.
PiB   Pittsburgh-B compound.
PKA   Protein kinase A.
PLP   Proteolipid protein.
PLP   Proteolipid protein peptide.
PP-2A   Protein phosphatase 2A.
PS1, 2   Presenilin 1, 2.
PSP   Progressive supranuclear palsy.
PV+   Parvalbumin-positive.
RRMS   Relapsing remitting multiple sclerosis.
rs-fMRI   Resting state functional magnetic resonance imaging.
RSN   Resting state network.
shRNA   Small hairpin RNA.
SHRSP (rat)   Spontaneously hypertensive rat stroke-prone.
siRNA   Small inhibitory RNA.
SN   Salience network.
SNP   Single nucleotide polymorphism.
SOD1   Superoxide dismutase one gene.
SPECT   Single photon emission computerized tomography.
SPMS   Secondary progressive multiple sclerosis.
STZ   Streptozotocin.
SUV   Standardized uptake value.

svPPA   Semantic variant primary progressive aphasia.
SWI   Susceptibility weighted imaging.
TDP-43   TAR DNA-binding protein 43.
THC   Δ9-Tetrahydrocannabinol.
TNF   Tumor necrosis factor.
ToM   Theory of Mind.
TREM-2   Triggering receptor expressed on myeloid cells gene.
VCP   Valosin-containing protein gene.
VEN   Von Economo neuron.
VOI   Volume of interest.
VTA   Ventral tegmental area.
WM   White matter.
YFP   Yellow fluorescent protein.

Index

'*Note*: Page numbers followed by "f" indicate figures and "t" indicate tables.'

Printed in the United States
By Bookmasters